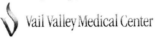

IMRT, IGRT, SBRT –
Advances in the Treatment Planning and
Delivery of Radiotherapy

Frontiers of Radiation Therapy and Oncology

Vol. 40

Series Editors

J.L. Meyer San Francisco, Calif.
W. Hinkelbein Berlin

IMRT, IGRT, SBRT – Advances in the Treatment Planning and Delivery of Radiotherapy

Volume Editor

John L. Meyer San Francisco, Calif.

Contributing Editors

B.D. Kavanagh Aurora, Colo.
J.A. Purdy Sacramento, Calif.
R. Timmerman Dallas, Tex.

237 figures, 174 in color, and 33 tables, online supplement material, 2007

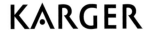

KARGER

Basel · Freiburg · Paris · London · New York ·
Bangalore · Bangkok · Singapore · Tokyo · Sydney

Frontiers of Radiation Therapy and Oncology

Founded 1968 by J.M. Vaeth, San Francisco, Calif.

John L. Meyer, MD FACR

Department of Radiation Oncology
Saint Francis Memorial Hospital
San Francisco, Calif. (USA)

Library of Congress Cataloging-in-Publication Data

IMRT, IGRT, SBRT : advances in the treatment planning and delivery of
radiotherapy / volume editor, John L. Meyer ; contributing editors, B.D.
Kavanagh, J.A. Purdy, R. Timmerman.
    p. ; cm. -- (Frontiers of radiation therapy and oncology, ISSN
0071-9676 ; v. 40)
 Includes bibliographical references and indexes.
 ISBN 978-3-8055-8199-8 (hard cover : alk. paper)
 1. Cancer--Radiotherapy. 2. Radiotherapy. I. Meyer, John, 1949- II.
Series.
 [DNLM: 1. Radiotherapy, Computer-Assisted--methods. W3 FR935 v.40 2007 /
WN 250.5.R2 I34 2007]
   RC271.R3I435 2007
   616.99'40642--dc22
                                                    2007013600

    Bibliographic Indices. This publication is listed in bibliographic services, including Current Contents® and Index Medicus.

© Copyright 2007 by S. Karger AG, P.O. Box, CH–4009 Basel (Switzerland)
www.karger.com
Printed in Switzerland on acid-free paper by Reinhardt Druck, Basel
ISSN 0071–9676
ISBN 978–3–8055–8199–8

Contents

II. IMRT / IGRT Clinical Treatment Programs

III. SBRT Concepts

IV. SBRT Clinical Treatment Programs

Frequently Used Abbreviations

3DCRT	Three-dimensional conformal radiation therapy
CTV	Clinical target volume
DVH	Dose-volume histogram
EPID	Electronic portal imaging device
GTV	Gross tumor volume
IGRT	Image-guided radiation therapy
IMRT	Intensity-modulated radiation therapy
kV	Kilovoltage
MV	Megavoltage
PTV	Planning target volume
RTOG	Radiation Therapy Oncology Group
SBRT	Stereotactic body radiation therapy
WEB	Online supplement material, www.karger.com/FRATO40_suppl

Meyer JL (ed): IMRT, IGRT, SBRT – Advances in the Treatment Planning and
Delivery of Radiotherapy. Front Radiat Ther Oncol. Basel, Karger, 2007, vol. 40, p IX–X

Preface

This text offers a guide to the new technologies of radiotherapy and their major applications in the modern radiotherapy clinic. It is intended to be a readable and practical resource, encompassing the several areas of concurrent development that have advanced this field. The volume is divided into three sections. The first offers explanations and discussions of the technologies themselves and technical methods for their implementation. The second section brings these technologies into the radiation clinic with presentations by noted physicians at major centers who have broad experience with these new treatment approaches. In each chapter, the authors offer specific guidelines for current clinical practice. The third section explores the use of these high-precision technologies in the developing field of stereotactic body radiotherapy.

I have planned and developed this volume based on presentations recently given at the San Francisco Radiation Oncology Conference, which is jointly sponsored by the Departments of Radiation Oncology of Stanford University; University of California at San Francisco; Saint Francis Memorial Hospital, San Francisco, and University of California at Davis. Drs. R. Hoppe, W. Wara and S. Vijayakumar joined me in organizing the conference, which carried the same name as this volume. In our planning, we were assisted by the physics directors at these centers, including Drs. A. Boyer, L. Verhey and J. Purdy. I wish to thank all of them. Papers were selected for publication from the conference presentations, and were supplemented by selected additional papers given at a recent meeting on Image-Guided Radiation Therapy held in Las Vegas, USA, and sponsored by the American Society of Radiation Therapists and Oncologists. All presentations have been expanded, updated and integrated for this volume.

Advances in radiologic imaging are the foundation of much of the current work explored in this text. Throughout the volume, examples of this are often presented in more than one format. In addition to the printed illustrations, a website (www.karger.com/FRATO40_suppl) allows the reader to view a number of the important figures in time-elapse video. This is especially useful in understanding the work presented by George Chen and colleagues in their chapter 'Four-Dimensional Imaging and Treatment Planning of Moving Targets' (p 59–71). Other illustrations are also posted on this website for greater clarity and dynamic visualization, and the website is an essential part of these presentations overall.

I wish to thank all of the authors, especially Drs. J. Purdy, B. Kavanagh and R. Timmerman for their excellent contributions and guidance on the volume. I wish to thank Dr. C. Burns for her assistance in the preparation of the manuscripts for publication. Finally I wish to thank Dr. Thomas Karger and Steven Karger, and the many associates of their fine publishing house.

John L. Meyer
San Francisco, Calif., USA

Meyer JL (ed): IMRT, IGRT, SBRT – Advances in the Treatment Planning and
Delivery of Radiotherapy. Front Radiat Ther Oncol. Basel, Karger, 2007, vol. 40, pp 1–17

New Technologies in the Radiotherapy Clinic

J.L. Meyer[a] · L. Verhey[b] · P. Xia[b] · J. Wong[c]

Departments of Radiation Oncology, [a]Saint Francis Memorial Hospital, [b]University of California,
San Francisco, Calif., [c]Johns Hopkins University, Baltimore, Md., USA

Abstract

What are the limitations to the accuracy of our current technologies in radiation oncology? The immobilization of the patient, definition of the target, motion of the target and localization of the target are the major concerns that must be addressed. Current approaches to meet these needs have brought new technical systems with greater precision and new clinical procedures with higher expectations of practice. This text offers discussions on these issues, including advances in intensity-modulated radiotherapy planning, clinical target definition for the major tumor sites, management of organ motion, target localization and image guidance systems, and the expanding applications of high-precision treatment with stereotactic body radiotherapy.   Copyright © 2007 S. Karger AG, Basel

The technologies of radiotherapy planning and delivery have undergone rapid change. While these changes have been welcomed and carefully nurtured for the benefit of the cancer patient, each change has carried with it a spectrum of new concerns about its appropriate application and efficient integration into radiotherapy practice. These technologies, and the clinical treatment programs that bring them into practical use, are the focus of this volume.

These technical achievements are closely interrelated: one development gives opportunity for another, but often necessitates the creation of a third, and then redefines the use of several others. Understanding this evolving world of new technologies and their applications requires broad perspectives from different vantage points. This volume first takes the viewpoint of computerized treatment planning and delivery with intensity-modulated radiotherapy (IMRT), an elaboration of three-dimensional conformal radiotherapy which has been the subject of prior comprehensive volumes in this series. This new level of treatment precision has brought requirements for image confirmation of the targets during treatment and even automated image guidance of the radiotherapy delivery (image-guided radiation therapy, IGRT). It has also brought an exciting new expansion of radiotherapy into the high-precision realm of accelerated stereotactic body radiotherapy (SBRT) for tumor sites outside the cranium. The practical concerns identified in each of these perspectives will be addressed in the sections of this volume.

Intensity-Modulated Radiation Therapy: Where Are We Now, Where Do We Need to Go?

The intensity modulation of radiation delivery has dramatically changed radiation oncology and greatly expanded the opportunities of the specialty. A little more than a decade ago, IMRT was a new and unconventional idea. Tomotherapy using the Nomos Peacock device was introduced around 1994 and entered use at a few research centers. It was a remarkable innovation, but operationally it carried limiting concerns, including the possible effects that any intratreatment patient motion might have on patient safety or tumor control. By 1996, multileaf collimation had been adapted for IMRT delivery. Its investigation was limited initially to academic centers that were required to develop and maintain appropriate resources in radiation physics not generally available in the community. By the early 2000s, the acquired experience brought confidence that IMRT could be carried out routinely at comprehensive radiotherapy facilities if the necessary quality assurance programs were provided.

To implement IMRT, the patient-specific quality assurance that must be done is additional but important work. Through these efforts, the number and types of patients benefiting from IMRT have expanded. Also, the time required to perform IMRT has decreased significantly, allowing clinics to treat more of their patients with this approach. Clinical results supporting the use of IMRT now exist for head and neck, prostate and other cancers. In many cases, they show that increasing the dose to the tumor can increase rates of local control while decreasing the dose to normal tissues can reduce complications. The clinical results with IMRT are actually occurring as many predicted they would. Yet the development of more precise means of delivering radiotherapy has brought new concerns, especially regarding patient stabilization, organ movement, tumor tracking, and treatment reproducibility.

What has changed? Most importantly, the efficiency of the clinical operations has changed. The efficiency of IMRT planning and delivery is approaching or even exceeding that of complex three-dimensional conformal therapy. Advancements

Table 1. Estimated decrease in planning and treatment times since 2002 for complex head and neck IMRT at UCSF

Contouring time	No change (estimated 2 h per case)
Planning time	Decrease by a factor of 2 (from 4 to 2 h) due to improved understanding of appropriate prescription information for optimization
Quality assurance[1]	Decrease by a factor of 2 (from 2 to 1 h) due to experience, better equipment
Treatment time	Decrease by a factor of 4 due to better delivery algorithm, better choice of angles, contour-based inverse planning algorithm (from 120 segments/40 min to 50 segments/10 min as of later in 2005)

[1] Measurements in phantom.

in treatment planning algorithms are now providing delivery of simpler treatments with equivalent quality. Image-guided radiotherapy, in one of its several available forms, offers the expectation that the treatment target can be localized as needed at the time of treatment, to decrease margins and make the dose delivery safer. The developing technologies for four-dimensional CT are now being used for planning and dose modification. Complex image-guided radiotherapy, as with daily megavoltage or kilovoltage cone beam CT imaging in the treatment room, can lead to a volumetric analysis of the actual dose delivered to the patient on a daily basis. It will be challenging to use and integrate all of this available information, called dose-guided radiotherapy, yet it offers a new level of understanding and quality assurance for every treatment delivered in a therapy course. Soon it may be an expected standard of care.

IMRT Efficiency and Benefit
IMRT planning and delivery can be examined in each of the work phases to show where efficiencies are improving (table 1). At the University of California, San Francisco (UCSF), the time required for contouring has not changed greatly over the past few years; the algorithms for contouring have improved, but the contouring of tissue volumes still requires about 2 h for an average head and neck case. The planning time itself has decreased by half, from about 4 to 2 h per case, largely because of a better understanding of what specific prescription information leads to the desired dose distributions for a given patient group. This efficiency can be attributed to the greater experience of the planners more than to the development of the planning systems. Quality assurance measurements require about 1 h per patient before the first treatment, again about half the time spent earlier. The actual treatment time, a precious commodity in the operation of any clinic, has diminished by almost a factor of four over the past 3 years. This reflects two

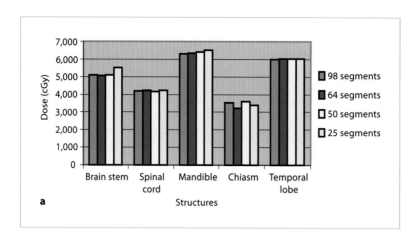

a

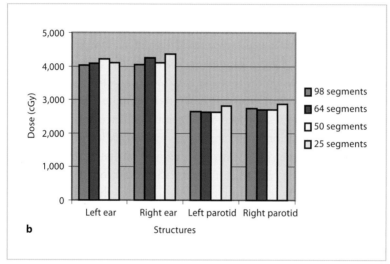

b

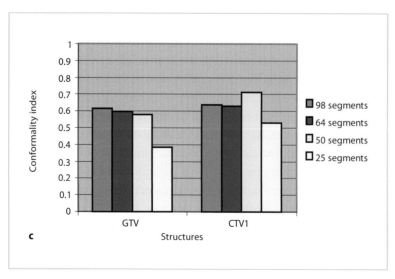

c

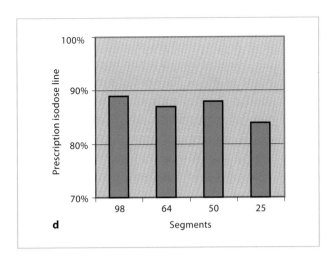

Fig. 1. Effect of the number of segments. Control of dose to normal tissues, conformality and uniformity indexes decrease below 50 segments. **a** Average maximum dose to 1 cc of serial structures. **b** Average mean dose for parallel structures. **c** Average conformality index. **d** Average uniformity index.

changes. First, the new algorithms for inverse planning that use optimization based on anatomic contours or apertures, instead of pixels, have reduced treatment time by half. Second, the number of treatment segments has been reduced by about 50% with no appreciable loss of quality. At UCSF, the most complex IMRT cases now use about 50 segments delivered over an average of 7 angles, which require about 10 min to deliver after the patient is set up. Previously, treatments required 25–35 min, and as long as 40 min for complex cases that were using 120–150 segments. This improvement is a breakthrough in efficiency, and anticipates a time in the near future when the most complex cases need only 15 min in the treatment room.

What level of IMRT complexity should be used? The balance between clinical efficiency and therapeutic benefit of IMRT segmentation has been approached in work at UCSF [1]. Their previous experience with pixel-based optimization algorithms showed that for simple head and neck cases, IMRT plans typically required 90 segments with 6–7 beam angles, but for complex head and neck cases as many as 130–160 segments with 9 beam angles were needed. The question is, can plans with equivalent quality be obtained with fewer segments? New planning algorithms have potentially made this possible. Using an aperture-based optimization algorithm implemented in the Pinnacle planning system, the maximum number of segments permitted in the optimized plan can be specified. Figure 1 shows the effect of 98, 64, 50 or 25 segments on several normal tissues, shown as serial or parallel organs.

As seen particularly for brain stem volumes, it is evident that there is a deterioration of the quality of the plan observed below 50 segments, whereas the results for 50 or more segments are similar. The conformality of the prescription dose line is significantly different at 25 segments than it is at 50–98. The uniformity index (the prescription isodose line that is used in the prescription) begins at about 89% for 98 segments, and is about the same for 50 segments. At 25 segments, it has diminished to around 84–85%, which is probably a significant decrease clinically. For the complex treatment plans in this study, the number of segments could be reduced by about half, from around 100 to around 50, without sacrificing quality.

Heterogeneity Correction

The manner of dose calculation is an essential aspect of accuracy in the planning process. The use of dose heterogeneity corrections for planning throughout the body is now considered standard in most radiation therapy clinics, and is especially important in thoracic sites. There are several different methods used to perform dose heterogeneity corrections, and some can approach (within a few percentage points) the results of exhaustive Monte-Carlo-based calculations. Convolution superposition has become a standard algorithm over the past few years. While the results obtained by these methods can vary, these differences are far smaller than the effects of not using heterogeneity corrections.

Image Guidance in Radiation Therapy

Tumor and normal tissues move with time, and this movement may be clinically significant from second to second, day to day, week to week, or longer. The movement may be periodic and predictable (like respiratory motion), irregular (like peristalsis), or even permanent (like tumor shrinkage). From a radiotherapy point of view, these variations may be considered *intratreatment* or *intertreatment*. In actuality, every tumor site will show both of these effects to varying degrees; some will be dosimetrically significant while others will not. For instance, a lung tumor may move with respiration; show three-dimensional rotational changes from day to day; be affected gradually by changing atelectasis, edema and fluid, and gradually shrink during a therapy course. Even repeated CT scanning will have difficulty in capturing all of these changes in each snapshot of imaging.

Each tumor site (and to some extent, every tumor) will have its own characteristics of movement. For thoracic tumors, periodic respiratory motion often predominates the pattern of change, while for head and neck tumors it is gradual tumor shrinkage over time. Prostate tumors may change position primarily day by day, though additional momentary and irregular changes can occur as a result of peristalsis in a minority of patients. However, no tumor appears to be immune from some combination of *all* of these momentary and more gradual changes, some of which may be complex and unpredictable. For all of these differences, how can the delivery of uniform radiotherapy dose to the targeted tissues be guaranteed? To embark on this journey, work in radiotherapy has begun to tame periodic motion through restriction of motion (e.g. breath hold, with or without assistance), prediction of motion (e.g. gating, four-dimensional CT reconstructions), or tracking of motion through robotics or other dynamic approaches, and will be discussed in this volume.

Intertreatment Changes

At present, radiation oncologists have the greatest opportunity to immediately improve therapy delivery through the identification and correction of change occurring between therapy fractions. Intertreatment motion can be studied by imaging the patient using megavoltage or kilovoltage cone beam systems referenced to the planning system or by other approaches. The imaging can be obtained on a regular, predefined basis or at specific points during a course of therapy.

Evaluation of intertreatment change is important in several areas, especially the head and neck region. Figure 2 projects the IMRT dose distributions for a head and neck cancer patient treated at UCSF; 70 Gy is planned to the gross tumor volume (GTV) and 59.4 Gy to the clinical target volume. In figure 2a, the treatment plan based on the initial CT is shown. After 21 treatment fractions were given, the tumor had markedly regressed and the patient had lost 5% of his body weight. A second CT was obtained, and figure 2b shows that the original plan now projects differently on the tissue structures, since some of the volumes have changed. For instance, the dose to the spinal cord is much higher than intended. Figure 2c shows the reoptimized plan based on the second CT.

Similar work was performed in a series of patients at UCSF; CT studies were repeated in head and neck cancer patients if their contour had noticeably changed, which is fairly common in this patient group [2]. The two CT studies were typically 4–5 weeks apart. For each case, a recalculation of the doses was performed, with endpoints being the dose to 95% of the target volumes, the maximum doses to the spinal cord and brain stem, the mean doses to parallel structures (mainly the parotid glands), and the total doses. Analysis of the normal and tumor tissue volumes indicates that the doses to the right and left parotid glands were reduced by 15.6 and 21.5%, respectively, and the clinical target volume dose decreased by 7.5%. Figure 3a illustrates the dose to 95% of the GTV that would have been delivered with or without replanning. Substantially lower doses would have been delivered to the GTV than intended by the initial plan in most cases. Figure 3b shows the spinal cord doses predicted by three plans for each case: an initial plan and a second reoptimized plan, and a third showing the first intensity patterns applied

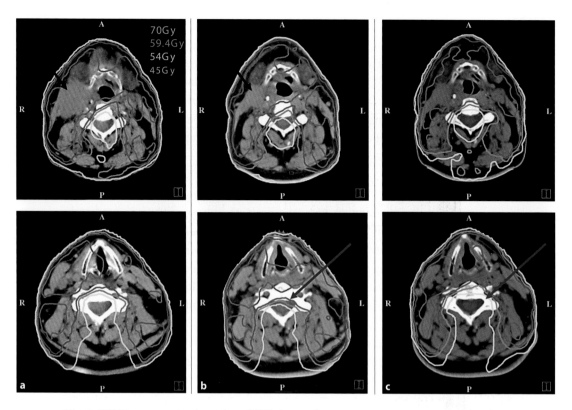

70Gy
59.4Gy
54Gy
45Gy

Fig. 2. IMRT treatment isodoses for a T4N2c base of tongue cancer in a 54-year-old male. Top row: level of hyoid bone; bottom row: lower neck. **a** CT 1: initial plan, before therapy. **b** CT 2: same plan shown on repeat CT scan after 21 fractions; tumor has regressed (black arrow) and patient has lost 5% of his body weight. Note that spinal cord dose has become unacceptable (blue arrow). **c** CT 2: reoptimized plan.

to the second CT scan. If replanning and reoptimization were not performed, significantly higher doses might have been given to the spinal cord than were intended. It is important to follow the patient and perform replanning when needed, and detection of significant soft tissue changes may be one of the most useful applications of image guidance with cone beam technology.

Intratreatment Motion and Tumor Tracking

The issues involved in imaging, tracking and managing motion during the treatment itself are challenging, though they may ultimately provide the best answers to treatment verification. Platforms now exist for three-dimensional radiographic tracking of passive implanted fiducial seeds and the radiofrequency tracking of implanted interactive seeds. Flat-panel technologies used in cone beam CT offer the potential for fluoroscopic monitoring of anatomy or fiducials at kilovoltage or

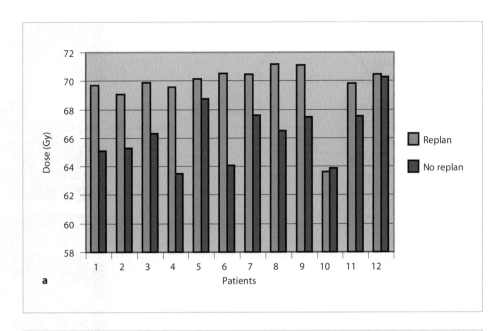

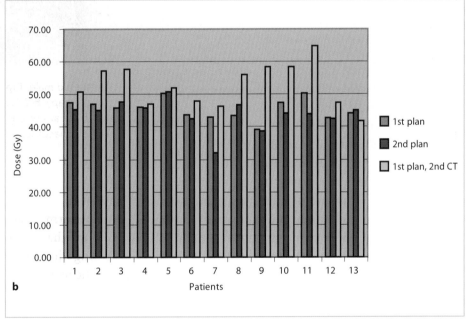

Fig. 3. Effect of replanning on head and neck cancer cases. **a** Dose to 95% of GTV (D95). Deterioration of tumor dose without replanning. **b** Maximum dose to spinal cord. Initial plan and replan doses to normal structures. Third bar shows doses to normal structures if replanning was not performed. Note potentially excessive doses to critical normal structures.

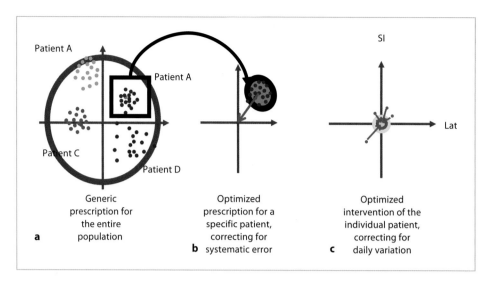

Fig. 4. ART strategies for correcting target positional variations. **a** Conventional radiotherapy, enlarging PTV for all patient variations. **b** ART, correction for systematic variations in a treatment course. **c** ART, correction for all systematic and random daily variations. Circle and elipse show required PTV expansion.

megavoltage energies. Algorithms are now being developed for on-line automated monitoring of targets or fiducials using cone beam technologies. These may even integrate a computer-directed decision about when to stop a treatment and make adjustments in the occasional cases that may require this. The quality of kilovoltage and megavoltage cone beam images is already sufficient for these processes, and the transfer of these technologies into the clinical setting in commercial products is a logical next step. This may include an evolution of the technologies to permit tracking of close tumor surrogates, perhaps adjacent bone contours, rather than implanted markers so that these may not be required in every case.

Adaptive Radiotherapy

Modern radiotherapy is all about defining the target – for clinical tumor delineation, treatment planning, and radiation delivery to the planning target volume (PTV). As new biologic methods and refinements of traditional imaging tools give better tumor delineations, and as greater efficiency and accuracy of treatment planning processes develop, the accurate delivery of the daily treatment itself emerges as a foremost concern. Imaging in the treatment room has provided extensive data documenting movement and anatomic change of targets during and between therapy sessions that can be clinically significant. We are challenged to represent, control and/or incorporate these changes in strategies to manage target movement and setup uncertainty.

The ability to develop automated mechanisms to identify and correct such treatment variations is a major objective, called adaptive radiation therapy (ART). Introduced by the William Beaumont Hospital group in 1997 [3], the concept of ART includes the following key features: it incorporates systematic measurements of treatment variations into a closed-loop radiation treatment process, provides feedback to reoptimize the treatment plan early on during the course of treatment, and delivers treatment that is customized to the daily patient target volumes.

The goals of ART are illustrated in figure 4. In figure 4a, the clusters of dots represent the actual daily setup positions for 4 patient treatment courses. In an ideal course, the patient would always be set up at the prescribed isocenter (the interception of the x- and y-axes in the figure). In practice, the actual daily setup positions are found to be distributed at distances away from this ideal position. If one wants to adjust the PTV expansion margins to accommodate for all such variations found for an entire treatment group (for instance, all prostate cancers treated with IMRT), then a quite large treatment margin would need to be added (represented by the shaded circle). Avoiding such large expansions requires on-treatment imaging of the individual patient, and is the reason for the image guidance of radiotherapy. This imagining information can reveal two types of variation that may be occurring: *systematic,* in which the mean of the observed positions is offset by a measured xyz amount from the prescribed position, or *random,* which can be measured as daily changes from this mean.

The systematic type of uncertainty is amenable to *off-line* analyses of imaging acquired at treatment. In figure 4b, patient A can be effectively treated with a smaller margin if the systematic error is identified early on during the treatment course and corrected, as demonstrated by the shift with the arrow. Now a smaller margin can be prescribed, since it only needs to account for the random variations specific to the patient. In general, a systematic error is the more detrimental, because the dose is being consistently delivered to an unintended location. Random errors are more forgiving, since any effects on the final dose distribution tend to smooth out during the treatment course, especially if it involves many fractions. However, when a treatment course involves high doses delivered using a small number of fractions, large random variations become unacceptable. Random errors can only be addressed with daily *on-line* imaging and modification. Figure 4c illustrates the example of a treatment course where every daily variation is observed and corrected, permitting the smallest PTV margins to be used.

It is estimated that the majority of treatment errors can be corrected through off-line analyses. For example, figure 5 shows the results for 300 prostate cancer patients that were treated at William Beaumont Hospital using an ART protocol. On-treatment imaging was obtained for each patient, the mean setup variation over the first week of therapy was determined, and an adjustment for any systematic error was made off-line. The figure shows that about 80% of treatments would

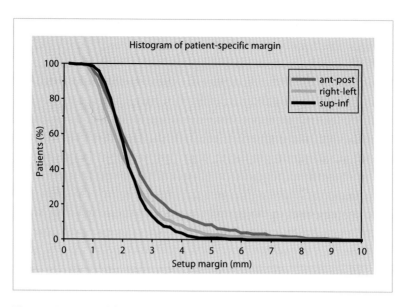

Fig. 5. ART protocol for prostate cancer cases (see text). After off-line correction of systematic error, about 80% of setup variations can be brought within 3 mm of the planned isocenter, and about 20% will gain from further on-line guidance. The gain in setup margin reduction is substantial and can be readily achieved by the general clinic.

then be within 3 mm of accuracy, and could be accurately accounted for by a PTV expansion of 3 mm or less. In only 20% of cases would daily on-line guidance be needed to bring treatments within this expansion margin.

The ART mechanism must identify setup errors and determine whether they represent systematic variation. If there is certainty of a change, then ART must drive a correction process, making the delivery system understand the referenced location of the isocenter. In the case of random setup differences, their magnitude must be identified in order to provide exact daily correction. Alternatively, ART may drive a change in the planning volume encompassing these daily variations or the delivery technique itself to reduce them. Ultimately, ART involves recognizing the daily treatment delivery process and adjusting it as required by identified positional or volumetric variations of the target.

To achieve these goals, ART integrates replanning and dose reconstruction tools. It requires infrastructure for distributing information and tools for off-line decision making to approve or disapprove actions. New skills must be learned to make better use of these new technologies, and the radiation treatment process must be redeveloped as an informatics system for the efficient management of imaging data for treatment control.

ART is patient, tumor site, equipment and institution specific. Practical development of ART requires an understanding of how the PTVs were developed for the individual patient or for a patient population as a class solution. These standards will be specific to each institution, which must then address fundamental questions. What should be the limits for on-line image-guided setup correction? How will these vary when imaging is directed by soft tissue contours, implanted markers or other surrogates? How reproducible is the clinic's management of breathing motion by gating or other strategies? What is the appropriate PTV after the introduction of a new IMRT method, which may be different than the PTV used before this technology? These decisions must be part of a directed process within the clinic's self-assessments, and an effective ART method will depend on having a well-established and continuing process of radiotherapy quality assurance overall.

Biology, Imaging and Image Guidance
Practical issues now confront the current treatment planner, whether physician, physicist or dosimetrist, that can only be answered in the realm of further biologic investigation. If one identifies shrinkage of a tumor during radiotherapy, what should be done? If a tumor appears to increase and edema is suspected, should the target be increased? How does a physical *anatomic* change in the tumor volume reflect a biologic *functional* change that permits a *target* change? As yet, few biological or clinical studies have addressed this issue. PET might be used; however, the significance of changes in its standard uptake value units is not understood, and indeed the tumor/blood ratios involved with this calculation may be altered during radiotherapy. Also, the measurement of the tumor size may vary based on the resolution or intensity adjustments used in the PET scan procedures. Perhaps molecular markers could be of help by allowing functional tracking of treatment-induced changes; however, biological and clinical evaluations are still needed to create useable clinical systems. At present, it is difficult to know how weekly radiographic changes in tumor volume reflect biologic changes. Many investigators feel that there is little scientific basis for modifying therapy volumes based on identified tumor changes during treatment, though treatment replanning may be important to correct for contour or soft tissue changes so that the originally intended dose distributions are achieved.

Stereotaxis and Radiotherapy Delivery

The field of stereotactic radiosurgery is not new, and is based on work by pioneering Swedish investigators led by L. Leksell (1907–1986). More than 50 years ago, he investigated combining stereotactic surgery techniques with external beam irradiation [4]. In 1956, about the same time that similar work began in the USA, Larsson and Leksell initiated proton radiosurgery in Uppsala, Sweden [5]. Some 12 years later, these two individuals led the development of Gammaknife cranial radiosurgery, and in 1972 Leksell and his son founded Elekta Instruments to manufacture this and other related devices. A linear accelerator alternative to gamma irradiation was described in 1983 [6]. Now cranial radiosurgery has become a standard of care for benign and malignant brain tumors of all histologies, and for numerous benign conditions including arteriovenous fistulas, trigeminal neuralgia and other pain conditions, and movement disorders including epilepsy and Parkinson's disease.

Based on the decades of experience with brain stereotaxis, investigators extended work to extracranial treatment using linear accelerator delivery systems. Workers at the Karolinska Institute, Stockholm, Sweden, presented a report on the stereotactic therapy of abdominal tumors in 1994 [7]. A body immobilization frame for thoracic radiosurgery was developed, which reported reproducibility within 5–8 mm for 90% of setups. At the same time, diaphragmatic movement could be limited to 5–10 mm with the use of an abdominal pressure device. The following year, an original clinical report described stereotactic radiotherapy of 31 patients with primarily solitary tumors in the liver and lung who received doses of 7.7–45 Gy in 1–4 fractions [8]. In the USA, spinal radiosurgery was reported in 1995 [9].

At the same time, essential work in SBRT was undertaken at the National Defense Medical College, Japan. Beginning in October 1994, 45 patients with primary or metastatic lung cancers were treated using a linear accelerator with in-room CT guidance. Radiation doses were 30–75 Gy in 5–15 fractions over 1–3 weeks, with or without conventional radiation therapy [10]. Careful protocol work commenced soon thereafter in the USA and is well reported in this volume.

The first SBRT investigations occurred during the same years that IMRT was introduced, and these concepts were logically married in new planning and delivery systems. In fact, the Cyberknife device was first conceived by J. Adler during work at the Karolinska Institute in the late 1980s, and practical development of the system began in 1990. Combining stereotaxis with image guidance and computer-controlled robotics, the Cyberknife was first cleared for use in the USA beginning in 1999. Extracranial treatments currently represent more than 50% of the procedures performed, including those for spine, lung, prostate, liver and pancreas sites. Currently, there are more than 100 Cyberknife centers in the USA, Japan, Europe and other areas of the world.

Concurrently, similar work developed a linear accelerator-based system for extracranial stereotactic radiosurgery using micromultileaf collimation. Founded in 1989, BrainLab developed commercial systems first available in 1993. Currently, the BrainLab Novalis system is open or planned for service in nearly 100 facilities worldwide. Since these initial specialized equipment developments, nearly all other manufacturers of radiation treatment systems have introduced features well-suited or easily adaptable for SBRT.

Current Concerns for SBRT

The technical progress in image-guided IMRT and dedicated radiosurgical delivery systems have assisted in the planning and delivery of SBRT, though effective SBRT work was performed prior to their introduction, and the safe use of this high-dose treatment method depends primarily on the advanced training of its personnel and their careful management of patients. While equipment is still developing for the accurate delivery of stereotactic radiosurgery for tumors outside the cranium, many fundamental biological and clinical questions remain regarding the use of these technologies in medical practice.

1. Dose

The cell survival curves that serve as the basis for conventional radiotherapy practice are derived from older laboratory studies characterizing in vitro cell survivals to single-fraction treatment over the first 2–3 logs of cell kill. These analyses fall short of the level of cell kill caused by the high fractions of SBRT, and the shapes of survival curves at higher fraction levels are not well understood. Therefore, the mathematical modeling of these curves, including their power series expansion coefficients, are not dependable either. Without this accurate modeling, it becomes difficult to extrapolate between the anticipated results of one fractionation scheme and another, and difficult to know whether any given treatment course may result in relative overtreatment or undertreatment in terms of tumor control or normal tissue preservation. What is known, in terms of the alpha/beta model that is currently understood, is that this model likely overpredicts the effectiveness of large-dose SBRT treatments.

2. Fractionation

Original investigations in Sweden used, on average, 3 treatment fractions for SBRT. While this selection may have merit, neither clinical nor biologic investigations have secured clear evidence for this choice. Since multiple treatments have been used, some element of biological effect has been recognized in these protocols. It is likely that this effect could be optimized through more careful analysis, giving physicians a clearer basis for their treatment specifications. From conventional radiobiology, it is probable that the host site of the tumor, whether liver, lung, bone or other tissue, will have different tolerance to the fraction size and total dose, as well as the field volume. This evidence can only be obtained through scientific studies using consistent treatment approaches and monitoring well-defined endpoints.

3. Patient Selection

There is no reason to suppose that all patients or tissue organs will tolerate SBRT equally well. From the science of radiotherapy, it is understood that toxicities to large radiation fractions are predominantly late occurrences. Though rare, these have been observed after SBRT in the bronchus, bowel, spinal cord, and other organs. Since these toxicities may occur late, longer follow-up will be required for wider acceptance of SBRT. At the same time, it is imperative that careful work be performed on the selection of appropriate candidates for therapy to establish a broader range of tumor-specific applications. Considerations may include the prior radiation history of the treatment tissues, treatment volume, organ function and capacity for recovery. Similarly, there is no reason to suppose that all patients will benefit equally from SBRT. Selection criteria might include the number of sites of disease, prior systemic therapy, histology, and many other individual cancer-related factors. Only through a consistent and monitored approach will optimal groups be identified for cancer treatment.

4. Treatment Availability

Finally, where will SBRT be delivered? At present, only a small number of radiotherapy centers offer this approach. Is this appropriate, or should it become widely available quickly, as IMRT has become? One aspect of SBRT to consider is the short duration of the treatment courses. This may be one of its chief advantages; for instance, as an alternative for prostate cancer therapy. In fact, the availability of SBRT at facilities offering service to more remote areas may be desirable, since lengthy stays away from home could be minimized. At the same time, it is essential to have a facility offering a high level of professional expertise and technical support. One must consider that the doses delivered by SBRT are the most highly accelerated and focused of any in radiation treatment, and may have the greatest potential for radiation injury. SBRT clearly requires management by radiation specialists well-trained and certified in its exacting requirements.

References

1 Ludlum E, Akazawa C, Xia P: IMRT plans can be simplified using one step optimization. Med Phys 2006;33:2111.

2 Hansen EK, Bucci MK, Quivey JM, Weinberg V, Xia P: Repeat CT imaging and replanning during the course of IMRT for head-and-neck cancer. Int J Radiat Oncol Biol Phys 2006;64:355–362.

3 Yan D, Vicini F, Wong J, Martinez A: Adaptive radiation therapy. Phys Med Biol 1997;42:123–132.

4 Leksell L: The stereotaxic method and radiosurgery of the brain. Acta Chir Scand 1951:102:316–319.

5 Larsson G, Leksell L, Rexed B, Sourander P, Mair W, Andersson B: The high energy proton beam as a neurosurgical tool. Nature 1958;182:1222–1223.

6 Betti O, Derechinsky V: Multiple-beam stereotaxic irradiation. Neurochirurgie 1983;29:295–298.

7 Lax I, Blomgren H, Naslund I, Svanstrom R: Stereotactic radiotherapy of malignancies in the abdomen. Methodological aspects. Acta Oncol 1994:33:677–683.

8 Blomgren H, Lax I, Naslund I, Svanstrom R: Stereotactic high dose fraction radiation therapy of extracranial tumors using an accelerator. Clinical experience of the first thirty-one patients. Acta Oncol 1995;34:861–870.

9 Hamilton A, Lulu B, Fosmire H, Stea B, Cassady J: Preliminary clinical experience with linear accelerator-based spinal stereotactic radiosurgery. Technique and application. Neurosurgery 1995; 36:311–319.

10 Uematsu M, Shioda A, Tahara K, Fukui T, Yamamoto F, Tsumatori G, Ozeki Y, Aoki T, Watanabe M, Kusano S: Focal, high dose, and fractionated modified stereotactic radiation therapy for lung carcinoma patients: a preliminary experience. Cancer 1998;82:1062–1070.

Dr. John L. Meyer
Department of Radiation Oncology
Saint Francis Memorial Hospital
900 Hyde Street
San Francisco, CA 94109 (USA)
Tel. +1 415 353 6420, Fax +1 415 353 6428
E-Mail JMeyerSF@aol.com

Meyer JL (ed): IMRT, IGRT, SBRT – Advances in the Treatment Planning and
Delivery of Radiotherapy. Front Radiat Ther Oncol. Basel, Karger, 2007, vol. 40, pp 18–39

From New Frontiers to New Standards of Practice: Advances in Radiotherapy Planning and Delivery

James A. Purdy

Department of Radiation Oncology, UC Davis Medical Center, Sacramento, Calif., USA

Abstract

Radiation therapy treatment planning and delivery capabilities have changed dramatically since the introduction of three-dimensional treatment planning in the 1980s and continue to change in response to the implementation of new technologies. CT simulation and three-dimensional radiation treatment planning systems have become the standard of practice in clinics around the world. Medical accelerator manufacturers have employed advanced computer technology to produce treatment planning/delivery systems capable of precise shaping of dose distributions via computer-controlled multileaf collimators, in which the beam fluence is varied optimally to achieve the plan prescription. This mode of therapy is referred to as intensity-modulated radiation therapy (IMRT), and is capable of generating extremely conformal dose distributions including concave isodose volumes that provide conformal target volume coverage and avoidance of specific sensitive normal structures. IMRT is rapidly being implemented in clinics throughout the USA. This increasing use of IMRT has focused attention on the need to better account for both intrafraction and interfraction spatial uncertainties, which has helped spur the development of treatment machines with integrated planar and volumetric advanced imaging capabilities. In addition, advances in both anatomical and functional imaging provide improved ability to define the tumor volumes. Advances in all these technologies are occurring at a record pace and again pushing the cutting-edge frontiers of radiation oncology from IMRT to what is now referred to as image-guided IMRT, or simply image-guided radiation therapy (IGRT). A brief overview is presented of these latest advancements in conformal treatment planning and treatment delivery.

An Evolution of Technology Redefining Clinical Practice

Three-dimensional conformal radiation therapy (3DCRT) is now well established in routine clinical practice as an effective means of achieving higher tumor doses without increasing doses to critical normal structures. The transition from this new frontier in radiation oncology in the late 1980s to early 1990s to a standard of practice today did not come easily and was met with some resistance. 3DCRT represented a radical change in practice for the radiation oncologist and treatment planner moving from the older two-dimensional treatment planning approach, which emphasized geometric beam portal design based on standardized techniques applied to whole classes of comparable patients. The two-dimensional approach was much less laborious than 3DCRT, particularly for the radiation oncologist; however, it greatly limited the ability to escalate dose. This transition to 3DCRT was well documented in a previous volume in this series [1]. Three-dimensional treatment planning emphasized the delineation of image-based tumor volume(s) and the associated microscopic disease volume(s), as well as the critical normal structures, for the individual patient – the gross tumor volume (GTV), clinical target volume (CTV), and organs at risk (OARs). Beam apertures could then be shaped to conform to the planning target volume (PTV) and avoid OARs using beam's eye view displays [2, 3]. This 'forward planning' approach to conformal therapy is now rapidly giving way to an 'inverse planning' approach referred to as intensity-modulated radiation therapy (IMRT), which can achieve even greater conformity by optimally modulating the individual beamlets that make up the radiation beams [4].

IMRT dose distributions can be created to conform much more closely to the PTV, particularly for those volumes having complex/concave shapes, and to avoid OARs. Sharp dose gradients near the boundaries of both the PTV and the OARs can be achieved, but this results in IMRT treatments being much more sensitive to geometric uncertainties than the two-dimensional or 3DCRT approaches. Also, during a single fraction, IMRT techniques treat only a portion of the PTV at any instance (i.e., beamlets or beam segments). Thus, there is the potential for significant dosimetric consequences if the patient and/or the GTV/CTV move during IMRT treatment (i.e., referred to as *intrafraction* geometric uncertainties as opposed to *interfraction* uncertainties associated with patient treatment setup). Furthermore, since IMRT treatments typically take longer than two-dimensional radiotherapy or 3DCRT treatments, the patient must remain in the fixed treatment position for a longer period of time, increasing the susceptibility to intrafraction geometric uncertainties. All of these factors contribute to IMRT being a 'less forgiving' form of radiation therapy with regard to the effects of geometric uncertainties, and this imposes more stringent requirements to account for both intrafraction and interfraction uncertainties.

This recognition of the need to better account for the spatial uncertainties when using IMRT has spurred the development of treatment machines with integrated planar and volumetric advanced imaging capabilities [5]. In addition, advances in both anatomical and functional imaging are providing improved ability to define the tumor volumes. These advances in treatment machine imaging technology and diagnostic imaging are occurring at a record pace and again pushing the edge of our frontiers in radiation oncology from IMRT to what is now referred to as image-guided IMRT, or simply image-guided radiation therapy (IGRT) [6].

Of course, the concept of image guidance is not new, and really should be viewed as evolutionary. We are all aware of the development and use of various systems to help better localize the patient for treatment, including dedicated simulators, megavoltage (MV) port films, electronic portal imaging devices, use of implanted radiopaque markers, ultrasound imaging systems, or optical tracking systems. Even the early cobalt-60 teletherapy machines could be equipped with a kilovoltage (kV) X-ray tube attached to the beam stop.

However, it is the development of the modern IMRT delivery system with integrated imaging capability that can provide three-dimensional volumetric imaging of soft tissues (including tumors) that has resulted in the term IGRT and the following IGRT hypothesis.

The IGRT hypothesis:

> *IGRT can reduce setup uncertainties and provide improved management of internal organ motion, and therefore will allow further dose escalation and/or conformal avoidance than IMRT alone, which will lead to improved treatment outcome.*

Like with the 3DCRT hypothesis, clinical trials should be conducted to test the IGRT hypothesis, but to date no such cooperative group studies specifically addressing this hypothesis are in place.

These new image-guided treatment machines are also spurring other exciting developments, including the further investigation of hypofractionation using what has been termed stereotactic body radiation therapy (SBRT) [7], which clinically integrates the results of new biologic studies looking at tumor responses to single high-dose fractionation [8] with the new technical capabilities to deliver highly focused therapy.

These are exciting developments and times for radiation oncology, but, as stated above, clinical trials should be initiated to validate and help determine the IGRT's most effective use. Certainly, its adoption should not be driven by reimbursement. A brief overview is presented of the latest advancements in three-dimensional treatment planning and delivery that are leading to our new standards of practice.

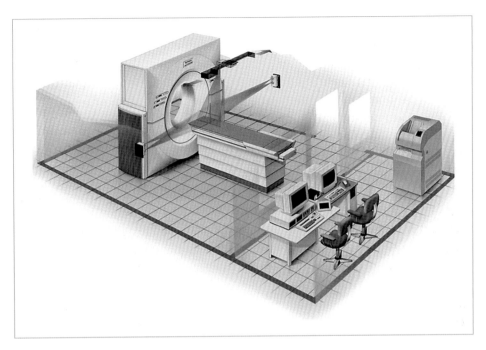

Fig. 1. CT simulator room layout consisting of a diagnostic CT scanner, external laser positioning system, and a virtual simulation software workstation. Courtesy of Philips Medical Systems, Cleveland, Ohio, USA.

CT Simulation and Three-Dimensional Treatment Planning

The radiation oncology community eagerly embraced the concept of virtual simulation and three-dimensional treatment planning in the early 1990s when robust commercial packages, including dedicated CT simulation systems, became available (fig. 1) [9]. Both CT simulation and three-dimensional treatment planning systems (3DTPS) have now matured to a point where they are the cornerstones of a modern radiation oncology facility [10]. Today's CT simulation systems incorporate large-bore CT scanners, especially designed for radiation oncology, with multislice capability, high-quality laser marking/patient positioning systems, and sophisticated virtual simulation software features. Also, many 3DTPS now include virtual simulation software features. The tremendous computational power of today's 3DTPS workstations permits near real-time interactivity for many of the treatment planning tasks. Beam's eye view displays (fig. 2) allow the treatment planner to efficiently develop plans, including those utilizing noncoplanar beams. Extremely high-quality digitally reconstructed radiographs (DRRs), in which the delineated contours and the projected beam apertures can be overlaid, can be quickly generated. Room's eye view displays (fig. 3) provide a powerful

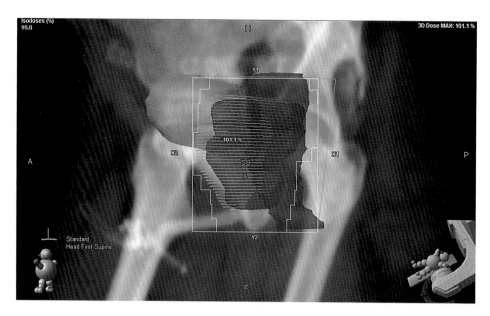

Fig. 2. 3DTPS beam's eye view display used to identify the best gantry, collimator and couch angles at which to irradiate target and avoid irradiating adjacent critical structures. Critical structures and target volumes outlined on patient's CT sections and outline of multileaf collimator aperture are shown (Varian Eclipse TPS).

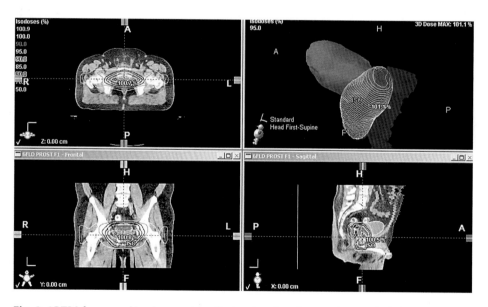

Fig. 3. 3DTPS four-panel isodose review display showing three orthogonal planes and room's eye view for planned dose distribution. The room's eye view display shown in the upper right panel is useful to quickly evaluate where the hot or cold spots occurred after dose-volume histogram review.

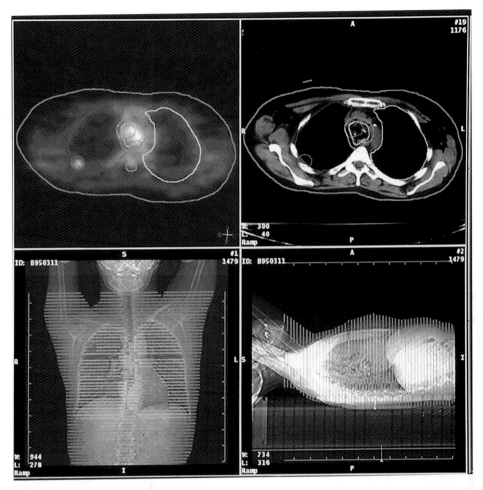

Fig. 4. 3DTPS software for contouring target volumes and organs at risk (image segmentation) continues to be improved, but is still not automated to the extent needed for IGRT. CT data are displayed and contours are drawn by the radiation oncologist around the tumor/target volumes, and organs at risk on a slice-by-slice basis, as seen in the upper right panel. At the same time, planar images from both anterior-posterior and lateral projections are displayed in the bottom right and left panels. The upper left panel shows PET scan data with overlying contours after image registration with the CT data. Continued development in automated image segmentation and image fusion (deformable registration) software should remain a high priority for the field.

plan evaluation tool in which a three-dimensional isodose volume can be viewed and rotated in real time, allowing evaluation of target volume coverage and search for excess dose hot spots to critical normal structure volumes. Unfortunately, even though software for contouring normal structures and target volumes (image segmentation) has been significantly improved in recent years, it is still not automated to the extent needed for IGRT (fig. 4). The contouring task remains too time consuming, and secondly complex sites such as head and neck are extremely challenging. Thus, continued development in automated segmentation and image fusion (deformable registration) software should remain a high priority for the field.

Those readers interested in more details regarding the historical development of CT simulators and 3DTPS are referred to the following references [10, 11].

Oncological Imaging

CT is still the principal source of imaging data used for defining the GTV for most sites, but this imaging modality presents several potential pitfalls. First, when contouring the GTV, it is essential that the appropriate CT window and level settings be used in order to determine the maximum dimension of what is considered potential gross disease. Secondly, for those treatment sites in which there is considerable organ motion, such as for tumors in the thorax, CT images do not correctly represent either the time-averaged position of the tumor or its shape [12–14]. This can be understood by appreciating the fact that today's single-slice CT simulators rely almost exclusively on the use of fast spiral CT technology, and thus acquire data essentially in two dimensions. This has the effect of capturing the tumor cross section images at particular positions in the breathing cycle. If the tumor motion is significant, different, and possibly noncontiguous, transverse sections of the tumor could be imaged at different points of the breathing cycle, leading to volume uncertainties [12–14]. The interpolation process in spiral CT technology adds further to the uncertainty. As a result, the three-dimensional reconstruction of the GTV from temporally variant two-dimensional images often results in a poor representation of the tumor and its motion. Thus, multislice CT technology (so-called *four-dimensional CT imaging*) is rapidly becoming the standard for CT simulators [15]. In addition, other technologies and methodologies to explicitly help manage respiratory motion (to the order of less than 5 mm during treatment) continue to be developed, including respiratory-gated techniques, respiration-synchronized techniques, breath-hold techniques, and forced shallow-breathing methods [16].

In some sites, MR is already known to be a better anatomic imaging modality for defining the boundaries of the target volume, e.g. prostate. This has led to the development of dedicated MR simulators for radiation oncology [17]. As IGRT matures, there is likely to be more interest in further developing MR simulators from the low tesla units that are available today.

Unfortunately, in many sites anatomic imaging techniques do not always distinguish malignant from normal tissues. There is growing use of the complementary information available from functional imaging studies, such as PET, when defining the GTV [18–20]. The benefit from such functional information has been pointed out by studies such as that by Caldwell et al. [21], who showed high observer variability in the CT-based definition of the GTV for non-small-cell lung cancer patients when compared with the GTV defined using FDG-hybrid PET images coregistered with CT. Integrated PET-CT units have already been implemented in some radiation oncology departments. It is very likely that over the next 5 years large-bore PET-CT simulators will be developed for radiation oncology. However, such dedicated radiation oncology imaging systems will not be as easily assimilated into the planning and follow-up process as was CT, and will require close collaboration with our imaging colleagues (both physicians and physicists).

Delineating the CTV is a much more complicated task than delineating either the GTV or most OARs. At this time, it is more of an art than a science, since current imaging techniques are not capable of detecting subclinical tumor involvement directly. When defining GTVs, CTVs and OARs on axial CT slices, particularly for sites such as head and neck cancer, assistance from a diagnostic radiologist is often helpful. Publications and symposiums addressing the problems of establishing consistent CTVs for the various clinical sites are now becoming commonplace [22, 23]. There is no question that image-based cross-sectional anatomy training should be a requirement in radiation oncology residency training programs. The radiation oncologist of the future will need to become much more expert in image recognition of normal tissue anatomy and gross tumor changes in order to take full advantage of the many advances in imaging. Research efforts that will allow a more accurate determination of the CTV (and facilitate a safe reduction in PTV margin when an appropriate motion management system is used) may be the single most important area to further advance the safe and effective use of IGRT.

Dose Calculations

Advanced three-dimensional algorithms that compute the photon beam dose distribution from more of a first-principle approach (i.e., convolution/superposition), rather than correcting parameterized dose distributions measured in a water phantom, are now commercially available [24]. These models utilize convolution energy deposition kernels that describe the distribution of dose about a single primary photon interaction site, and provide accurate results even for complex heterogeneous geometries. It is the author's opinion that heterogeneity-corrected treatment plans generated using such advanced algorithms should be the standard of practice for IGRT. The study by Frank et al. [25] provides a clear methodology for safely transitioning clinical use from one based on planning that assumes a homogeneous unit density patient, to one using a heterogeneous patient model.

Even the convolution/superposition dose calculation algorithms will eventually be replaced by the Monte Carlo technique [26–28]. Monte Carlo is, in principle, the only method capable of computing the dose distribution accurately for all situations encountered in radiation therapy. This includes being able to accurately predict the dose near interfaces of materials with very dissimilar atomic number such as near metal prostheses, or different densities such as tumors in lung tissue. I believe that accurate Monte-Carlo-based dose calculations, combined with the advantages of IGRT for managing motion uncertainties, hold great promise in the treatment of lung cancer.

Treatment Plan Optimization

Presently, most (if not all) optimization engines in IMRT treatment planning systems utilize dose- and/or dose-volume-based objective functions in which the failure to achieve the prescribed dose distribution is proportional to the dose difference (or the square of the difference) between the planned and prescribed doses. The limitations of dose- or dose-volume-based criteria have led a number of investigators to propose dose response models, such as tumor control probabilities and normal tissue complication probabilities (see the review by Brahme [29]). More recently, Niermierko [30] and Wu et al. [31] have proposed IMRT optimization based on a dose response using equivalent uniform dose. Such work should be encouraged, as the development of robust dose response models that accurately predict clinical outcome is an important research area for radiation oncology, particularly for furthering the automation of the IGRT planning process.

Image-Guided Treatment Machines

Cone Beam CT Linear Accelerator IGRT
The first commercially available cone beam CT (CBCT) IGRT system was the Elekta Synergy™ (Elekta, Crawley, UK) [5, 32]; the other medical linear accelerator (linac) manufacturers have also now embraced the IGRT concept and have either produced their own version of an IGRT linac, Varian Trilogy™ (Varian Medical Systems, Palo Alto, Calif., USA), or are in the process of such developments, Siemens ARTÍSTE™ (Siemens Medical Solutions USA, Inc., Malvern, Pa., USA). The Synergy (fig. 5) consists of a retractable kV X-ray source, an amorphous silicon flat panel imager mounted on the linear accelerator perpendicular to the radiation beam direction, and a software module (referred to as the XVI system). The system provides planar, motion, and volumetric images. Figure 6 depicts the IGRT data flow and work process currently used at UC Davis. For CBCT image acquisitions, the gantry is rotated around the patient for a preset angle (between 180 and 360° to allow sufficient data acquisition) and images are acquired via an

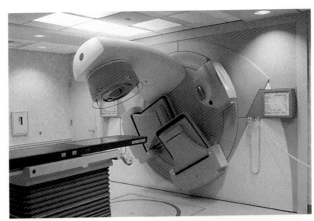

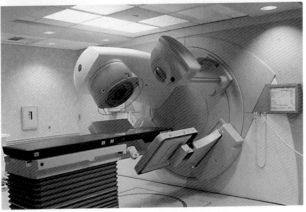

Fig. 5. Elekta Synergy consists of a conventional multi-modality medical linac with a retractable kV X-ray source, an amorphous silicon flat panel imager mounted on the linear accelerator perpendicular to the radiation beam direction, and a software module (referred to as the XVI system). The upper panel shows the X-ray tube amorphous silicon flat panels retracted and the lower panel shows them extended.

amorphous silicon panel. Volumetric image reconstruction is performed simultaneously with the acquisition to expedite the process. The reconstructed three-dimensional geometry is subsequently registered with the reference geometry planning image, either manually or automatically (using either soft tissue or bone mode). For some disease sites, such as prostate cancer, the soft tissue mode is conceptually ideally suited, since the prostate often moves relative to the bones. However, at present, it is difficult to visualize the prostate in all cases, and thus implanted radiopaque seeds are used to make the registration process more efficient. Based on the registration, the difference between the data sets is calculated and displayed as translation along and rotation about the three axes. Subsequent treatment table adjustments are made (fig. 7) and the patient treated. One can clearly appreciate that CBCT-based IGRT shows great potential for objective, precise positioning of patients for treatment, matching the treatment setup image model to that of the planning image model. It remains to be determined exactly which imaging features on the integrated CBCT linacs (i.e., kVp CBCT, planar, motion, and MV electronic portal imaging device) are best suited for a particular disease site.

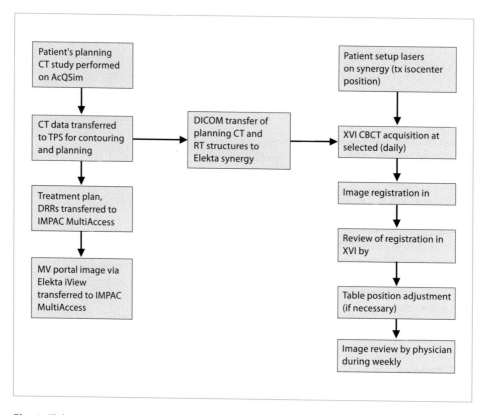

Fig. 6. Elekta IGRT data flow and work process used at UC Davis. Physician performs initial reviews and later delegates to therapists after communicating objectives and verifying registration success in initial sessions.

Helical Tomotherapy IGRT

Helical tomotherapy was first proposed by Mackie et al. in 1993 and is now commercially available as the TomoTherapy HI-ART system (TomoTherapy, Inc., Madison, Wisc., USA) [33–36]. A short in-line 6-MV linac (Siemens Oncology Systems, Concord, Calif., USA) rotates on a ring gantry at a source-axis distance of 85 cm. Figure 8 shows the unit installed at UC Davis. The IMRT treatment is delivered while the patient support couch is translated in the y-direction (toward the gantry) through the gantry bore, in the same way as a helical CT study is conducted. In the patient's reference frame, the treatment beam is angled inwards along a helix with the midpoint of the fan beam passing through the center of the bore. Similar to helical CT, the treatment beam pitch is defined as the distance traveled by the couch per gantry rotation, divided by the field width in the y-direction. The width of the beam in the y-direction is defined by a pair of jaws that is fixed, for any particular patient treatment, to one of three selectable values (1, 2.5 or 5 cm).

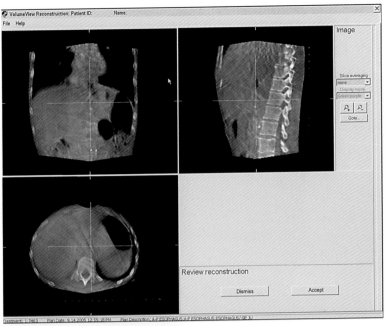

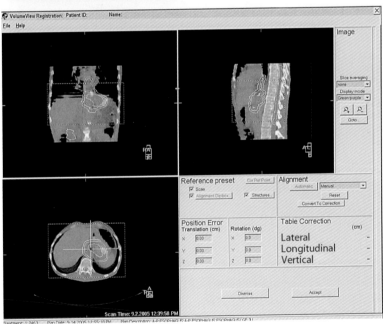

Fig. 7. Elekta Synergy XVI display screens showing the image registration process. The difference between the prescription and CBCT data sets is calculated and displayed as translation along and rotation about the three axes; subsequent treatment table adjustments are made and then the patient is treated.

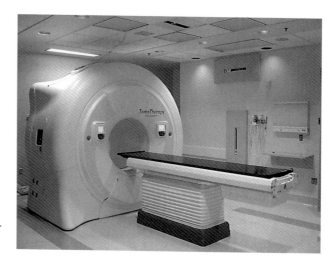

Fig. 8. TomoTherapy HI-ART system installed at UC Davis.

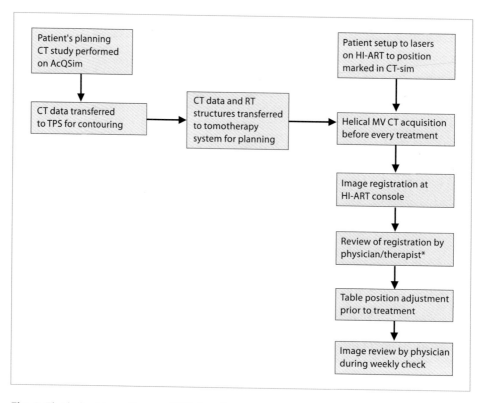

Fig. 9. The helical tomotherapy IGRT data flow and work process used at UC Davis. Physician performs initial reviews and later delegates to therapists after communicating objectives and verifying registration success in initial sessions.

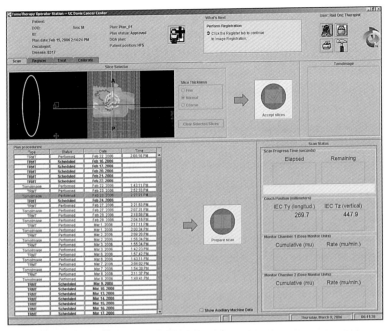

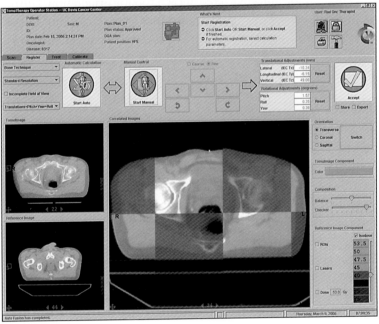

Fig. 10. TomoTherapy HI-ART display screens showing the image registration process after which table adjustments are automatically made and the patient treated.

Laterally, the treatment beam is modulated by a 64-leaf binary multileaf collimator, whose leaves transition rapidly between open and closed states providing a maximum possible open lateral field length of 40 cm at the bore center. Highly modulated treatments can achieve great conformality, though they inevitably take longer to deliver. The IGRT process in use at UC Davis is shown in figure 9. A helical MV CT image is acquired prior to treatment each day using the on-board xenon CT detector system and the 6-MV linac (detuned to 3.6 MV). Registration software is provided to compare the daily patient setup image with the stored prescription CT planning image. After image registration, table adjustments are then automatically made and the patient is then treated (fig. 10).

Cyberknife IGRT

The use of a small X-band linear accelerator mounted on an industrial robot was first developed for radiosurgery [37]. The robot provides the capability of aiming beamlets with any orientation relative to the target volume. The system uses two ceiling-mounted diagnostic X-ray sources, and amorphous silicon image detectors mounted flush to the floor. The treatment is specified by the trajectory of the robot and by the number of monitor units delivered at each robotic orientation. During the patient's treatment, the Cyberknife System correlates live radiographic images with preoperative CT or MRI scans in real time to determine patient and tumor position repeatedly over the course of treatment. More details are provided by users of this system in subsequent articles in this volume.

Image-Guided Intensity-Modulated Proton Therapy and Beyond

Establishing the optimum clinical use of the above-described IGRT machines (and their continued development) will require considerable effort over the next several years. Many practical questions need answering.

Questions in the applications of IGRT:

(1) *Which anatomical sites are best suited for IGRT treatments?*
(2) *Which type of IGRT is the most efficient, and is this site dependent?*
(3) *What are the optimum treatment time periods required for IGRT?*
(4) *What is the optimum use of daily imaging in the IGRT planning/treatment process?*
(5) *What are the most effective periodic technical quality assurance (QA) methodologies and patient-specific QA methodologies including weekly chart rounds for IGRT?*
(6) *What are the components of a dedicated radiation oncology picture archive communication system (RO-PACS)?*

Particularly important will be the development of accurate and efficient deformable registration tools that will allow image-guided adaptive radiation therapy to become a routine standard of practice [38–40].

Even after we gain considerable experience with photon-based image-guided IMRT and further development of it occurs, other technological advances in treatment modalities will continue to take place. Those already involved in proton beam therapy are developing image-guided intensity-modulated proton therapy. Also, there is promising work going on at the *Gesellschaft für Schwerionenforschung* in Darmstadt, Germany, where they are treating patients with carbon ions and using a PET scanner to monitor the individual patient treatments [41].

The point is that technology is going to continue to advance in radiation oncology. It is particularly exciting to contemplate the potential synergy resulting from the progress being made in image-guided planning/delivery systems and the progress being made in molecular and cancer biology. Such advances are likely to lead to optimized radiation therapy for the individual patient [42]. This will require many types of professionals – clinicians, physicists, biologists and computer scientists – all working together to develop what will eventually evolve into the next frontier of cancer therapy. This may in turn become a new standard of practice, as we repeat this cycle as advances continue, until cancer is finally eliminated or at least turned into a chronic disease in which a high quality of life can be maintained.

Radiation Oncology Informatics

The amount of digital data transferred and stored (and thus the available information) in a radiation oncology department has drastically increased with the development/implementation of IGRT treatment machines. Daily kV CBCT images or MV helical CT images are acquired during a patient's treatment course and add several dozen megabytes to gigabytes of information, which needs to be stored in a manner that permits efficient accessing when needed. At the same time, the patient's treatment planning data, which often exist only in a system-specific proprietary format, need to be similarly stored and readily accessible. In addition, cancer biology imaging techniques currently used (or those under development) generate huge digital data files that require storage. But storage is not the only issue. New software tools to effectively use the imaging data (for clinical workflow issues, outcome research, and basic research) are needed if we are to take full advantage of the new information. IGRT clearly points to the need for a new type of picture archive communication system (PACS) specifically designed for radiation oncology, i.e., RO-PACS. The development of a robust RO-PACS will be one of the most important developments for radiation oncology, as the use of information technology will be 'mission critical' in order to make radiation oncology more effective and efficient [43].

Another important informatics effort in radiation oncology is that being led by the Image-Guided Therapy QA Center (ITC) as part of the Advanced Technology QA Consortium (ATC) (http://atc.wustl.edu/) [44]. NCI-sponsored advanced technology trials in several sites are now in progress in which the patient's three-dimensional planning and verification digital data are submitted via the Internet. All target volumes and designated critical structure contours (superimposed on CT display), first-day portal films on all patients, and the three-dimensional dose distributions are all reviewed using web-based tools. The data are stored in a treatment planning verification database. This database resource is allowing researchers to mine the data so as to better understand the relationship between dose and outcomes of 3DCRT/IMRT, and ultimately to develop robust tumor control probability and normal tissue complication probability models.

Collaborative Working Groups

During the 1980s and early 1990s, the Radiation Research Program of the NCI supported several multi-institutional collaborative working groups (CWG) research contracts that focused research efforts on translating advanced technologies that were available only in a few academic institutions to the radiation oncology community as a whole. These efforts included the Photon 3D Treatment Planning CWG (1984–1987), Electron 3D Treatment Planning CWG (1986–1989), and the Radiotherapy Treatment Planning Tools CWG (1989–1994) [45]. Even IMRT benefited from a consensus paper developed using the CWG approach [46]. A parallel for university and industry collaboration can be drawn from the Elekta Research Consortium, which led to the development of the Elekta Synergy. It is now time to re-embrace the CWG concept for IGRT and address the clinical use of IGRT. This effort should combine both NCI and industry support to establish an IGRT CWG to help answer the many questions posed by IGRT.

Education and Training Requirements in the Image-Guided Radiation Therapy Era

In this new image-guided IMRT era, it should be recognized that the complexity of treatment planning and delivery is increased. The level of precision needed for planning target volume localization is amplified, as well as the requirement to preserve this geometrical precision during treatment. These requirements will impact the roles of the radiation therapy team members, and their education and training requirements to meet these new challenges. In addition to the ever-increasing needs for training in cancer medicine and cancer biology, the radiation oncologist will need to develop much more expertise in using multimodality imaging studies (e.g.

CT, CBCT, MRI, PET). Cross-sectional imaging training should be an essential component of the training programs of radiation oncologists in the IGRT era. In addition, they must be much more computer literate as the electronic medical record, RO-PACS and associated software tools become ubiquitous throughout the clinic.

The radiation oncology physicist also needs much more training in imaging physics, as four-dimensional spiral CT and multimodality imaging become the foundation of the planning process and integrated kV and/or MV imaging (including CBCT) become the foundation of the treatment verification process. Data accessibility and networking issues are extremely important to radiation oncology clinics implementing IGRT capability. Just as high-energy accelerator physicists were critical to radiation oncology in the 1970s, physicists with strong imaging and computer backgrounds, particularly with regard to networking and integration of peripheral devices, are essential for the IGRT clinic.

The medical dosimetrist also needs much more training in cross-sectional imaging anatomy. Delineating OARs continues to be too time-consuming. Dosimetrists should also become much more familiar with the inverse planning optimization approach.

The radiation therapist in the IGRT era also needs much more training in image-based anatomy, and in dealing with the very complex treatment delivery systems including the positional tracking systems likely to become standard in IGRT treatment rooms. Current IGRT systems should be thought of only as first-generation systems, as some have as many as 4 or 5 monitors and keyboards for the radiation therapist to deal with. While these cumbersome arrangements will probably continue for quite a while, eventually these components will become integrated. Ultimately, after the patient is repositioned and fixated, the treatment delivery will be highly automated using image-guided IMRT techniques without doubt. The radiation therapist will continue to play a key role in monitoring patient position and system operation in the IGRT era.

Implementing Image-Guided Radiation Therapy in the Clinic

This section is intended to briefly review lessons learned over my career in implementing advanced technologies such as IGRT. These remarks are based on my experience in implementing multimodality medical linacs in the 1970s; three-dimensional treatment planning and conformal therapy in the 1980s to early 1990s; IMRT in the 1990s to 2000s, and IGRT in the mid 2000s to the present day.

When first considering implementing an IGRT program, the department leadership must do adequate homework to fully understand the resources needed. Complex new technology places increased demands on the radiation therapy team; all members are typically affected to some degree whether it is increased contouring effort, new and more detailed plan prescriptions, more complex treatment planning, change in workflow, i.e., daily image registration, and/or new QA efforts. It is prudent to assign key physician and physicist teams as the initial clinical users who will eventually become the teachers/mentors of the other new users in the department. The initial team should visit and learn from clinical groups already expert in use of the new technology, and also attend vendor training in use of the technology, particularly the planning system and the treatment delivery system.

Once the technology is in place and the team leaders have acquired initial training, the focus should be on building a strong clinical foundation. This is best accomplished by starting with disease sites in which there is already published experience, or in which there is local disease site expertise that fits well with the use of the new technology. Typically, these include such sites as prostate, head and neck, and brain. During the initial use period, try to limit weekly starts (2–3 a week) in order for all members of the team to gain experience and coordinate workflow, technology use, and QA issues. The initial team should build up a large number of clinical cases before training other new users. Also, they should provide an ample number of in-service training sessions to the various groups involved.

It is extremely important to establish strong QA and preventive maintenance inspection programs for the use of the new technology. Utmost importance is making sure that appropriate physics staffing and appropriate QA instrumentation and phantoms are provided. The QA program should incorporate redundant checks and involve all members of the team. It is essential to have written use and QA procedures. The preventive maintenance program should include vendor training classes and adequate support to maintain spare parts and appropriate test instrumentation. These points are often missed by administrators as they focus only on the purchase and not the support needed for the new technology. The bottom line is this: when implementing advanced technologies, there must be a strong commitment from the hospital administration with no shortcuts taken.

Once the new technology is in place, the goal should be to develop efficient use, i.e., class solutions. This is best accomplished by establishing weekly conferences to discuss plans and develop written procedures, review pertinent literature, and surface issues for discussion with the entire group. These weekly conferences will help establish disease site consistency in target volume and critical structure specifications, in dose prescription (including critical organ dose-volume constraints), and target volume doses. It is advised to start with simpler sites such as prostate.

A useful tool implemented at UC Davis is the use of benchmark dose-volume histograms (DVHs) for making treatment decisions in prostate cancer therapy [47]. These benchmark DVHs (for the rectum and bladder) were developed by creating both 3DCRT and IMRT plans for a certain number of patients during our initial implementation of IMRT and treating with IMRT only if its DVH profile was judged better than 3DCRT.

Finally, when implementing advanced technologies, it is essential to monitor progress in the program. This is done by establishing a quality improvement program for the new technology: (1) define and record treatment planning metrics (e.g. number plans, time required for planning per site); (2) monitor changes in volumes/prescriptions; (3) track outcomes, and (4) and most importantly, record monthly treatment planning/treatment machine uptime as reliability is key in the clinic.

Summary and Conclusion

I am going to conclude this paper with some comments that I wrote for an editorial that was published in the year 2000 in the journal *International Journal of Radiation Oncology Biology Physics* [48]. At the time, I had been invited to envisage (from a physics perspective) where radiation oncology would be in the year 2035. Today it is clear that in some areas things are developing at an even faster pace than I predicted, while other areas remain problematic.

IGRT systems are providing an integrated approach to radiation oncology treatment planning, dose delivery, and treatment verification. However, these are first-generation systems and most of the tasks in the IGRT process are not fully automated.

The ability to more accurately define the volumes containing the gross disease is improving with the use of advanced multimodality imaging. However, little progress has been made in providing a solution for accurately defining subclinical disease, i.e., the CTV.

Significant progress has been made in technologies that account for or minimize patient setup error and organ motion. However, caution is urged when reducing the PTV margins as it is essential to fully appreciate the still large uncertainty associated with the CTV specification in most disease sites.

Physicists are currently struggling with the planning and QA challenges posed by image-guided IMRT. New instrumentation and methodology that minimizes the human steps needed to plan, treat, and verify a cancer patient's radiation therapy are still needed.

In summary, these first-generation IGRT systems are truly exciting, but improvements in image quality, data storage, data import/export, and software tools (for specific workflow tasks and for data mining) are needed. Most importantly, IGRT machine reliability (i.e., 99% uptime) is absolutely critical.

While there is considerably more research and developmental work to do, as we move from these new frontiers to new standards of practice, I repeat exactly what I said in the year 2000: 'I strongly believe that this next generation of radiation oncology clinicians and scientists have a unique opportunity to significantly improve treatment outcomes and lower costs thus making high quality radiation therapy available the world over.'

References

1 Meyer JL, Purdy JA (eds): 3-D Conformal Radiotherapy: A New Era in the Irradiation of Cancer. Front Radiat Ther Oncol. Basel, Karger, 1996, vol 29.

2 International Commission on Radiation Units and Measurements: ICRU Report 50: Prescribing, Recording, and Reporting Photon Beam Therapy. Bethesda, International Commission on Radiation Units and Measurements, 1993.

3 International Commission on Radiation Units and Measurements: ICRU Report 62: Prescribing, Recording, and Reporting Photon Beam Therapy (Supplement to ICRU Report 50). Bethesda, International Commission on Radiation Units and Measurements, 1999.

4 Webb S: The physical basis of IMRT and inverse planning. Br J Radiol 2003;76:678–689.

5 Jaffray DA, Siewerdsen JH, Wong JW, et al: Flat-panel cone-beam computed tomography for image-guided radiation therapy. Int J Radiat Oncol Biol Phys 2002;53:1337–1349.

6 Ling CC, Yorke E, Fuks Z: From IMRT to IGRT: frontierland or neverland? Radiother Oncol 2006;78:119–122.

7 Kavanagh BD, Timmerman RD (eds): Stereotactic Body Radiation Therapy. Philadelphia, Lippincott Williams & Wilkins, 2005, pp 1–159.

8 Fuks Z, Kolesnick R: Engaging the vascular component of the tumor response. Cancer Cell 2005; 8:89–91.

9 Coia LR, Schultheiss TE, Hanks G (eds): A Practical Guide to CT Simulation. Madison, Advanced Medical Publishing, 1995, p 209.

10 Mutic S, Palta JR, Butker EK, et al: Quality assurance for computed-tomography simulators and the computed-tomography-simulation process: report of the AAPM Radiation Therapy Committee Task Group No 68. Med Phys 2003;30:2762–2792.

11 Purdy JA: 3-D radiation treatment planning: a new era; in Meyer JL, Purdy JA (eds): 3-D Conformal Radiotherapy: A New Era in the Irradiation of Cancer. Front Radiat Ther Oncol. Basel, Karger, 1996, pp 1–16.

12 Caldwell CB, Mah K, Skinner M, et al: Can PET provide the 3D extent of tumor motion for individualized internal target volumes? A phantom study of the limitations of CT and the promise of PET. Int J Radiat Oncol Biol Phys 2003;55:1381–1393.

13 Chen GTY, Kung JH, Beaudette KP: Artifacts in computed tomography scanning of moving objects. Semin Radiat Oncol 2004;14:19–26.

14 Rietzel E, Chen GTY, Choi NC, et al: Four-dimensional image-based treatment planning: target volume segmentation and dose calculation in the presence of respiratory motion. Int J Radiat Oncol Biol Phys 2005;61:1535–1550.

15 Rietzel E, Pan T, Chen GT: Four-dimensional computed tomography: image formation and clinical protocol. Med Phys 2005;32:874–889.

16 Bortfeld TR, Chen GTY: High-precision radiation therapy of moving targets. Semin Radiat Oncol 2004;14:1–100.

17 Mah D, Steckner MC, Palacio E, et al: Characteristics and quality assurance of a dedicated open 0.23 T MRI for radiation therapy simulation. Med Phys 2002;29:2541–2547.

18 Chapman JD, Bradley JD, Eary JF, et al: Molecular (functional) imaging for radiotherapy applications: an RTOG symposium. Int J Radiat Oncol Biol Phys 2003;55:294–301.

19 Ling CC, Humm J, Larson S, et al: Towards multidimensional radiotherapy (MD-CRT): biological imaging and biological conformality. Int J Radiat Oncol Biol Phys 2000;47:551–560.

20 Munley MT, Marks LB, Hardenbergh PH, et al: Functional imaging of normal tissues with nuclear medicine: applications in radiotherapy. Semin Radiat Oncol 2001;11:28–36.

21 Caldwell CB, Mah K, Ung YC, et al: Observer variation in contouring gross tumor volume in patients with poorly defined non-small-cell lung tumors on CT: the impact of [18]FDG-hybrid PET fusion. Int J Radiat Oncol Biol Phys 2001;51:923–931.

22 Gregoire V, Coche E, Cosnard G, et al: Selection and delineation of lymph node target volumes in head and neck conformal radiotherapy. Proposal for standardizing terminology and procedure based on the surgical experience. Radiother Oncol 2000;56:135–150.

23 Martinez-Monge R, Fernades PS, Gupta N, et al: Cross-sectional nodal atlas: a tool for the definition of clinical target volumes in three-dimensional radiation therapy planning. Radiology 1999;211:815–828.

24 Ahnesjö A, Aspradakis MM: Dose calculations for external photon beams in radiotherapy. Phys Med Biol 1999;44:R99–R155.

25 Frank SJ, Forster KM, Stevens CW, et al: Treatment planning for lung cancer: traditional homogeneous point-dose prescription compared with heterogeneity-corrected dose-volume prescription. Int J Radiat Oncol Biol Phys 2003;56:1308–1318.

26 Verhaegen F, Seuntjens J: Monte Carlo modeling of external radiotherapy photon beams (topical review). Phys Med Biol 2003;48:R107–R164.

27 Fraass BA, Smathers J, Deye JA: Summary and recommendations of a National Cancer Institute workshop on issues limiting the clinical use of Monte Carlo dose calculation algorithms for megavoltage external beam radiation therapy. Med Phys 2003;30:3206–3216.

28 Cygler JE, Daskalov GM, Chan GH, et al: Evaluation of the first commercial Monte Carlo dose calculation engine for electron beam treatment planning. Med Phys 2004;31:142–153.

29 Brahme A: Optimized radiation therapy based on radiobiological objectives. Semin Radiat Oncol 1999;9:35–47.

30 Niemierko A: A generalized concept of equivalent uniform dose (EUD) (abstract). Med Phys 1999;26:1100.

31 Wu Q, Mohan R, Niemierko A, et al: Optimization of intensity-modulated radiotherapy plans based on the equivalent uniform dose. Int J Radiat Oncol Biol Phys 2002;52:234–235.

32 Jaffray DA, Drake DG, Moreau M, et al: A radiographic and tomographic imaging system integrated into a medical linear accelerator for localization of bone and soft-tissue targets. Int J Radiat Oncol Biol Phys 1999;45:773–789.

33 Jeraj R, Mackie TR, Balog J, et al: Radiation characteristics of helical tomotherapy. Med Phys 2004;31:396–404.

34 Mackie TR, Holmes T, Swerdloff S, et al: Tomotherapy: a new concept for the delivery of dynamic conformal radiotherapy. Med Phys 1993;20:1709–1719.

35 Mackie TR, Kapatoes J, Ruchala K, et al: Image guidance for precise conformal radiotherapy. Int J Radiat Oncol Biol Phys 2003;56:89–105.

36 Welsh JS, Patel RR, Ritter MA, et al: Helical tomotherapy: an innovative technology and approach to radiation therapy. Technol Cancer Res Treat 2002;1:311–316.

37 Adler JR, Chang SD, Murphy MJ, et al: The CyberKnife: a frameless robotic system for radiosurgery. Stereotact Funct Neurosurg 1997;69:124–128.

38 Martinez AA, Yan D, Lockman D, et al: Improvement in dose escalation using the process of adaptive radiotherapy combined with three-dimensional conformal or intensity-modulated beams for prostate cancer. Int J Radiat Oncol Biol Phys 2001;50:1226–1234.

39 Yan D, Ziaga E, Jaffray D: The use of adaptive radiation therapy to reduce setup error: a prospective clinical study. Int J Radiat Oncol Biol Phys 1998;41:715–720.

40 Yan D, Lockman D: Organ/patient geometric variation in external beam radiotherapy and its effects. Med Phys 2001;28:593–602.

41 Jakel O, Kramer M, Schulz-Ertner D, et al: Treatment planning for carbon ion radiotherapy in Germany: review of clinical trials and treatment planning studies. Radiother Oncol 2004;73(suppl 2):S86–S91.

42 Coleman CN: Linking radiation oncology and imaging through molecular biology (or now that therapy and diagnosis have separated, it's time to get together again!). Radiology 2003;228:29–35.

43 Purdy JA: Data management in radiation oncology. Semin Radiat Oncol 1997;7:1–94.

44 Purdy JA, Harms WB, Michalski JM, Bosch WR: Initial experience with quality assurance of multi-institutional 3D radiotherapy clinical trials. Strahlenther Onkol 1998;174(suppl II):40–42.

45 Zink S: 3D radiation treatment planning: NCI perspective; in Purdy JA, Emami B (eds): 3D Radiation Treatment Planning and Conformal Therapy. Madison, Medical Physics Publishing, 1995, pp 1–10.

46 Intensity Modulated Radiation Therapy Collaborative Working Group: Intensity-modulated radiation therapy: current status and issues of interest. Int J Radiat Oncol Biol Phys 2001;51:880–914.

47 Vijayakumar S, Narayan S, Yang C, et al: Use of benchmark dose-volume histograms in radiotherapy treatment planning for prostate cancer; in Meyer JL (ed): Advances in the Treatment Planning and Delivery of Radiotherapy. Front Radiat Ther Oncol. Basel, Karger, 2006, vol 40, pp 180–192.

48 Purdy JA: Future directions in 3-D treatment planning and delivery: a physicist's perspective. Int J Radiat Oncol Biol Phys 2000;46:3–6.

Prof. James A. Purdy, PhD
Department of Radiation Oncology, UC Davis
Medical Center
4501 X Street, Suite G140
Sacramento, CA 95816 (USA)
Tel. +1 916 734 3932, Fax +1 916 454 4614
E-Mail james.purdy@ucdmc.ucdavis.edu

I. IMRT and IGRT Techniques and Technology

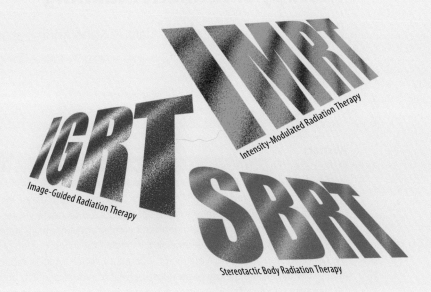

Meyer JL (ed): IMRT, IGRT, SBRT – Advances in the Treatment Planning and
Delivery of Radiotherapy. Front Radiat Ther Oncol. Basel, Karger, 2007, vol. 40, pp 42–58

Obstacles and Advances in Intensity-Modulated Radiation Therapy Treatment Planning

Joseph O. Deasy · James R. Alaly · Konstantin Zakaryan

Siteman Cancer Center and Department of Radiation Oncology, Washington University School
of Medicine, St. Louis, Mo., USA

Abstract

In this paper, the current state of intensity-modulated radiation therapy (IMRT) treatment planning systems is reviewed, including some inefficiencies along with useful workarounds and potential advances. Common obstacles in IMRT treatment planning are discussed, including problems due to the lack of scatter tails in optimization dose calculations, unexpected hot spots appearing in uncontoured regions, and uncontrolled tradeoffs inherent in conventional systems. Workarounds that can be applied in current systems are reviewed, including the incorporation of an 'anchor zone' around the target volume (including a margin of separation), which typically induces adequate dose falloff around the target, and the use of pseudostructures to reduce conflicts among objective functions. We propose changing the planning problem statement so that different dosimetric or outcome goals are prioritized as part of the prescription ('prioritized prescription optimization'). Higher-priority goals are turned into constraints for iterations that consider lower-priority goals. This would control tradeoffs between dosimetric objectives. A plan review tool is proposed that specifically summarizes distances from a structure to hot or cold doses ('dose-distance plots'). An algorithm for including scatter in the optimization process is also discussed. Lastly, brief comments are made about the ongoing effort to use outcome models to rank or optimize treatment plans.

Basic Concepts in Intensity-Modulated Radiation Therapy Treatment Planning

In this first part of our report, basic principles of intensity-modulated radiation therapy (IMRT) treatment planning systems will be briefly reviewed. We will discuss the components of a typical IMRT planning system, how it works, and common problems encountered during planning. The second part will focus on issues our group is concerned with, relevant to improving IMRT planning. For the reader, good introductions are available elsewhere [1–3] and we will high-light important points while emphasizing our own experience and views in this report.

A Typical IMRT Treatment Planning System Today

In IMRT treatment planning, the computer spends a lot of time trying to improve the best beam weight solution previously found. But what is a better solution? The answer is: the one with a lower defined mathematical objective function consistent with the constraints.

In a typical commercial system, some mathematical statements should always hold. These are called *constraints;* for example, 'no more than 45 Gy should be delivered to the spinal cord'. Other mathematical functions, or some of the functions, should be made as small or as large as possible. For instance, 'the average square difference between the target prescription doses and the computer-predicted doses should be as small as possible'. Such statements are added together, with relative weights, resulting in the *objective function.*

The objective function includes terms for normal tissues as well as the target volume, and is usually a weighted sum. This is called a *linear sum objective function.* Different terms have different multiplying weights. This represents a way of specifying the relative importance of these terms, though it may be fuzzy and imprecise.

The state-of-the-art treatment planning system typically has other inputs called *dose-volume constraints,* where the planner does not want any more than x percent of an organ, by volume, to receive y dose. The treatment planning system will try to match or exceed the goal dose-volume histogram (DVH) parameters for target volumes and normal tissues.

A mathematical equation that is often used in IMRT treatment planning as an objective function term is the *generalized equivalent uniform dose* (GEUD). The GEUD, as it has been named by André Niemierko [4], is a volumetric power law average of the dose distribution over a given structure:

$$\text{GEUD} = \left\{ \frac{1}{N} \sum_{i=1}^{N} d_i \times d_i^{(a-1)} \right\}^{1/a} ,$$

where a is the user-defined parameter. It is written this way to emphasize that it is just a power law weighting of the dose distribution. This is very similar, in fact it is mathematically equivalent, to the DVH reduction step in what is called the Lyman-Kutcher-Burman normal tissue complication probability model [5, 6]. The advantage of this simple equation is that, depending upon what the value of the parameter a is chosen to be, the GEUD tends towards the minimum dose, or maximum dose, or something between. If a is negative and large in magnitude, the GEUD tends toward (but does not quite reach) the minimum dose for that structure. If a is positive and large in magnitude, the GEUD tends toward the maximum dose. This might be appropriate for so-called serial structures. If a is close to 1, the GEUD is similar to the mean dose, which might be appropriate for parallel structures [7, 8].

After the objective function is specified, the incident beams are typically idealized by mapping them into small discrete elements, called *beamlets* [3, 9]. Each beam is mathematically modeled, comprised of a sum of these beamlets. Typically, thousands of such beamlets are used in the first part of the optimization process. The aim is for the computer to determine the best or 'optimal' beamlet weights.

In the computer, beamlets are represented as dose contributions to different voxels for a given level of beam monitor units (for example, dose for 1 monitor unit). The overall dose to a volume, for instance a target volume, will be the weighted contributions of all of the beamlets from all beams. Most commercial systems take the approach wherein beamlet fluences are first optimized and afterwards multileaf collimator (MLC) settings are derived as a deliverable sequence. This is the most common approach, although some companies are considering an approach that starts with apertures, and directly modifies or optimizes the aperture shapes.

Once all the terms are put together into an objective function, and the beamlet matrices are computed, the computer is asked to iterate the beamlet weights until objective function progress between iterations falls to a specified low level. In actual practice, it is always a problem to tell when you should cut off the optimization iterations, and it is often not very clear at all when you are done.

After the beam fluence maps have been derived, they must be broken up (decomposed) into deliverable segments for each beam that the MLC can deliver in a stepwise fashion. For some systems, the beam can be on when the segment is delivered, even when the MLC leaves are moving (dynamic delivery). Otherwise, the beam is off when the MLC leaves are moving between segments (static or step-and-shoot delivery). The many resulting segments together comprise the full delivery of the fluence map. An attempt is made to reconstruct that fluence map (as well as possible) by the superposition of these segments, but there is always some discretization error (usually but not necessarily small).

Problems with Today's IMRT Treatment Planning Systems
There are multiple problems with this state-of-the-art system, and some of these we will discuss here:

(1) Do DVH Constraints Derived in the Pre-IMRT Era Apply to IMRT Dose Distributions?
It is often difficult to know what the clinical outcome effect of input DVH parameters will be. This is especially important because much of the outcome literature is based on an analysis of three-dimensional conformal radiation therapy data.

If you specify DVH constraints from data derived from three-dimensional conformal radiation therapy, the resulting IMRT plan will of course be different. There is a fundamental problem here of walking into unknown territory and extrapolating, at least until we gather more outcome data based upon IMRT dose distributions [10].

(2) The Weight Paradox

A related issue is what we will call the *weight paradox:* the planner desires to give the target a high enough weight such that the target coverage is excellent, but the planner also wants to give enough weight to nearby normal structures so that they are avoided as much as possible. These often conflict, and must be balanced. The best balance is unfortunately unknown, resulting in expensive trial-and-error tests that never authoritatively resolve the issue. This leads to an uncertain answer to the ubiquitous question: 'Are we finished planning?'

Even if the clinical implications of DVH input parameters were clear (typically not the case), there is still a guessing game of what DVH dose-volume cut points should be input. The reason is that the planner should specify DVH goals that push the system to perform better by reducing normal tissue dose-volume levels. But DVH goals that are much too aggressive may overly affect the target dose distribution, or the planner may be forced to reduce the DVH weight so low that it is effectively ignored. On the other hand, because the best performance (i.e., best dose distributions) are unknown before planning takes place, the DVH constraints may often be chosen to be too lenient. Typically, initial parameters are used that worked for the last treatment plan. This strategy often works for prostate tumors where the patients often look similar (from a planning perspective). But this strategy typically fails for head and neck tumors, where the whole process is iterated: the planner puts in some inputs, a new plan is generated, inputs are changed, a new plan is generated, etc. Thus, there is nearly always uncertainty in terms of what the best input parameters are.

(3) Hard-to-Control Tradeoffs and the Lack of Clear Priorities

Again, the planner wants the target to receive a high uniform dose, but nearby normal structures should be avoided. If the normal tissue structures are close enough, and they are given high weights, this would compromise the target dose coverage. There is no perfect compromise between conflicting goals, and it is almost always impossible for the planner to determine if the 'right' compromise has been achieved.

Hence, there is frequently heard a conversation that goes something like this:
Physician, 'This is the prescription I would like to give.'
Dosimetrist, comes back later and says, 'I tried it, and tried to fix it, here is the plan.'

Physician (thinking to himself, 'is that the best that they can do?') says, 'Well, thanks. Uh, how busy are you? Can you try to improve this part?'

Dosimetrist, 'I am busy but I will try, if you really want me to.'[1]

This illustrates the near-universal inability, with current IMRT planning systems, to determine if the best tradeoffs between target and normal tissue dosimetric goals have been achieved. Another approach, which is sometimes adopted, is to relax planning goals to make the problem easier without many cycles of changing inputs and rerunning the planning system.

(4) Dosimetric Modeling Problems

There are always issues with the dosimetric modeling of the delivery system because the requirement is (typically) to do fast beamlet optimization and then convert to deliverable leaf sequences. As mentioned above, during the leaf sequence creation based on the fluence maps, there is a degradation in dose distribution quality because it is impossible to match the fluence map exactly with a limited number of static segments. Another important issue is that simplified dose calculation methods are often used during the optimization step. This usually means that a so-called optimal solution was derived based on beamlets that have the scattered radiation tails cut off. Thus, the long tails of radiation are not correctly added into the solution. This has some consequences for target coverage, further discussed below. This issue is highly planning system specific.

(5) Hot Spots outside the Target

Sometimes the planner ends up with hot spots outside the target but in regions that were not contoured. Planners often create pseudostructures, either after the fact where a hot spot has shown up, or before the planning run where hot spots are known to often show up. Below, we discuss our approach to this issue.

(6) The Lack of Dose Tweaking Tools

The lack of tools to make small, limited changes to an IMRT treatment plan ('tweaking tools') is a problem because often there is a dose distribution that is almost what is desired, but not quite. With almost all of the commercial systems available now, the planner is basically forced to rerun the whole process. This continues to be a missing element of most commercial planning systems. However, some of the systems will do a so-called 'hot start' where you do not have to go all the way back to the beginning. The NOMOS company has recently introduced an interesting tweaking tool based on dragging isodose lines.

---

[1] During the conference, attendees (mostly physicians) were asked by a show of hands how many had previously had such a conversation. I estimate 80–90% of hands were raised. Individuals believing that research into IMRT treatment planning is 'done' should carefully consider this present inefficient status of the current systems.

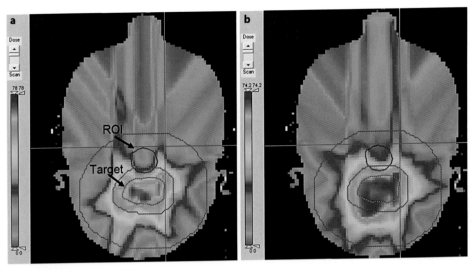

Fig. 1. The effect of increasing the target weight. **a** Target compromised; ROI highly spared. Target = 1 × ROI. **b** Target takes precedence, but ROI is still somewhat spared. Target = 20 × ROI.

Treatment Planning Workarounds: Some Suggestions

To illustrate a few of these issues and demonstrate strategies, we show results of some simple simulations. The treatment plan setup uses just five photon beams (6 MV) with a weighted quadratic objective function, in our research treatment planning system (CERR) [11]. The geometry is that of an oval cross section target in the brain (the inner oval) and a nearby (green) dose-limiting normal structure region of interest (ROI) (fig. 1). We emphasize that these are not treatment quality results, but rather illustrations of the effects seen in many of today's commercial planning systems.

If we start with the target objective function term having the same weight as the normal tissue ROI, the dose will typically be compromised in the target (fig. 1a). So, the weight of the target is typically increased (fig. 1b). Of course, this lesson does not have to be learned for every plan. In figure 1b, the target has a weight of 20 times the normal tissue ROI. The target takes precedence where it is close to the ROI, but the ROI is still spared somewhat. This works in this case because there is a gap between the ROI and the target.

The outer region in figure 2, marked 'AZ' (anchor zone), is a workaround/solution to avoid hot spots outside of the target. We create a 'moat' or margin around the target where there is no weighted contour, allowing for dose falloff. Inner and outer boundaries comprise an anchor zone. The anchor zone acts to squeeze down the dose outside of the target in a relatively uniform way without overly affecting the dose at the edge of the target volume. Some clinics, such as The Fox Chase

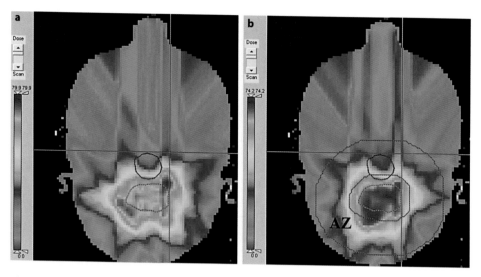

Fig. 2. The effect of adding an anchor zone. **a** No anchor zone. Hot spots outside target up to 80 Gy. **b** Anchor zone (AZ). Hot spots outside target reduced to 74 Gy or less.

Cancer Center, introduce concentric shells that are structures contiguous to the target. The shells are weighted to induce rapid dose falloff. The anchor zone technique, however, leaves a gap to allow the dose to fall off gradually in voxels immediately adjacent to the target. With the anchor zone (fig. 2b), the hot spot dose outside the target is reduced. To induce falloff superior and inferior to the target volume, it is also useful to put caps/ROIs superior and inferior to the target (fig. 3).

What if the problem is made harder by moving the normal tissue ROI closer to the target (fig. 4)? Here in figure 4a, the ROI is in contact with the target. The ROI is spared, but the target gets compromised somewhat. If the ROI is made to overlap the target significantly (fig. 4b), it is important to establish the *priority* of the two structures. If not, the optimizer will make a compromise among unachievable objectives. Either the target will receive a good dose distribution, or the optimizer will spare the ROI. One option is to crank up the weight to the target to 100 times the ROI, but then the ROI volume even far from the target will be poorly spared (fig. 5).

Another option, used by planners fairly routinely, is to take the ROI volume minus the target volume and create a new volume. There is a slight improvement in the target DVH when a nonoverlapping structure is created (fig. 6). Although it does not have a big impact in this particular example, this workaround is often used to keep the conflict down for the optimizer, so that it will still work effectively on both the ROI and the target. At Washington University, this is fairly common practice. For example, the bladder minus the planning target volume (PTV) is often specified in prostate plans.

Deasy · Alaly · Zakaryan

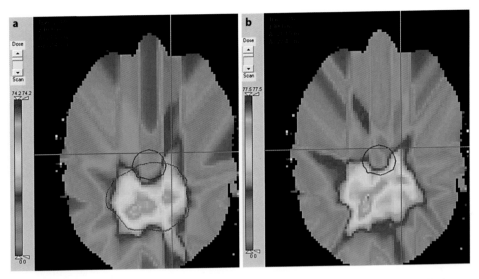

Fig. 3. The effect of adding superior and inferior end caps to the target volume. **a** End caps superior/inferior to target. Hot spot outside target up to 70 Gy. **b** No superior/inferior end caps. Hot spot superior to target goes up to 78 Gy.

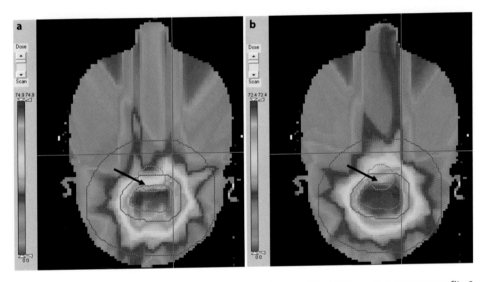

Fig. 4. The problem of geometrically conflicting volumes. What if there is a greater conflict? **a** ROI in contact with target. ROI spared; target compromised. **b** ROI overlaps target. Target takes precedence, but some compromise.

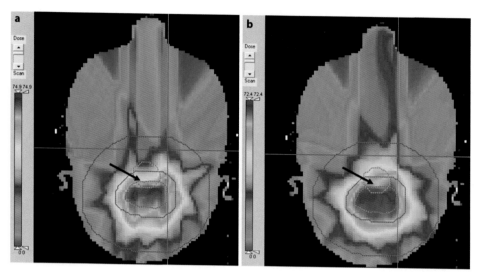

Fig. 5. The effect of making the target weight huge. **a** Target is compromised. Target = 20 × ROI. **b** ROI is effectively ignored. Target = 100 × ROI.

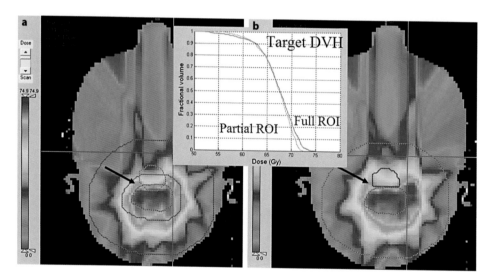

Fig. 6. Redefining the normal tissue ROI. **a** ROI overlaps target. ROI spared, but target compromised. **b** ROI minus target. Slightly better target coverage.

Deasy · Alaly · Zakaryan

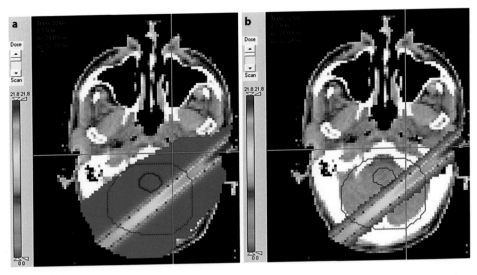

Fig. 7. The scatter tail of an IMRT beamlet. Beamlets are usually simplified for the optimization phase. **a** Beamlet with a 4-cm tail. **b** Beamlet with a 1-cm tail.

Workaround for Chopped Beamlets

Beamlets are usually dosimetrically simplified for the optimization phase, as previously mentioned. The algorithm designer will often chop off the scatter tails for each beamlet, so that the data structures are reduced in size (fig. 7). In figure 7, we compare beamlets with the scattered tail included (fig. 7a) and with the tails chopped off (fig. 7b). The scatter tail does fall off rapidly with distance from the beamlet center axis. However, those tails do have significant effects. One effect of not including scatter tails in the optimization algorithm that we see clinically occurs when you start out with just a PTV and optimize to that. When you look at the final computed dose distribution, computed with a dose calculation algorithm that includes scatter, the superior and inferior slices will typically not be well covered. The reason (we believe) is that the 'final' dose calculation includes scatter (i.e., a more complete version of each beamlet's influence), but during the optimization process itself the influence of coplanar beamlets on other slice planes is somewhat neglected. Hence, the optimizer infers that fluence is not required superior and inferior to the target to contribute dose to the target end slices. At Washington University, we often add a pseudo-PTV target on slices superior and inferior to the real PTV. After optimization to that pseudo-PTV, the desired dose coverage to the original PTV is achieved, after the good (final) dose calculation.

Figure 8 sketches an algorithm we are using that allows for the optimization process to be based on chopped beamlets, while correcting periodically based on full-scatter corrections so that overall solution converges to a good result that

An iterative scatter correction method

(1) Estimate the scatter dose using full dose (primary plus scatter) beamlet matrices and best current estimate of beam weights. Initially assume uniform fluence from all beams.
(2) Adjust prescription dose, on a voxel-by-voxel basis, to reflect the expected scatter contribution.
(3) Solve for optimal beam weights using primary-only beamlet matrices.
(4) Recompute full dose using beamlet matrices stored on disk.
(5) If full dose is close enough to prescription, terminate; otherwise go to step 1. Typically, two to three iterations are sufficient.

Fig. 8. A method for including scatter in the optimization phase [12].

accounts for scatter. Typically, the full-scatter correction needs only to be done two or three times. This is quite similar to an algorithm used at Memorial Sloan Kettering Cancer Center [13]. The only important difference is that we start with an estimate of the scattered dose assuming uniform intensity from all beams.

Approaches to Improving Intensity-Modulated Radiation Therapy Treatment Planning

Here are some approaches to improving IMRT treatment planning we have been investigating.

Prioritized Prescription Optimization
As mentioned, in conventional linearly weighted optimization the problem of uncontrolled tradeoffs between objective function terms will always exist. The conventional workflow is shown in figure 9. The IMRT problem is stated, the computer solves the optimization problem, and the planner reviews the result. If the plan is judged to be not good enough to terminate, then (based on the experience and intelligence of the treatment planner) the input is changed, and another plan is run. We believe we should move to a solution paradigm that is described in figure 10, which we call *prioritized prescription optimization* [14, 15]. This is known as *preemptive goal programming* or lexicographic goal programming in the operations research field [16]. The University of Michigan group has developed a clinically useful implementation of this paradigm, which they presented at the AAPM meeting in 2004 [17]. This is a paradigm where the physician first specifies the priorities of the competing clinical objectives. First, the optimizer tackles the highest-priority objective (such as best target coverage), along with any high-pri-

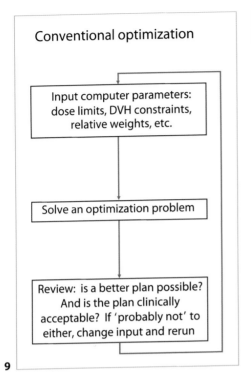

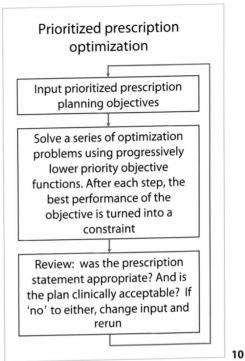

Fig. 9. The conventional IMRT planning workflow.

Fig. 10. Prioritized prescription IMRT planning workflow.

ority constraints (such as no more than 45 Gy to the spinal cord), and determines the best performance. Then, the algorithm turns that performance into a constraint for lower-priority iterations, and the optimizer then solves with the next lower-priority prescription objective. In this iterative fashion, the optimizer works through all the less important objectives. Some objectives may be placed on the same priority level if there is no concern about how they might trade off against each other. Objectives like smooth weights might be less important, though still clinically useful, but only if they do not degrade something like target coverage. This way, more important objectives are never corrupted by less important objectives. Yet, less important objectives are considered in an effective way, so long as they do not corrupt more important objectives.

Figure 11 shows an example result of prioritized treatment planning derived using our research treatment planning system (CERR) [11] and the Mosek optimization toolbox. In this head and neck treatment plan, the most important objective is to have good target coverage. Next, the risk of xerostomia should be reduced as much as possible. Lastly, the dose falloff should be good in all direc-

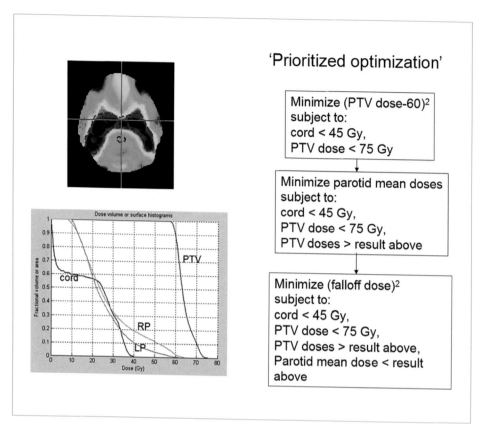

Fig. 11. A head and neck prioritized prescription example.

tions (something that also encourages smooth beam weights). In the first step, the dose variation in the PTV was minimized given the hard constraint on the spinal cord dose. In the second step, dose was reduced to the parotid glands, but the optimizer did not ruin the target coverage, which had been turned into a constraint. In this paradigm, the optimizer appears able to better avoid the parotid glands compared to the conventional alternative of using a linearly weighted objective function, giving the parotid glands a very low weight, and expecting them to come out well. Finally, we minimized the average square dose in the anchor zone. This serves to facilitate dose falloff outside the target and actually smoothes out beam weights as well (a more complete report has been submitted [18]).

Prioritized optimization has many benefits. (1) Physicians tend to have a natural prioritization that they would be able to elucidate, but the commercial systems do not allow that right now. (2) Prioritized optimization avoids clinically undesirable tradeoffs among objectives that are difficult to control. (3) Prioritized optimization avoids fixing hard constraints to be more restrictive than necessary,

Deasy · Alaly · Zakaryan

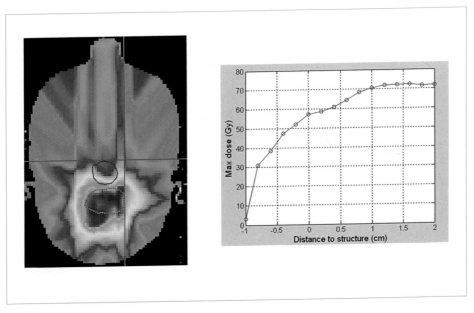

Fig. 12. The dose-distance plot for a normal tissue structure.

something that often happens when you are guessing the inputs into these treatment planning systems. (4) More factors can be included in the optimization process in a reliable way. (5) There is more certainty that better plans are unobtainable compared with conventional linearly weighted formulations. This last issue is extremely important, as the planning team gets away from guessing whether the planning process (changing inputs and running new plans) has reached diminishing returns.

There are two main drawbacks to prioritized optimization: (1) more optimization problems need to be solved, and (2) it is possible that a better solution may actually exist with a different prioritization scheme. However, with prioritized optimization, there may often be fewer instances of changing inputs and rerunning the optimizer, so total planning time is likely to be reduced on average. Ultimately, future clinical experience will determine the value of this framework. Nonetheless, due to its advantages, we believe prioritized optimization (or something like it) is likely to end up in most commercial planning systems.

Summarizing Locational Information about Hot and Cold Spots:
Dose-Distance Plots
Tools for examining or interrogating the dose distributions can be significantly improved. Figure 12 shows something we have named the *dose-distance plot.* It answers the question of how far hot spots are from a critical normal structure, or

how far cold spots are from the surface of a target volume. For a normal structure ROI (fig. 12), the zero x-axis point represents the surface of the displayed ROI (negative values are inside the structure), and the corresponding data point is the maximum dose anywhere on the surface of that structure. Similarly, the 0.5-cm data point is the maximum dose *anywhere* at a minimum distance of 0.5 cm outside the structure (this is a 'differential' plot). Dose-distance plots can give a clear idea of the setup accuracy that is required for the treatment,[2] something that is missing from DVHs. In this case, the dose-distance plot indicates that a shift of only 4 mm could potentially increase the ROI surface dose to 60 Gy. Dose-distance plots are highly complementary to DVHs, and are simple graphical summaries of important, yet currently inaccessible plan information. We hope they find their way into commercial systems soon.

Biologically Based Treatment Planning

Finally, we briefly discuss the inevitable move towards more biologically based treatment planning using models to predict the complication risk of a given treatment plan, or even using the models as computerized objective functions. After all, the goal is to get local/regional control while avoiding complications insofar as possible. An increasing number of data sets have been published that have been used to refine or reinforce the outcome models, and thus support the idea that ranking individual treatment plans is not just 'pie in the sky' [19]. It might be 10 years or more, for some endpoints, before we have well-validated and reliable models that can rank treatment plans, but this is the clear direction.

As one example, figure 13 shows a result from a clinical study of xerostomia at Washington University which was begun by Dr. Clifford Chao [20, 21]. This is stimulated relative whole-mouth salivary flow as a function of right parotid mean dose and left parotid mean dose (fig. 13a is 6 months after radiotherapy, fig. 13b is 12 months after radiotherapy), taken from our second publication on this subject [20]. From these data, it appears likely that if even just one parotid gland gets significantly less than a 20-Gy mean dose, there is a good chance of preserving relative salivary function greater than 25% (the technical threshold of xerostomia). However, the data imply that whole parotid gland function improves as the mean dose is decreased, even below 20 Gy.

These data show that we can predict salivary function, though with some uncertainty [22]. It appears we can clearly group some patients into high risk and low risk, based on a model of the data using mean dose alone [20]. Other data sources and endpoint analyses relevant for IMRT have recently become available, for example for rectal bleeding and small bowel complications [7].

---

[2]   An exception when the dose-distance plot is not useful for understanding setup error is when the structure is near the skin, and the dose falloff is due to anatomy, rather than fluence falloff alone.

Deasy · Alaly · Zakaryan

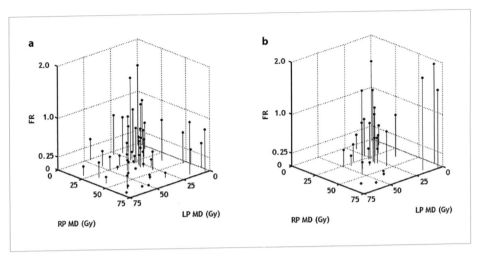

Fig. 13. Stimulated whole-mouth salivary flow as a function of left and right parotid mean doses. Salivary flow is a strong function of parotid gland mean doses. FR = Flow relative to pre-RT; RP MD = right parotid mean dose; LP MD = left parotid mean dose. **a** Six months after RT. **b** Twelve months. Reproduced with permission of Blanco et al. [19].

Conclusion

In summary, IMRT treatment planning needs further developments, including greater efficiency and improved dosimetric accuracy especially within the optimization phase. The systems need to have improved 'clinical steerability', meaning that when the clinician has a goal that is feasible, the system can be directed to go there in a straightforward way. Above all, tradeoffs between clinical goals should be made controllable, because, as Goethe said: 'More important things should never be at the mercy of less important things.'

Acknowledgments

We gratefully acknowledge useful discussions with Mark Wiesmeyer (Washington University and Siteman Cancer Center) and Rudi Bertrand (Barnes-Jewish Hospital and Siteman Cancer Center). This work was supported by NIH grants R01 CA85181 and R01 CA90445 and a grant from Computerized Medical Systems, Inc.

References

1 Galvin JM, Ezzell G, Eisbrauch A, Yu C, Butler B, Xiao Y, Rosen I, Rosenman J, Sharpe M, Xing L, Xia P, Lomax T, Low DA, Palta J: Implementing IMRT in clinical practice: a joint document of the American Society for Therapeutic Radiology and Oncology and the American Association of Physicists in Medicine. Int J Radiat Oncol Biol Phys 2004;58:1616–1634.

2 Ezzell GA, Galvin JM, Low D, Palta JR, Rosen I, Sharpe MB, Xia P, Xiao Y, Xing L, Yu CX: Guidance document on delivery, treatment planning, and clinical implementation of IMRT: report of the IMRT Subcommittee of the AAPM Radiation Therapy Committee. Med Phys 2003;30:2089–2115.

3 Langer M, Lee EK, Deasy JO, Rardin RL, Deye JA: Operations research applied to radiotherapy, an NCI-NSF-sponsored workshop February 7–9, 2002. Int J Radiat Oncol Biol Phys 2003;57:762–768.

4 Niemierko A: A generalized concept of equivalent uniform dose (abstract). Med Phys 1999;26:1100.

5 Deasy JO: Comments on the use of the Lyman-Kutcher-Burman model to describe tissue response to nonuniform irradiation. Int J Radiat Oncol Biol Phys 2000;47:1458–1460.

6 Kutcher GJ, Burman C, Brewster L, Goitein M, Mohan R: Histogram reduction method for calculating complication probabilities for three-dimensional treatment planning evaluations. Int J Radiat Oncol Biol Phys 1991;21:137–146.

7 Deasy JO, Fowler JF: The radiobiology of intensity-modulated radiation therapy; in Mundt AJ (ed): Intensity-Modulated Radiation Therapy: A Clinical Perspective. Hamilton, Decker, 2005.

8 Moiseenko V, Deasy JO, Van Dyk J: Radiobiological modeling for treatment planning; in van Dyk J (ed): Modern Technology of Radiation Therapy. Madison, Medical Physics Publishing, 2005, vol 2.

9 Webb S: Intensity-Modulated Radiation Therapy. Bristol, Institute of Physics Publishing, 2001.

10 Deasy JO, Niemierko A, Herbert D, Yan D, Jackson A, Ten Haken RK, Langer M, Sapareto S: Methodological issues in radiation dose-volume outcome analyses: summary of a joint AAPM/NIH workshop. Med Phys 2002;29:2109–2127.

11 Deasy JO, Blanco AI, Clark VH: CERR: a computational environment for radiotherapy research. Med Phys 2003;30:979–985.

12 Zakarian C, Lindsay PE, El Naqa I, Deasy JO: 46th Annu Meet Am Soc Ther Radiol Oncol, Atlanta, 2004. Int J Rad Oncol Biol Phys 2004;60:S629.

13 Spirou S, Chui C: IMRT plan optimization; in Fuks Z, Leibel S, Ling C (eds): A Practical Guide to Intensity-Modulated Radiation Therapy. Madison, Medical Physics, 2003, pp 53–70.

14 Deasy JO: Prioritized treatment planning for radiotherapy optimization. World Congr Med Phys Biomed Eng (proceedings on CD-ROM), Chicago, 2000.

15 Deasy JO: The IMRT optimization problem statement. Operations Res Appl Radiat Ther, Dulles, 2002. http://www2.isye.gatech.edu/nci-nsf.orart.2002/talks.php.

16 Ignizio JP: Introduction to Linear Goal Programming. Beverly Hills, Sage Publications, 1985, vol 56.

17 Jee K, McShan D, Fraass B: Intuitive multicriteria IMRT optimization using a lexicographic approach. Med Phys 2004;31:1715–1715.

18 Wilkens JJ, Alaly JR, Zakaryan K, Thorstad WL, Deasy JO: A method for IMRT treatment planning based on prioritizing prescription goals. Phys Med Biol, accepted.

19 Ten Haken RK: Partial Organ Irradiation. Sem Rad Oncol 2001, vol 11.

20 Blanco AI, Chao KSC, El Naqa I, Franklin GE, Zakarian K, Vicic M, Deasy JO: Dose-volume modeling of salivary function in patients with head-and-neck cancer receiving radiotherapy. Int J Radiat Oncol Biol Phys 2005;62:1055–1069.

21 Chao KS, Deasy JO, Markman J, Haynie J, Perez CA, Purdy JA, Low DA: A prospective study of salivary function sparing in patients with head-and-neck cancers receiving intensity-modulated or three-dimensional radiation therapy: initial results. Int J Radiat Oncol Biol Phys 2001;49:907–916.

22 Deasy JO, Chao KS, Markman J: Uncertainties in model-based outcome predictions for treatment planning. Int J Radiat Oncol Biol Phys 2001;51:1389–1399.

Dr. Joe Deasy
WUSM Radiation Oncology, Division of
Bioinformatics and Outcomes Research
4921 Parkview Place, Box 8224
St. Louis, MO 63110 (USA)
Tel. +1 314 362 1420, Fax +1 314 362 8521
E-Mail jdeasy@radonc.wustl.edu

Meyer JL (ed): IMRT, IGRT, SBRT – Advances in the Treatment Planning and
Delivery of Radiotherapy. Front Radiat Ther Oncol. Basel, Karger, 2007, vol. 40, pp 59–71

Four-Dimensional Imaging and Treatment Planning of Moving Targets

George T.Y. Chen · Jong H. Kung · Eike Rietzel

Department of Radiation Oncology, Massachusetts General Hospital, Boston, Mass., USA

Abstract

Four-dimensional CT acquisition is commercially available, and provides important information on the shape and trajectory of the tumor and normal tissues. The primary advantage of four-dimensional imaging over light breathing helical scans is the reduction of motion artifacts during scanning that can significantly alter tumor appearance. Segmentation, image registration, visualization are new challenges associated with four-dimensional data sets because of the overwhelming increase in the number of images. Four-dimensional dose calculations, while currently laborious, provide insights into dose perturbations due to organ motion. Imaging before treatment (image guidance) improves accuracy of radiation delivery, and recording transmission images can provide a means of verifying gated delivery.

Precise knowledge and control of the three-dimensional dose distribution is considered to be essential for a favorable therapeutic outcome. The ability to deliver highly conformal dose distributions through intensity-modulated radiotherapy has become common for sites such as head and neck and prostate. When the target moves due to respiration, precise delivery of dose becomes more challenging and of concern. This is due in part to inadequate knowledge of the detailed dose delivered during motion [1, 2]. This article reviews three aspects of the irradiation of moving targets: (1) the imaging of moving objects, and understanding of such images; (2) the impact of respiratory motion on dose, and (3) a clinical example of image-guided/gated radiotherapy delivered to a moving target. For the interested reader, additional information on the irradiation of moving targets appeared in 2004 [3].

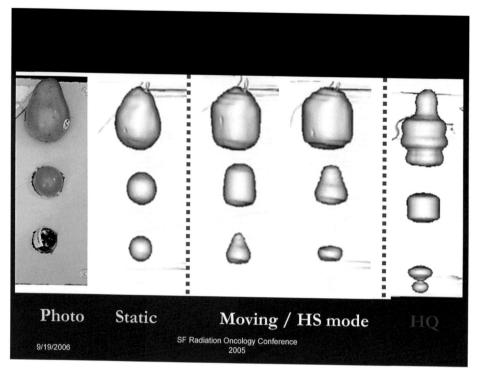

Fig. 1. Temporal aliasing resulting from helical scanning of moving objects. From left to right: photograph of static phantom objects, followed by surface rendering of objects after CT scan under static conditions. The next three columns of images show distortions when the object moves simulating respiration. The mid two columns of images are under conditions of high-speed mode; the rightmost column shows different artifacts when the object is scanned in the high-quality mode, where the pitch is one half that of the high-speed mode.

Artifacts in Imaging of Moving Objects

Artifacts due to motion during tomographic scans have been appreciated for many years [4, 5]. A common observation in scans of the thorax is the irregularity of beam's eye view of a target in the lung due to motion during scanning. Discontinuities in the diaphragm/lung interface are also commonly observed when scans are taken during light breathing. In 2002, one of the authors (J.H.K.) proposed an experiment to scan a phantom moving on a mechanical stage that simulated motion during respiration. He built a mechanical stage that sinusoidally oscillated along the longitudinal axis of the body with a periodicity of 4 s, and an amplitude of 1 cm; spherical objects (balls) placed in a block of Styrofoam rested on the stage. The left column in figure 1 shows a photograph of a portion of the phantom, where several rubber balls are visible. The second column is a surface rendering of these

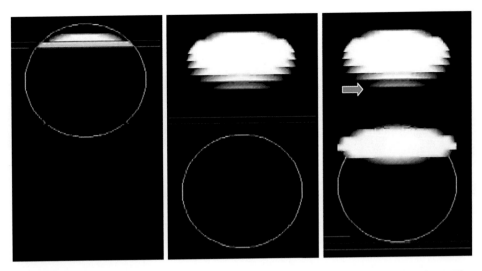

Fig. 2. Frames of a computer animation illustrating formation of images of a moving object. The white circle represents a sphere moving up/down sinusoidally. The white objects are CT slices formed during the intersection of the imaging plane with the spherical object. Note the lowest slice of the upper object (arrow) is actually the top of the sphere (see animation online at *WEB*).

objects when the phantom was scanned in the static mode. This surface rendering shows a geometrically accurate image of the objects. When the mechanical stage is set in motion and scans are acquired in the conventional helical mode, the resulting images of the spherical objects are significantly distorted as shown in the next three columns. The direction of the oscillatory motion is up/down along the columns. In one experiment, a 6-cm diameter ball was imaged during motion (2 cm peak to peak) as a distorted sphere with a longitudinal axis dimension of 4 cm, a full 2 cm smaller than its actual physical size. The technical term for this distortion is temporal aliasing.

A computer program was written to simulate the scanning process of moving objects, in order to improve our understanding of the effect [6]. Figure 2 is a composite image of the dynamic simulation. The sphere, which is represented by a thin white circle, is imaged in the simulation as two separate objects. The sphere moves over a much larger range than the objects imaged (see animation online at *WEB*). Notice the shape of the bottom slice of the upper object. This can be recognized as the top of the sphere by its curvature. The simulation graphically illustrates the presence of shuffling of the axial slices of the object. The asynchronous motions of organ/target and the monotonically advancing axial imaging of the object by the scanner can result in unusual perturbations in the imaging of a known object. Object parameters such as the size, shape, amplitude of motion, periodicity asyn-

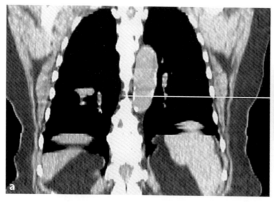
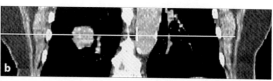

Fig. 3. a Coronal section through the patient scanned for lung tumor in the right lung. Section is through a light breathing CT scan. **b** One phase of a 4DCT scan through the same plane. Note the difference in tumor shape. Coverage longitudinally differs to spare the normal lung from dose, and focuses primarily on tumor motion.

chronously interact with scan parameters (slice thickness, pitch) through the respiratory phase at which the scanner intersects the moving object. Note in figure 1 that in the displayed coronal plane, it is possible for some objects to be lengthened while others are shortened. The effect depends on the specific phase of object motion as the scan plane intersects the sphere.

Temporal aliasing artifacts are also frequently observed in patient scans. Figure 3a is the coronal multiplanar reconstruction of a thorax scanned in the helical mode under the commonly applied condition of light breathing. One clearly sees the lung/diaphragm discontinuity artifacts. In comparison, figure 3b shows a comparable coronal section that has been reconstructed from a four-dimensional CT (4DCT) scan at a specific phase of the respiratory cycle. The difference in shape and size of the tumor between the two scanning techniques is apparent.

Four-Dimensional CT Scanning

Proof of the principle of respiration-correlated CT was shown by early investigators [7–9] in 2003, and 4DCT became commercially available in 2004. Respiration-correlated CT uses a surrogate signal, such as the abdominal surface, respiratory air flow, or internal anatomy to provide a signal that permits resorting of the reconstructed image data, resulting in multiple coherent spatiotemporal data sets at different respiratory phases. The scan time for 4DCT with multislice scanners is on the order of a few minutes, and postprocessing takes an additional 30 min if manual phase selection is required. The output of this process is typically 10 CT

Chen · Kung · Rietzel

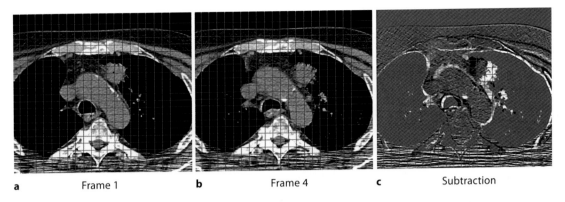

Fig. 4. Frames 1 (**a**) and 4 (**b**) are at the extrema of tumor motion. Subtracted (difference) image in **c** shows little bone motion, but significant motion of the tumor in the left-right axis (see animation of tumor motion online at *WEB*).

volumes, each with a temporal resolution of approx. 1/10 of the respiratory period. At Massachusetts General Hospital (MGH), we have used the GE/Varian 4D acquisition system, and have scanned about 150 patients to date. The 4DCT implementation relies on sensing the respiratory phase by using the Varian RPM system. Technical details of the approach are described elsewhere [10–12].

4DCT thus provides an imaging tool to quantify and characterize tumor and normal tissue shape and motion as a function of time. This provides the radiation oncologist and treatment planner with information essential in the design of an aperture that more adequately covers the internal target volume (assuming respiration during treatment is reproducible to that during CT simulation). 4DCT data can also be used as input in making treatment decisions on when to intervene with gating or other motion management strategies. In addition, the 4DCT data can be used as direct input into four-dimensional treatment planning, and to generate time-varying dose-volume histograms or isodose distributions [13, 14].

An effective method of conveying the utility of 4DCT is through computer animation. Typically, as used in the clinic at MGH, animations are played to display the position of tumor and normal anatomy over a respiratory cycle. In this print version, we display several static frames from the animation as well as difference images to show differences in anatomy as a function of time.

Figure 4 shows an interesting case provided by Dr. Noah Choi, thoracic radiation oncologist at MGH. As can be seen, the lesion is near the aortic arch. An animation shows tumor motion is primarily from left to right rather than craniocaudal; the magnitude of the lateral motion is approximately ±1 cm. Figure 4a, b shows the lesion in the extreme lateral positions; figure 4c shows the difference image. Regions of dark and light highlight areas of greatest motion. As can be seen, there is relatively little motion of the bony anatomy, and a slight shifting of the trachea between respiratory extrema. Dr. Choi et al. [pers. commun., 2005] have found that approximately one half of patients with early-stage disease have motion of less than 10 mm during quiet breathing (in approx. 100 cases). Seppenwoolde et al. [15] reported on the motion of 21 lesions in 20 patients and found a mean motion of 5.5 mm in the craniocaudal direction (data ranged from 0 to 2.5 cm). Average periodicity was observed to be 3.5 s, and ranged from 2.8 to over 6 s. The clinical importance of 4DCT is that it provides insight into patient-specific organ motion.

Challenges Posed by Four-Dimensional CT

The value of four-dimensional imaging is in its use to make clinical treatment decisions. There are typically three options considered in treating a moving tumor. One is to treat the internal target volume; under this circumstance, the role of 4DCT is to define the extent of tumor motion and design an aperture that includes the target trajectory. The second approach is to gate treatment; a number of groups have chosen to gate beam on at exhale. The role of four-dimensional imaging here is to initially determine that the magnitude of motion is sufficiently large to require gating, and then to ascertain the accurate shape of the tumor near exhale. The third option is to track the tumor during its motion as proposed by some investigators [14, 16]. In principle, four-dimensional imaging and dose calculations can provide data on the suitability of these treatment strategy options. At the current time, such calculations remain a practical challenge because of the volume of image data generated.

There is nearly an order-of-magnitude increase in the amount of image data available in 4DCT. One cannot expect radiation oncologists or treatment planners to contour 10 sets of tumor and normal anatomy in treatment planning. Alternative automated methods must be developed, validated and implemented.

After synthesizing multiple volumetric anatomic data sets from 4DCT, tools are needed to effectively browse and visualize the data. Approximately 500 MB of image data are available for visualization. Figure 5 shows one approach we have pursued in collaboration with the Scientific Computing Institute at the University of Utah (http://www.sci-utah.org). Bioimage displays gradients in the data that can show four-dimensional anatomy at near-interactive frame rates. An animation can be seen online at *WEB*. Additional Bioimage tools can be used to measure the trajectories of points of interest.

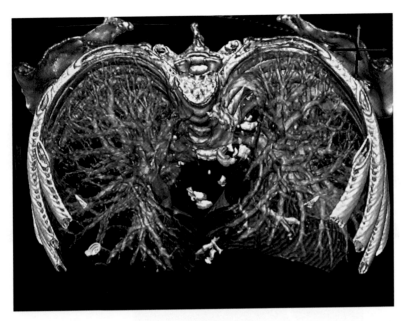

Fig. 5. Volume-rendered frame of a 4DCT scan, showing the tracheobronchial tree from a superior anterior view. A version of Bioimage was used to generate the four-dimensional volume rendering (see animation online at *WEB*).

Four-Dimensional Dose Calculations

A number of questions arise in considering how delivered dose to each voxel is affected by motion. These include: (1) the magnitude of isodose perturbations by motion with three-dimensional conformal radiation therapy; (2) the specific impact of motion on intensity-modulated radiation therapy (IMRT) delivery; (3) how to use 4DCT to decide if a motion mitigation strategy is needed, and (4) the primary factors that determine the magnitude of dose changes from motion. These questions are technically challenging to answer because of the complexities of four-dimensional treatment planning and the assumptions about breathing patterns during treatment itself. However, some insights can be gained by initial planning studies, and will be described.

Figure 6 shows (static images; see animation online at *WEB*) the consequences of applying a treatment plan designed for a 'static' geometry, but applied to 4DCT data. A static fluence pattern of photons (designed from a helical scan) is applied to the 10 respiratory phases of the 4DCT data in the irradiation of a lung target. Upon careful inspection, there are perturbations in the isodose lines of the treatment plan. In this example, the radiation fields are sufficiently large so that within the motion of the 4DCT, there is no obvious geometric miss of the gross tumor

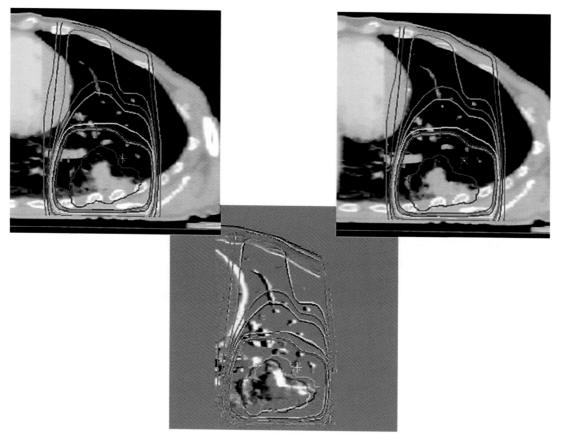

Fig. 6. Selected frames of isodose animation and the difference image, showing motion of the pericardium and tumor shift as well as isodose line shifts (see animation online at *WEB*).

volume. In addition to instantaneous isodose distributions for each respiratory phase, corresponding dose-volume histograms can be calculated. To calculate the cumulative dose-volume histograms over the various time phases, deformable image registration, in principle, can be used. This calculational tool provides the voxel displacement map from one respiratory state to another, thus permitting the summation over time. An overview and application of deformable registration is described in greater detail in Rietzel et al. [13]. Deformable registration is an active area of study, with several distinct approaches. Validation of such methods of deformable registration is still being developed.

We have qualitatively shown effects of tumor and normal tissue motion on conformal dose distributions. These perturbations are calculated based on a synthesized single respiratory cycle. Variations in respiration occur, principally in the amplitude and frequency of breathing. Furthermore, anatomical images as a function of time from 4DCT do not necessarily characterize breathing during the multiple fractions of treatment. In addition, beam delivery uncertainties can be present. A slow multileaf collimator (MLC) leaf during IMRT delivery may occur. In such a scenario, the beam may be gated off, until all MLC leaves are again at the correct synchronized position. During this time, the patient continues to breath, perturbing the synchronization between beam delivery and breathing. What is the magnitude of such effects? Another variable is the patient's respiratory state at beam on: is he inhaling or exhaling? These temporal uncertainties make a deterministic dose calculation challenging.

One specific aspect of asynchronous motion relevant to IMRT delivery to moving targets is the interaction between MLC leaf motion and respiration. Theoretical studies and experiments done by MGH investigators and others show that on average, interplay of MLC motion with target motion does not show a large effect in fractionated treatment. Studies [17–21] have shown the mean dose to the moving target is within a few percent of the planned dose given at random starting phases. However, the interplay effects can be much larger for single or a few fractions.

Case Study

We present a case study that integrates many facets of the discussion on 4DCT, treatment planning, and delivery. The case involves a patient with a 7-cm diameter liver lesion. A 4DCT was obtained and showed that the liver tumor was moving approximately 2 cm craniocaudally. It was decided to treat this patient with image-guided/gated radiotherapy, using conformal radiation therapy (not IMRT). Coaching was performed to train the patient to breathe more regularly; this is facilitated by the patient viewing his breathing pattern through LCD glasses, and following a pattern that reproduced the point of exhale. Four-dimensional imaging studies showed that by gating around a 30% window centered at exhale, the residual motion was reduced to 5 mm peak to peak as seen by animation of the 30% duty cycle around exhale. A treatment plan was designed for the exhale anatomical state, using three-dimensional conformal fields. Imaging by diagnostic X-rays on the treatment linear accelerator was performed before every treatment to align the patient with isocenter at exhale.

In fig. 7 (see animation online at *WEB*), representative axial and coronal planes are shown. Figure 7a, c shows organ motion throughout the entire respiratory cycle, while figure 7b, d shows anatomy in the gated interval. It can be seen in the gated interval that the liver and tumor appear relatively static. There is a residual motion over the duty cycle of approximately 5 mm.

The dome and the inferior tip of the liver are approximately static. When viewed in a volume-rendered mode, as seen in figure 8a, the radiopaque clips implanted around the tumor are seen to move significantly (approx. 2 cm) when the entire breathing cycle is animated. In figure 8b, only the 30% duty cycle centered at exhale is shown. This is the interval in which the tumor is planned to be irradiated, and the clips seem to be approximately static (residual motion within approx. 5 mm).

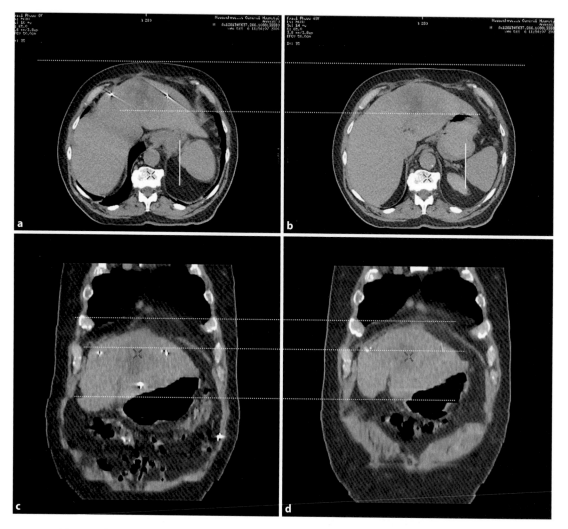

Fig. 7. a, **b** Axial image of the liver tumor. Radiopaque clips denote tumor margins. **a** Ungated complete respiratory cycle. **b** Gated CT animation, showing only frames between 40 and 60% respiratory phase (around exhale). Significant reduction in motion is achieved through gating. **c**, **d** Coronal image of a 4DCT scan: full respiration cycle (**c**) and gated scan (**d**) (see animation online at *WEB*).

Fig. 8. Volume-rendered image of a liver tumor case. **a** Patient breathes normally. The region of interest ellipses identify the clips surrounding the tumor. The circular regions of interest show the position of the Bbs (small metallic spheres used as fiducials) used to align the patient to scanner lasers. **b** Volume-rendered image during gated frames only. The clips and BBs are both static in comparison to **a**. See animation of the exit beam online at *WEB*.

Chen · Kung · Rietzel

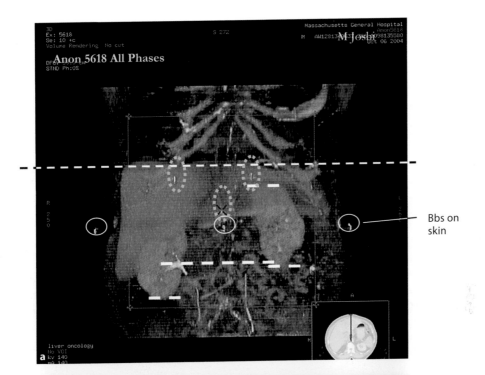

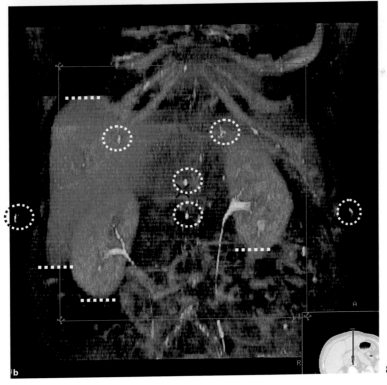

Bbs on skin

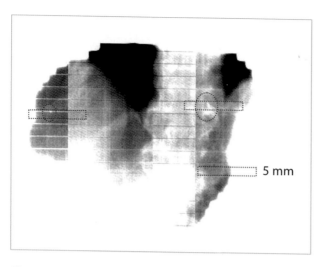

Fig. 9. Transmission radiation animation showing clips in the liver tumor from the anterior-posterior field. The clips in the circular regions of interest move by an amount comparable to the size of the MLC leaves, i.e. 5 mm. The amount of motion is consistent with that observed in a gated 4DCT scan in the 40–60% gate window. Only gated frames during treatment are shown (see animation online at *WEB*).

The image-guided therapy treatment unit used in this irradiation, IRIS [22], has two X-ray tubes and two amorphous silicon panels. By stereoscopic visualization, diagnostic quality images can be obtained at a gated respiratory position (exhale based upon RPM), and then aligned to the CT digitally reconstructed radiographs generated at the same respiratory phase. The electronic portal imaging device on this linear accelerator is set to the cine acquisition mode, during which it acquires images continuously. Because the beam is on only over 3/10ths of the time, during 7/10ths of the time the images are blank. During the gated treatment interval, the electronic portal imaging device will capture the exit radiation and provide documentation of the position of the radiopaque clips during treatment.

Figure 9 is an exit beam image captured by the electronic portal imaging device during gated radiotherapy. If you focus on the two regions of interest, identified by small circles, you see that a radiopaque clip is visible within each region of interest and moves about 5 mm as judged by the MLC vane height. This is evidence that we are delivering gated radiotherapy as planned, with a residual motion of approximately 5 mm over the 30% duty cycle around exhale.

Acknowledgements

The authors wish to acknowledge the valuable discussions and contributions of the MGH Radiation Oncology Department staff members, including Drs. Noah Choi, Paul Busse, Steve Jiang, Ross Berbeco, and Thomas Bortfeld. We also wish to thank the radiation therapists involved in IGRT. Early work in 4DCT was supported in part by Varian Medical Systems and General Electric Medical Systems. Discussions with T.S. Pan of GE were very valuable. We thank Dr. David Weinstein and McKay Davis for generation of the four-dimensional volume-rendered image.

Chen · Kung · Rietzel

References

1 National Cancer Institute: NCI IMRT Guidelines, 2002.
2 National Cancer Institute: Revised NCI IMRT Guidelines, 2005.
3 Bortfeld T, Chen GT: Irradiation of moving targets SRO. Semin Radiat Oncol 2004;14:1.
4 Balter JM, Ten Haken RK, Lawrence TS, Lam KL, Robertson JM: Uncertainties in CT-based radiation therapy treatment planning associated with patient breathing. Int J Radiat Oncol Biol Phys 1996;36:167–174.
5 Balter JM, Lam KL, McGinn CJ, Lawrence TS, Ten Haken RK: Improvement of CT-based treatment-planning models of abdominal targets using static exhale imaging. Int J Radiat Oncol Biol Phys 1998;41:939–943.
6 Chen GT, Kung JH, Beaudette KP: Artifacts in computed tomography scanning of moving objects. Semin Radiat Oncol 2004;14:19–26.
7 Ford EC, Mageras GS, Yorke E, Ling CC: Respiration-correlated spiral CT: a method of measuring respiratory-induced anatomic motion for radiation treatment planning. Med Phys 2003;30:88–97.
8 Low DA, Nystrom M, Kalinin E, et al: A method for the reconstruction of four-dimensional synchronized CT scans acquired during free breathing. Med Phys 2003;30:1254–1263.
9 Vedam SS, Keall PJ, Kini VR, Mostafavi H, Shukla HP, Mohan R: Acquiring a four-dimensional computed tomography dataset using an external respiratory signal. Phys Med Biol 2003;48:45–62.
10 Pan T, Lee TY, Rietzel E, Chen GT: 4D-CT imaging of a volume influenced by respiratory motion on multi-slice CT. Med Phys 2004;31:333–340.
11 Pan T: Comparison of helical and cine acquisitions for 4D-CT imaging with multislice CT. Med Phys 2005;32:627–634.
12 Rietzel E, Pan T, Chen GT: Four-dimensional computed tomography: image formation and clinical protocol. Med Phys 2005;32:874–889.
13 Rietzel E, Chen GT, Choi NC, Willet CG: Four-dimensional image-based treatment planning: target volume segmentation and dose calculation in the presence of respiratory motion. Int J Radiat Oncol Biol Phys 2005;61:1535–1550.
14 Keall PJ, Joshi S, Vedam SS, Siebers JV, Kini VR, Mohan R: Four-dimensional radiotherapy planning for DMLC-based respiratory motion tracking. Med Phys 2005;32:942–951.
15 Seppenwoolde Y, Shirato H, Kitamura K, et al: Precise and real-time measurement of 3D tumor motion in lung due to breathing and heartbeat, measured during radiotherapy. Int J Radiat Oncol Biol Phys 2002;53:822–834.
16 Murphy MJ: Tracking moving organs in real time. Semin Radiat Oncol 2004;14:91–100.
17 Kung JH, Zygmanski P, Choi N, Chen GT: A method of calculating a lung clinical target volume DVH for IMRT with intrafractional motion. Med Phys 2003;30:1103–1109.
18 Bortfeld T, Jokivarsi K, Goitein M, Kung J, Jiang SB: Effects of intra-fraction motion on IMRT dose delivery: statistical analysis and simulation. Phys Med Biol 2002;47:2203–2220.
19 Bortfeld T, Jiang SB, Rietzel E: Effects of motion on the total dose distribution. Semin Radiat Oncol 2004;14:41–51.
20 Jiang SB, Pope C, Al Jarrah KM, Kung JH, Bortfeld T, Chen GT: An experimental investigation on intra-fractional organ motion effects in lung IMRT treatments. Phys Med Biol 2003;48:1773–1784.
21 Chui CS, Yorke E, Hong L: The effects of intra-fraction organ motion on the delivery of intensity-modulated field with a multileaf collimator. Med Phys 2003;30:1736–1746.
22 Berbeco RI, Jiang SB, Sharp GC, Chen GT, Mostafavi H, Shirato H: Integrated radiotherapy imaging system (IRIS): design considerations of tumour tracking with linac gantry-mounted diagnostic X-ray systems with flat-panel detectors. Phys Med Biol 2004;49:243–255.

Dr. George T.Y. Chen
Department of Radiation Oncology
Massachusetts General Hospital
Boston, MA 02114 (USA)
Tel. +1 617 726 8153, Fax +1 617 643 0848
E-Mail gchen@partners.org

Meyer JL (ed): IMRT, IGRT, SBRT – Advances in the Treatment Planning and
Delivery of Radiotherapy. Front Radiat Ther Oncol. Basel, Karger, 2007, vol. 40, pp 72–93

Image Guidance: Treatment Target Localization Systems

Michael B. Sharpe · Tim Craig · Douglas J. Moseley

Department of Radiation Oncology, University of Toronto and Radiation Medicine
Program, Princess Margaret Hospital, Toronto, Canada

Abstract

Highly conformal radiation therapy tailors treatment to match the target shape and position, minimizing normal tissue damage to a greater extent than previously possible. Technological advances
such as intensity-modulated radiation therapy, introduced a decade ago, have yielded significant
gains in tumor control and reduced toxicity. Continuing advances have focused on the characterization and control of patient movement, organ motion, and anatomical deformation, which all introduce geometric uncertainty. These sources of uncertainty limit the effectiveness of high-precision
treatment. Target localization, performed using appropriate technologies and frequency, is a critical
component of treatment quality assurance. Until recently, the target position with respect to the
beams has been inferred from surface marks on the patient's skin or through an immobilization device, and verified using megavoltage radiographs of the treatment portal. Advances in imaging technologies have made it possible to image soft tissue volumes in the treatment setting. Real-time
tracking is also possible using a variety of technologies, including fluoroscopic imaging and radiopaque markers implanted in or near the tumor. The capacity to acquire volumetric soft tissue
images in the treatment setting can also be used to assess anatomical changes over a course of
treatment. Enhancing localization practices reduces treatment errors, and gives the capacity to monitor anatomical changes and reduce uncertainties that could influence clinical outcomes. This review
presents the technologies available for target localization, and discusses some of the considerations
that should be addressed in the implementation of many new clinical processes in radiation oncology.

From its origins, radiation oncology has striven to limit damage in healthy organs
when treating tissues burdened with cancer. Important technological advances
help in subverting some of the limitations imposed by normal tissue toxicity. Now,
intensity-modulated radiation therapy (IMRT) maximally avoids normal tissues
and has become both feasible and effective, with the aid of robotic treatment con-

trol systems and software to simulate and optimize more conformal dose distributions [1, 2]. Anatomically conformal approaches, such as IMRT, require treatment planning simulations based on increasingly sophisticated patient models, which are formulated from accurate volumetric anatomical and physiological data generated from a host of imaging modalities [3]. CT and other imaging modalities have shifted the focus of simulation: from inferring disease location from radiographic landmarks, to the localization of explicit targets and normal organs delineated from soft tissue images in three dimensions. The value of volumetric imaging for radiotherapy treatment planning cannot be overemphasized.

Treatment planning establishes the relationship between the target and the isocenter of the treatment machine. This relationship is used to assure that the planned patient geometry can be reproduced for each fraction delivered. The addition of safety margins around the target forms the planning target volume (PTV) and assures dosimetric coverage, in spite of setup uncertainties in patient position from fraction to fraction, anatomical variations, or physiologic motion. Clearly, the PTV must be as small as possible to maximize normal tissue protection.

Target localization is the process of maintaining the planned relationship to the isocenter for each subsequent treatment session. Target localization, performed using appropriate technologies and frequency, is a critical component of any treatment quality assurance strategy. It assures that the accuracy and precision of each fraction meet predetermined error tolerance criteria that are appropriate for the PTV margin selected. There is a range of technologies to consider in the design of localization procedures. This paper reviews the general characteristics of available systems by presenting some specific examples. For an additional perspective on the issues involved with motion uncertainties and target localization, the reader is referred to the bibliography, and especially to a number of seminal full-issue reviews [4–7].

The Treatment Planning and Delivery Process

In addition to imaging, high-precision radiotherapy requires procedures and nomenclature to implement clear clinical goals. The treatment process is divided broadly into distinct planning and delivery activities. Planning begins with patient positioning and the fabrication of devices to provide patient comfort, aid in the robust and efficient setup of patients, and to provide the degree of immobilization appropriate to the objectives of therapy. A CT scan acquired in the treatment position is then registered with any supplemental imaging [MRI, positron emission tomography (PET), or single photon emission tomography] to enhance the delineation of targets and normal structures. Treatment planning proceeds based on the patient model formed from these images, organs delineated using manually drawn contours, and image processing to extract relevant quantitative information, such as tissue density; or more recently, parameters indicating physiological activity, such as the creatine/choline ratio, or fluorodeoxyglucose uptake [8–11]. Following the segmentation of images into anatomical regions, the dose distribution is optimized by adjusting the number and orientation of beams, and in the case of IMRT, the distribution of the energy fluence, or 'intensity' within each beam [12].

The clinical objectives are communicated by adhering to the standardized prescription guidelines. Over the past decade, International Commission on Radiological Units and Measurements reports 50 and 62 have served as a framework for defining target volumes and prescribing dose in image-based treatment planning protocols [13, 14]. The reports also outline the accepted conventions for dealing with patient setup uncertainties and organ movement over the course of treatment using a PTV. While there are acknowledged limitations to its application, the target volume terminology recommended by the International Commission on Radiological Units and Measurements has become central to the practice of modern radiation oncology [15]. When the plan is accepted and exported to the treatment unit, the focus of the process shifts to the treatment delivery phase. Under ideal circumstances, the daily patient setup for each fraction follows the nominal patient model developed in the planning phase. In practice, a number of uncertainties must be factored into the planning [16]. Clinical uncertainties, such as the risk of undetected microscopic spread and metastases, are addressed during the treatment planning process by determining the clinical target volume and prescribing an appropriate dose and fractionation.

Sources of Geometric Uncertainty

Physical uncertainties related to setup variation, organ movement, and tissue deformation are controlled using target localization systems. Setup variations arise from gross inconsistencies in the patient's treatment position. Organ motion is related to physiological processes, such as breathing motion, organ filling, and peristalsis, all of which can lead to shifts in organ and target position from fraction to fraction, or even within a treatment session [17]. As the patient progresses through the treatment, target and normal tissue response can lead to volume changes and deformation. As a result, the relative position, size, or shape of the tumor as well as the normal tissues can deviate from the organ models defined in the planning phase of the process.

The effects of these variations are classified as a *random* variation around a mean, and as a *systematic* variation manifested by an average shift in a landmark's position, relative to its position at simulation [18]. Systematic errors may accumulate and form a time trend, for example if the average position or volume of a struc-

Table 1. Time scale of the processes leading to geometric uncertainties

Intrafraction	Seconds	Cardiac cycle Breathing		
	Minutes	Organ filling Peristalsis	Patient movement Setup variation	
Interfraction	Hours		Patient movement Setup variation	
	Days		Patient movement Setup variation	Anatomical changes Normal tissue and tumor response
	Months		Patient movement Setup variation	Anatomical changes Normal tissue and tumor response

ture drifts with time. Systematic and random errors can occur within a treatment and over longer time intervals, as summarized in table 1. Clearly, the factors leading to random and systematic uncertainties vary in relative importance for a particular disease site, or even a particular patient. Effective implementation of conformal and IMRT treatment techniques requires an objective understanding of these sources of uncertainties, and the adoption of appropriate strategies to control them.

Target Localization Technologies

Several technologies are available to reestablish the patient setup with respect to the machine isocenter prior to each fraction, and to monitor the patient's position during treatment delivery. Target localization technologies can be classified according to the surrogate that is used to infer the location of the target. For example, surface landmarks, stereotaxy, radiographic landmarks, implanted markers, and soft tissue localization with ultrasound and in-room CT systems are candidates for target localization surrogates. Some of these systems are represented in figure 1. As was seen within the treatment planning process, there is an emerging shift from localization inferred from surface marks or radiographs, to the more direct use of implantable markers and soft tissue localized via volumetric imaging in the treatment suite.

Surface Markers and Optical Tracking
Landmarks based on surface anatomy are commonly used to infer the location of internal anatomy, usually in concert with mechanical fixation devices used to aid in patient setup and to reduce uncertainties. Fixation is accomplished using

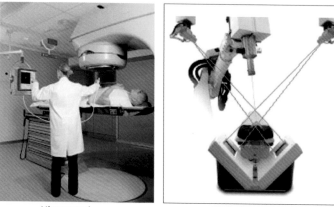

Ultrasound

kV Radiographic

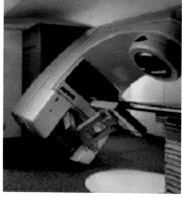

Portal imaging

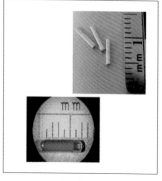

Markers
(active and passive)

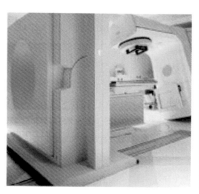

CT 'on rails'

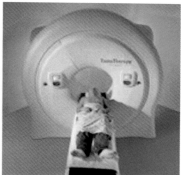

Tomo Therapy
MV CT

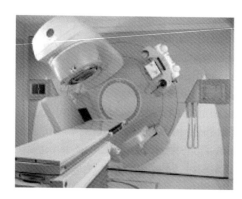
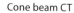

Cone beam CT

Fig. 1. Examples of systems used for target localization.

patient-specific positioning molds constructed from various materials, including expanding polyurethane foam, vacuum cushions filled with polystyrene beads, and thermoplastic masks [19, 20]. The target is aligned by triangulating surface points, delineated with tattoos, to a set of laser-defined cross hairs aligned to the machine isocenter. Optical tracking has emerged as a means of monitoring surface landmarks objectively in real time. Most systems track infrared-reflecting markers attached to the patient's external surface. The position of reflecting landmarks is determined within the field of view of a pair of stereoscopic cameras, which are calibrated with respect to the machine isocenter [21].

Target localization is achieved by establishing the positions of several optical markers relative to the target volume in a CT simulator. In the treatment room, the marker positions are measured relative to the isocenter to assess the need for setup correction, and to monitor with real-time feedback. Real-time tracking offers the possibility to detect setup changes during treatment delivery and interrupt treatments in the event of a gross misalignment of the treatment beam. Optical tracking systems can be integrated with other target localization technologies, such as bite plates used in stereotactic radiotherapy, or ultrasound or radiographic X-ray imaging, which are discussed below. In some body sites, the influence of organ motion caused by breathing, organ filling and interabdominal pressure can confound target localization using surface landmarks [22, 23]. When dealing with mobile internal anatomy, great care must be taken to assure the external surface marks are a valid surrogate for target position.

Stereotaxy

Stereotaxy is the methodology involved in the three-dimensional localization of structures using a mechanical frame and precise coordinate system to align and direct surgical instruments. Stereotactic radiosurgery uses stereotaxy adopted from neurosurgery applications to localize small brain tumors and certain benign brain disorders [24, 25]. Recently, radiosurgery principles have been extended to extracranial disease, using a stereotactic body frame [26, 27]. This approach incorporates a variety of technologies with the aim of controlling lung and other organ movement that would otherwise require large PTV margins to compensate for target motion. This approach allows a dramatic reduction of treatment volumes, which opens the avenue of hypofractionation with distinctly increased daily doses and very short courses of treatment.

Megavoltage Electronic Portal Imaging

This widely available localization technology has long been used to create radiographic images using the therapy X-ray beam. Decades of development have led to the current generation of electronic portal imaging devices (EPIDs) [28, 29]. State-of-the-art portal imaging is based on amorphous silicon panels, which contain millions of photodetectors coupled to switching transistors and fast readout electronics. These devices produce good image quality, sufficient for detecting bone structures and implanted radiographic markers. Modern EPIDs offer advantages over film-based megavoltage (MV) radiography, mainly because of the capacity to adjust display contrast, and to assess target position and adjust the patient promptly.

While MV EPID technologies have achieved a presence in commercial treatment systems, a number of factors have impeded the widespread adoption of frequent portal imaging in clinical practice, including the inherently low contrast of radiographs made at MV energies, field of view limitations and a lack of tools and computer networking infrastructure to permit integration in the clinical environment. In spite of these limitations, EPID technologies have spawned a large body of inquiry into the utility of frequent imaging, appropriate strategies for intervention, and the design of PTV margins [18]. MV portal images have served as a foundation for developing modern principles for localization and intervention, and continue to yield significant benefits in assuring correct treatment delivery of the radiation dose. Using MV radiographs, however, it is difficult to infer field placement with respect to soft tissue structures. The desire to further improve normal tissue sparing and shorten fractionation schemes is driving requirements for greater accuracy in target localization.

Radiopaque Markers

A number of studies have demonstrated a lack of correlation between prostate position and the localization of pelvic bony anatomy, and the ability to improve target localization using implanted markers as a surrogate [23, 30, 31]. Many institutions implant multiple gold seeds into the prostate under transrectal ultrasound guidance, usually a few days prior to CT simulation. The seeds are identified on the planning CT, as well as on a pair of orthogonal digitally reconstructed radiographs. Radiation therapists acquire MV portal images on a daily basis, and align the seeds with the corresponding digitally reconstructed radiographs. Setup discrepancies exceeding a predefined threshold are corrected by adjusting the couch.

The practice of using radiographic markers may not be restricted to passive seeds or wires. Some innovative emerging technologies include a solid-state radiation dosimeter hermetically sealed in a glass tube [32]. The marker includes a Mosfet dosimeter, which integrates radiation exposure, and is visible on radiographs and on CT images. The integrated dose can be interrogated using an external radio frequency antenna to energize the sensor, which radiates back a signal reporting the dose information. The capability of confirming dose delivery in concert with target localization is intriguing. However, the benefits of implanting any form of marker for guidance should be weighed against the risk of infection or tumor seeding along the needle track [33–35].

Sharpe · Craig · Moseley

Kilovoltage Imaging

Because of the more pronounced photoelectric absorption in the lower energy range, radiographic imaging with kilovoltage (kV) X-rays offers higher contrast than MV imaging. This translates into greater visibility of bones or implanted markers at a lower imaging dose, and simplified interpretation of images. Several kV imaging systems are offered commercially. These systems frequently offer fluoroscopic imaging capability for real-time monitoring and include two or more imaging systems to permit real-time three-dimensional localization of markers, or bony anatomy. Figure 2a is an example of an independently developed system installed at Hokkaido University, in Japan [36]. Four X-ray tubes and image intensifiers are organized in the room to provide stereoscopic fluoroscopy or radiographs for all accelerator orientations. Figure 2b is an example of a marker that has been isolated, and is being tracked dynamically during fluoroscopy. Dynamic tracking of a radiopaque marker in real time gives the option to adopt treatment gating strategies, and the possibility to limit the margins required to compensate for breathing motion. However, the benefit of real-time tracking must be weighed against the possibility of delivering an excessive skin dose due to the fluoroscopy procedure [37].

Ultrasound

In some situations, imaging of soft tissue contrast can provide a better targeting surrogate than implanted markers, or skeletal landmarks on radiographs. Ultrasound systems are relatively inexpensive and offer soft tissue visualization capability in some clinical situations. Transabdominal systems for guiding prostate cancer treatment have received a large amount of attention [38]. Images of the prostate and adjacent organs are acquired in the treatment position by placing a transducer on the patient's abdomen. The transducer is calibrated and coregistered with the isocenter using an additional localization technology, such as optical tracking, possibly in both the CT scanner and treatment rooms [21].

Contours from the planning system are displayed in the ultrasound context and correctly aligned to the position of the prostate with respect to the isocenter, as depicted in figure 3. Placement of the transabdominal imaging transducer requires a degree of technical skill and training to acquire suitable images and to avoid displacing the prostate with extra-abdominal pressure [39, 40]. While ultrasound systems have been employed successfully for prostate cancer and upper abdominal treatment, difficulties are encountered with sites where bone or large air cavities generate reflections that overwhelm the ultrasound signal from soft tissue targets.

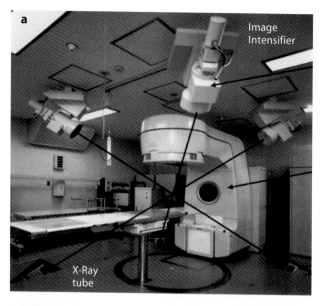

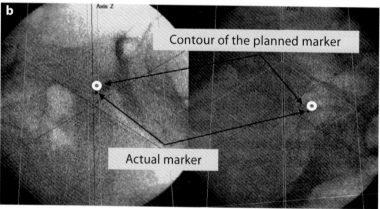

Fig. 2. a A motion-gated linear accelerator system with a fluoroscopic tumor tracking system.
b Fluoroscopic real-time marker tracking. The actual marker position can be seen on the fluoroscopic images. The planned position of the marker is projected as a contour on each image [36].

CT Imaging in the Treatment Room

There is growing interest in the use of CT for the localization of soft tissue targets. CT images are geometrically accurate and applicable to a broad range of anatomical sites. CT images are acquired without contact with the patient, but require exposure to additional ionizing radiation. Most CT systems provide an accurate measure of tissue attenuation, i.e., Hounsfield numbers, which is important for

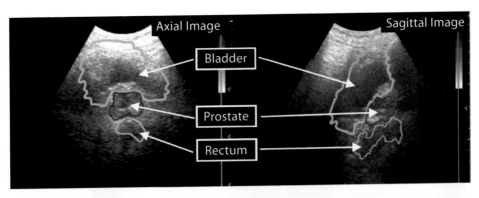

Fig. 3. An example of ultrasound-guided target localization. Contours imported from the treatment planning CT are overlaid as a reference for aligning the ultrasound images acquired inside the treatment room [38].

dose calculations in treatment planning. This may be an advantage in adaptive treatment strategies, when a midcourse reoptimization of the treatment plan is required. Several implementations bring CT capability to the treatment suite, and are briefly outlined here.

CT on Rails

One of the first systems to provide CT imaging in the treatment room was the so-called 'CT-on-rails' device [41–44]. A conventional scanner is located within the treatment room, adjacent to a linear accelerator. The treatment couch has been modified to minimize CT artifacts, and to transit patients between the CT scanner and accelerator. Images are acquired by translating the scanner along the rails and along the stationary patient. Images acquired prior to treatment are compared with the planning CT and couch movements are calibrated so that the patient can be correctly repositioned from the scanning position to the treatment isocenter following the evaluation of images. This affords a high degree of accuracy and precision in setup correction based on soft tissue anatomy.

Frequent CT imaging during the course of therapy has opened the door to assess how organs move and deform, how to properly assess the dose distribution in light of these anatomical changes, and when to replan treatment. CT-on-rails systems have demonstrated the implications of frequent volumetric imaging for image guidance, including dramatic changes in tumor shrinkage that can occur over the course of treatment, especially in head and neck cancer patients [45], and the capacity for frameless stereotactic treatment for early-stage lung cancer [46].

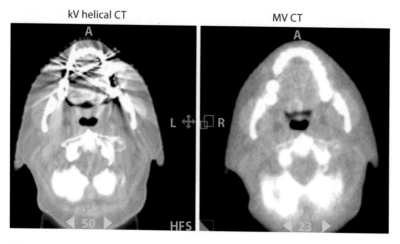

kV helical CT

MV CT

Fig. 4. MV CT images are immune from artifacts produced by high-atomic-number materials, like dental amalgam or metal prostheses. Images are courtesy of Ken Ruchala, Tomotherapy, Inc.

Tomotherapy Imaging

The tomotherapy device (Madison, Wisc., USA) includes an MV CT imaging system based on a fan beam and helical acquisition paradigm [47, 48]. Volumetric MV CT images are acquired in the treatment position, just prior to treatment delivery, using a detuned linear accelerator producing 3.5 MV X-rays and a reduced photon output. An array of xenon ion chambers separated by thin tungsten septa forms the detector system, and photons interacting in the septa release electrons that ionize the xenon gas [49]. This process is very 'photon efficient' compared with MV portal imaging devices. As a result, imaging doses can be acquired at doses in the range of 0.5–3 cGy, which is competitive with conventional CT systems. Because MV photons interact via Compton scattering, MV CT images are immune from artifacts produced by high-atomic-number materials, like dental amalgam or metal prostheses, as shown in figure 4.

Cone Beam CT

Cone beam CT systems enable volumetric imaging on a conventional medical linear accelerator. Cone beam CT differs in the source-detector geometry for image acquisition, compared with the conventional fan beam geometry. Like the tomotherapy system, cone beam CT reconstructions are acquired in the treatment position, just prior to treatment delivery. In a single gantry rotation, volumetric images are reconstructed by back-projection of hundreds of two-dimensional radiographs acquired from using a large-area amorphous silicon detector. The field of view can approach a 50-cm diameter in the transverse plane, and 25 cm in the

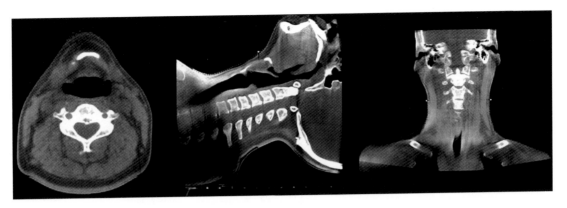

Fig. 5. kV cone beam CT images of the head and neck.

craniocaudal direction. Jaffray [50], McBain et al. [51] and Oldham et al. [52] have reported on kV cone beam CT systems, and clinical experience is emerging. The imaging dose associated with a volumetric image is typically less than 3 cGy with kV cone beam CT systems. MV cone beam CT systems have also been described [53, 54], and the dose used for volumetric imaging is comparable with portal imaging using contemporary MV EPIDs. Objective comparisons of imaging doses require consideration of the associated image contrast, resolution, and noise characteristics [54]. kV systems tend to be more flexible in terms of dose, and support planar radiographs and real-time fluoroscopy for patient monitoring over the course of treatment delivery. At this time, three of the leading radiotherapy vendors are offering cone beam CT technology, all of which appear capable of producing high-resolution volumetric images of soft tissue anatomy at reasonable doses (<5 cGy).

Transverse, coronal and sagittal images of a patient with head and neck cancer, shown in figure 5, illustrate the utility of kV cone beam CT for image guidance based on soft tissues. Good contrast is seen between fat, vessels, and muscle groups. Figure 5 also illustrates typical artifacts seen on cone beam CT images, in particular shading caused by X-ray scatter, and beam hardening in the vicinity of the shoulders. It should also be pointed out that cone beam CT systems do not yield proper calibration relating CT numbers to attenuation coefficients at this time, i.e., Hounsfield numbers. Artifacts and quantitative attenuation in cone beam CT are areas of continuing investigation, which are beyond the scope of this paper and are addressed in more detail by Jaffray [50].

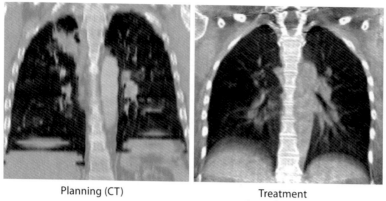

Planning (CT)

Treatment
(cone beam CT)

Fig. 6. Artifacts arising from breathing motion in a fan beam CT (planning), and a cone beam CT (treatment). Images are courtesy of J.J. Sonke, Netherlands Cancer Institute, Amsterdam.

Organ Motion Occurring within a Treatment Session

Organ movement during treatment can be a source of residual uncertainties in target localization procedures. In particular, thoracic and abdominal treatments are affected by breathing, which can introduce substantial organ displacements (i.e., >3 cm) [5, 55]. Organ movement can be monitored in real time using fluoroscopy and implanted markers, for example, to provide data for the design of appropriate margins, or to employ in treatment gating strategies [18, 56–58]. Alternatively, the complexities caused by breathing motion can be reduced using breath-hold immobilization, and if repeated, the patient can better tolerate these maneuvers. Breath-hold immobilization has been explored for patients with liver cancer, Hodgkin's lymphoma, lung cancer, and breast cancer [59–63].

Addressing breathing motion begins with treatment planning, where fluoroscopy and cinegraphic MRI can provide real-time information about temporal change in the tumor and normal tissues, but not necessarily volumetric data. Organ movement can introduce imaging artifacts on slice-based CT scanners, which confound the delineation of targets and normal tissues, as illustrated in figure 6 [64]. Modern multislice CT scanners have been adapted to rapidly observe temporal changes due to breathing [65, 66]. The periodic nature of breathing motion is exploited in reconstructions by using the phase or amplitude of the respiratory cycle to sort images and construct a sequence of respiratory-correlated CT volumes. This results in a four-dimensional animation of periodic breathing, or '4D CT'. Respiratory sorting of PET images leading to '4D PET' scans is also under investigation [67, 68].

Sharpe · Craig · Moseley

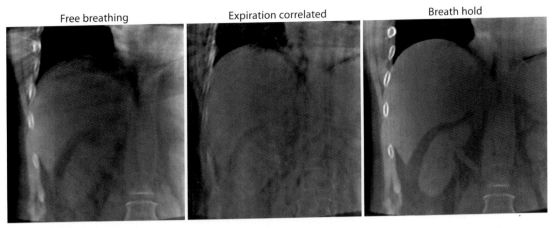

Free breathing   Expiration correlated   Breath hold

Fig. 7. Comparison of cone beam CT scans of the liver and diaphragm region. Scans are acquired under free breathing (325 projections), reconstructed using only expiration-correlated projections (68 projections), and a scan acquired using three repeated breath-hold maneuvers (327 projections).

Figure 6 also shows the effect of free breathing on a cone beam CT scan. In this case, breathing motion causes blurring artifacts, rather than the distortions and tearing associated with slice-based acquisition under free breathing. The periodic nature of breathing motion can also be exploited for target localization. Respiratory-correlated, or four-dimensional, cone beam CT techniques have also been described [69], as well as cone beam CT imaging combined with breath-hold immobilization [70]. The coronal images shown in figure 7 compare cone beam CT scan of the liver and diaphragm region, acquired under free breathing, reconstructed using expiration-correlated projections, and a scan acquired using three repeated breath-hold maneuvers.

In addition to volumetric imaging, kV fluoroscopic imaging can be employed to monitor high-contrast anatomy or implanted markers, as alluded to previously [56–58]. Using fluoroscopy with implanted markers or respiratory-correlated cone beam CT for treatment guidance can address the systematic errors in the planned position of the target, as observed during patient setup, and assure that PTV margins provide appropriate target coverage after the systematic error has been corrected. Some components of organ motion occur within the interval of treatment delivery, but are not necessarily periodic. Peristalsis and the presence of bowel gas could generate undetected shifts in the target position, if there is a delay in between the localization procedure and treatment delivery [17, 71]. In the absence of real-time information, guided interventions to improve target positioning should be performed with consideration of how random intrafraction movements could affect the validity of the measurements, and thus the underlying decision to apply a correction. In some cases, patient education that gives advice related to diet, as well as bowel and bladder filling, can help to reduce the risk of random intrafaction motion [17, 72].

Recently, a novel system has been reported for real-time localization of radio frequency transponders that are energized and monitored with an external antenna array [73]. Each marker resonates a unique frequency, and its position is determined with respect to the array. The transponders are implanted prior to the CT simulation and are linked to the treatment isocenter in the planning phase. In the treatment room, the array is positioned over the target, to monitor the positions of the transponders with respect to the array. The array is integrated with an optical tracking system, which, in turn, links the transponder location to the treatment isocenter. This system offers the unique capability to monitor implanted markers in real time, without fluoroscopy, within a 15-cm cubic volume. At the time of writing, this system was not commercially available, but preclinical testing and experience was being reported for prostate cancer [71]. The current field of view of this system is suitable for this application, and further development may refine it for localization of larger volumes.

Designing an Image-Guided Intervention Strategy

Target localization technologies permit frequent assessment of treatment to minimize patient setup uncertainties, and in some cases, provide a record of anatomical changes over a treatment course. In particular, the potential for frequent volumetric CT imaging during the course of therapy generates a number of opportunities and challenges. Fortunately, the experience gained in the MV EPID era has led to a framework for the continuing development of clinical guidance strategies [18]. Implementation of target localization falls broadly into *on-line* and *off-line* approaches for assessment and intervention. On-line approaches evaluate information acquired immediately prior to each fraction, and simple couch translations are applied to correct for observed deviations in treatment position that exceed a predefined threshold. An off-line approach refers to the frequent acquisition of setup information at the start of a treatment course (e.g. first 3 fractions), followed by an off-line statistical analysis to determine the patient's systematic (mean offset) and random (standard deviation) setup errors. A correction of the systematic error, the most important component of geometric uncertainties, is then made for future fractions. On-line correction strategies tend to lead toward a larger reduction in geometric errors than an off-line approach, but action thresholds must be set to control the time and effort spent in 'chasing' random setup errors. On-line correction strategies appear to be most appropriate when the tumor is relatively unaffected by uncharacterized organ movement and in close proximity to critical normal tissues, where small errors in setup could compromise toxicity or local control. On-line approaches also seem appropriate when high-dose radiation is delivered in one or very few fractions, where there is little opportunity to obtain statistical information to detect systematic positioning errors. However, the impact of geometric uncertainties on tumor control may be small, depending on the size of the PTV margins [74]. An off-line analysis may also be useful to identify and address the random and systematic uncertainties due to breathing motion in hypofractionated treatment [75].

More complex on-line and off-line approaches can be envisioned. Over the course of treatment, volume changes and organ deformation can arise in response to radiation therapy, adjuvant medications, or the overall well-being of the patient. Simple isocenter and margin adjustments may not account for these changes adequately. When based on volumetric soft tissue imaging, strategies can be designed to estimate and accommodate the impact of organ motion and anatomical deformation [7, 76–78]. Strategies that involve replanning of a patient in response to anatomical changes observed under treatment are broadly referred to as 'adaptive' radiation therapy. Currently, 'adaptive' terminology is used casually to describe a wide variety of correction and replanning strategies. Yan et al. [79, 80] and Martinez et al. [81] have gained a large experience in using formal adaptive control principles in the off-line setting. This approach begins with generic population-based PTV margins, but nearly eliminates systematic errors and tailors PTV margins specifically to the random variations observed for each individual patient in the second week of treatment.

Adaptive control principles are expected to have broad implications in the emerging relationship between target localization and the replanning of patients under treatment. Currently, replanning is rarely conducted in clinical practice, because appropriate anatomical information is not available, and because it is labor and time intensive. Furthermore, the optimal frequency, or even the clinical need, for replanning is unknown in many disease sites. Ideally, when clinically indicated, temporal and volumetric imaging would be obtained while the treatment is delivered with the opportunity for efficient adaptation of therapy during and between radiation treatments. It may be tempting to embark on fully on-line adaptive replanning, but the desire for submillimeter technical precision should be balanced with the risk of chasing only the modest clinical gains, and with the possibility of imposing an unacceptable workload on clinical planning, treatment delivery and review process. The continuing development of tools and algorithms will assist in target and normal tissue contouring, planning, deformable registration of images, and decision support for determining corrections are required before replanning can be investigated properly in clinical practice [82–85]. The computer networking and data storage involved in the management and visualization of large quantities of image-based information must be considered in the early adoption and continuing development of image-based localization technologies.

Conclusion

Advances in target localization systems promise the combined advantages of volumetric imaging and real-time monitoring of the patient during treatment, and can be expected to enhance the quality of radiation therapy delivery significantly. Novel target localization systems are creating new avenues for innovative applications of radiation therapy through dose escalation, new fractionation schemes, and the use of disease-specific markers in multimodality imaging for treatment design. An ideal target localization system supports accurate and precise treatment by rapidly reporting volumetric soft tissue information in a form that is explicit and objective. It would be integrated into the treatment delivery process to reduce the cost of the guidance procedure, at least in terms of treatment time. Soft tissue imaging over a large field of view would support broad application to a large number of anatomical sites. The ideal system is also capable of assessing organ movement noninvasively and continuously in real time. It would avoid exposure to additional ionizing radiation, and has minimal impact on patient comfort, staffing workload, clinical information management infrastructure, or treatment time. At this time, none of the technologies under review spans the complete range of these requirements.

Table 2 attempts to classify the target localization systems discussed in this paper in order to render a comparison. In-room CT and ultrasound solutions offer soft tissue imaging. Some CT solutions can demonstrate breathing motion using breathing-correlated reconstructions, but real-time updates are not feasible with CT. Alternatively, volumetric CT images can be used in concert with fluoroscopy systems to monitor targets in real time, but the formation of images in both systems requires the administration of additional dose. The extra dose delivered to the patient from more frequent imaging appears clinically insignificant in the radiotherapy context, but long-term follow-up of patients is not available. The benefit of imaging should be weighed against any perceived risk of second malignancies, especially in young patients. Alternatively, optical tracking of surface markers report data in real time. This surrogate may be too remote to be used alone for targets influenced by internal organ movement, but this deficiency can be addressed by combining optical tracking with implanted transponders, ultrasound, or CT to establish a valid relationship with the target location. The real-time aspects of optical tracking could then use surface makers to detect gross setup changes and breathing motion. A number of other scenarios can be considered. Clearly, there are a number of tradeoffs to consider in the implementation of a target localization procedure. To be safe and effective, the selection and commissioning of equipment must be done in the context of the clinical requirements for target and normal tissue localization.

Table 2. A summary of the features and limitations of target localization systems

Method	Dimensions (x, y, z)	Evaluated features	Time frame	Cons
Radiography (MV/kV)	2D/3D	bones/markers	snapshot	dose?
Fluoroscopy (kV)	2D/3D	bones/markers	real time	dose?
Tomography	3D	soft tissue	snapshot	dose
Ultrasound	2D/3D	soft tissue	snapshot/real time?	expertise
Optical	1D/2D/3D	skin surface	real time	remote surrogate
Implantable sensors	0D/3D	markers	real time	invasive, FOV?

Adapted from Dr. H. Sandler, University of Michigan. FOV = Field of view.

Continuing technological developments must lead to practical solutions for meaningful clinical problems, while operating within the constraints imposed by time and treatment resources, especially the limitations of human workload, skill training, and our capacity to deal with complex systems. Further development of decision support tools and robust correction algorithms will facilitate more complex adaptive guidance strategies, which include accuracy replanning throughout the course of treatment. Implementation of localization technologies is likely to have indirect implications beyond the treatment room. Certain image-based guidance strategies, for example, may be accompanied by the need to address the capacity of data storage, archiving, and retrieval systems. Perhaps the most substantial potential limitation of target localization systems is the potential for false reassurance it may provide when used inappropriately, leading to inappropriate margin reduction and overconfidence. Quality assurance procedures and education programs need to be formalized with broad community input, to avoid inappropriate use of image-guided radiation therapy as it is rapidly disseminating into clinical practice.

Acknowledgements

The authors wish to acknowledge the contributions of the staff and faculty of Princess Margaret Hospital. We are especially grateful to David Jaffray, Laura Dawson, Tom Purdie, and Elizabeth White for their contributions and suggestions. For generously sharing slides used in the preparation of this material, we also wish to thank Michael Herman, Howard Sandler, Jan Jakob Sonke, Marcel van Herk, Ken Ruchala, Hiroki Shirato, Luc Beaulieau, James Balter, Lei Dong, Jean Pouliot, and Kara Bucci.

References

1 Leibel SA, Fuks Z, Zelefsky MJ, Wolden SL, Rosenzweig KE, Alektiar KM, et al: Intensity-modulated radiotherapy. Cancer J 2002;8:164–176.

2 Eisbruch A, Ship JA, Dawson LA, Kim HM, Bradford CR, Terrell JE, et al: Salivary gland sparing and improved target irradiation by conformal and intensity modulated irradiation of head and neck cancer. World J Surg 2003;27:832–837.

3 Brock KK, Dawson LA, Sharpe MB, Moseley DJ, Jaffray DA: Feasibility of a novel deformable image registration technique to facilitate classification, targeting, and monitoring of tumor and normal tissue. Int J Radiat Oncol Biol Phys 2006; 64:1245–1254.

4 Mageras GS: Introduction: management of target localization uncertainties in external-beam therapy. Semin Radiat Oncol 2005;15:133–135.

5 Langen KM, Jones DT: Organ motion and its management. Int J Radiat Oncol Biol Phys 2001; 50:265–278.

6 Bortfeld T, Chen GTY: Introduction: intrafractional organ motion and its management. Sem Radiat Oncol 2004;14:1.

7 Mackie TR, Kapatoes J, Ruchala K, Lu W, Wu C, Olivera G, et al: Image guidance for precise conformal radiotherapy. Int J Radiat Oncol Biol Phys 2003;56:89–105.

8 Pickett B, Kurhanewicz J, Coakley F, Shinohara K, Fein B, Roach M 3rd: Use of MRI and spectroscopy in evaluation of external beam radiotherapy for prostate cancer. Int J Radiat Oncol Biol Phys 2004;60:1047–1055.

9 Van Dyk J, Battista JJ, Cunningham JR, Rider WD, Sontag MR: On the impact of CT scanning on radiotherapy planning. Comput Tomogr 1980;4:55–65.

10 Bradley J, Thorstad WL, Mutic S, Miller TR, Dehdashti F, Siegel BA, et al: Impact of FDG-PET on radiation therapy volume delineation in non-small-cell lung cancer. Int J Radiat Oncol Biol Phys 2004;59:78–86.

11 Black QC, Grills IS, Kestin LL, Wong CY, Wong JW, Martinez AA, et al: Defining a radiotherapy target with positron emission tomography. Int J Radiat Oncol Biol Phys 2004;60:1272–1282.

12 Galvin JM, Ezzell G, Eisbrauch A, Yu C, Butler B, Xiao Y, et al: Implementing IMRT in clinical practice: a joint document of the American Society for Therapeutic Radiology and Oncology and the American Association of Physicists in Medicine. Int J Radiat Oncol Biol Phys 2004;58:1616–1634.

13 International Commission on Radiation Units and Measurements: Prescribing, recording, and reporting photon beam therapy (supplement to ICRU report 50). Washington, International Commission on Radiation Units and Measurements, 1999, report No 62.

14 International Commission on Radiation Units and Measurements: Prescribing, recording, and reporting photon beam therapy. Washington, International Commission on Radiation Units and Measurements, 1993, report No 50.

15 Purdy JA: Current ICRU definitions of volumes: limitations and future directions. Semin Radiat Oncol 2004;14:27–40.

16 Urie MM, Goitein M, Doppke K, Kutcher JG, LoSasso T, Mohan R, et al: The role of uncertainty analysis in treatment planning. Int J Radiat Oncol Biol Phys 1991;21:91–107.

17 Ghilezan MJ, Jaffray DA, Siewerdsen JH, Van Herk M, Shetty A, Sharpe MB, et al: Prostate gland motion assessed with cine-magnetic resonance imaging (cine-MRI). Int J Radiat Oncol Biol Phys 2005;62:406–417.

18 Van Herk M: Errors and margins in radiotherapy. Semin Radiat Oncol 2004;14:52–64.

19 Bentel GC: Patient Positioning and Immobilization in Radiation Oncology. New York, McGraw-Hill, 1999.

20 Misfeldt J, Chessman M: Advances in patient positioning. J Oncol Manag 1999;8:14–16.

21 Meeks SL, Tome WA, Willoughby TR, Kupelian PA, Wagner TH, Buatti JM, et al: Optically guided patient positioning techniques. Semin Radiat Oncol 2005;15:192–201.

22 Hoisak JD, Sixel KE, Tirona R, Cheung PC, Pignol JP: Correlation of lung tumor motion with external surrogate indicators of respiration. Int J Radiat Oncol Biol Phys 2004;60:1298–1306.

23 Schallenkamp JM, Herman MG, Kruse JJ, Pisansky TM: Prostate position relative to pelvic bony anatomy based on intraprostatic gold markers and electronic portal imaging. Int J Radiat Oncol Biol Phys 2005;63:800–811.

24 Podgorsak EB, Pike GB, Olivier A, Pla M, Souhami L: Radiosurgery with high energy photon beams: a comparison among techniques. Int J Radiat Oncol Biol Phys 1989;16:857–865.

25 Wu A: Physics and dosimetry of the gamma knife. Neurosurg Clin N Am 1992;3:35–50.

26 Timmerman RD, Kavanagh BD: Stereotactic body radiation therapy. Curr Probl Cancer 2005; 29:120–157.

27 Kavanagh BD, Timmerman RD: Stereotactic radiosurgery and stereotactic body radiation therapy: an overview of technical considerations and clinical applications. Hematol Oncol Clin North Am 2006;20:87–95.

28 Antonuk LE: Electronic portal imaging devices: a review and historical perspective of contemporary technologies and research. Phys Med Biol 2002;47:R31–R65.

29 Herman MG, Balter JM, Jaffray DA, McGee KP, Munro P, Shalev S, et al: Clinical use of electronic portal imaging: report of AAPM Radiation Therapy Committee Task Group 58. Med Phys 2001;28:712–737.

30 Chung PW, Haycocks T, Brown T, Cambridge Z, Kelly V, Alasti H, et al: On-line aSi portal imaging of implanted fiducial markers for the reduction of interfraction error during conformal radiotherapy of prostate carcinoma. Int J Radiat Oncol Biol Phys 2004;60:329–334.

31 Wu J, Haycocks T, Alasti H, Ottewell G, Middlemiss N, Abdolell M, et al: Positioning errors and prostate motion during conformal prostate radiotherapy using on-line isocentre set-up verification and implanted prostate markers. Radiother Oncol 2001;61:127–133.

32 Briere TM, Beddar AS, Gillin MT: Evaluation of precalibrated implantable MOSFET radiation dosimeters for megavoltage photon beams. Med Phys 2005;32:3346–3349.

33 Haddad FS, Somsin AA: Seeding and perineal implantation of prostatic cancer in the track of the biopsy needle: three case reports and a review of the literature. J Surg Oncol 1987;35:184–191.

34 Rodgers MS, Collinson R, Desai S, Stubbs RS, McCall JL: Risk of dissemination with biopsy of colorectal liver metastases. Dis Colon Rectum 2003;46:454–458.

35 Clayman G, Cohen JI, Adams GL: Neoplastic seeding of squamous cell carcinoma of the oropharynx. Head Neck 1993;15:245–248.

36 Shirato H, Shimizu S, Kitamura K, Nishioka T, Kagei K, Hashimoto S, et al: Four-dimensional treatment planning and fluoroscopic real-time tumor tracking radiotherapy for moving tumor. Int J Radiat Oncol Biol Phys 2000;48:435–442.

37 Valentin J: Avoidance of radiation injuries from medical interventional procedures. Ann ICRP 2000;30:7–67.

38 Kuban DA, Dong L, Cheung R, Strom E, de Crevoisier R: Ultrasound-based localization. Semin Radiat Oncol 2005;15:180–191.

39 Artignan X, Smitsmans MH, Lebesque JV, Jaffray DA, van Her M, Bartelink H: Online ultrasound image guidance for radiotherapy of prostate cancer: impact of image acquisition on prostate displacement. Int J Radiat Oncol Biol Phys 2004;59: 595–601.

40 Van den HF, Powell T, Seppi E, Littrupp P, Khan M, Wang Y, et al: Independent verification of ultrasound based image-guided radiation treatment, using electronic portal imaging and implanted gold markers. Med Phys 2003;30:2878–2887.

41 Uematsu M, Fukui T, Shioda A, Tokumitsu H, Takai K, Kojima T, et al: A dual computed tomography linear accelerator unit for stereotactic radiation therapy: a new approach without cranially fixated stereotactic frames. Int J Radiat Oncol Biol Phys 1996;35:587–592.

42 Shiu AS, Chang EL, Ye JS, Lii M, Rhines LD, Mendel E, et al: Near simultaneous computed tomography image-guided stereotactic spinal radiotherapy: an emerging paradigm for achieving true stereotaxy. Int J Radiat Oncol Biol Phys 2003;57:605–613.

43 Yenice KM, Lovelock DM, Hunt MA, Lutz WR, Fournier-Bidoz N, Hua CH, et al: CT image-guided intensity-modulated therapy for paraspinal tumors using stereotactic immobilization. Int J Radiat Oncol Biol Phys 2003;55:583–593.

44 Paskalev K, Ma C, Jacob R, Price R: Clinical evaluation of a CT gantry on rails as a daily target localization tool. Int J Radiat Oncol Biol Phys 2003;57(2 suppl):S266.

45 Barker JL Jr, Garden AS, Ang KK, O'Daniel JC, Wang H, Court LE, et al: Quantification of volumetric and geometric changes occurring during fractionated radiotherapy for head-and-neck cancer using an integrated CT/linear accelerator system. Int J Radiat Oncol Biol Phys 2004;59: 960–970.

46 Uematsu M, Shioda A, Suda A, Fukui T, Ozeki Y, Hama Y, et al: Computed tomography-guided frameless stereotactic radiotherapy for stage I non-small cell lung cancer: a 5-year experience. Int J Radiat Oncol Biol Phys 2001;51:666–670.

47 Ruchala KJ, Olivera GH, Schloesser EA, Mackie TR: Megavoltage CT on a tomotherapy system. Phys Med Biol 1999;44:2597–2621.

48 Ruchala KJ, Olivera GH, Kapatoes JM, Schloesser EA, Reckwerdt PJ, Mackie TR: Megavoltage CT image reconstruction during tomotherapy treatments. Phys Med Biol 2000;45:3545–3562.

49 Keller H, Glass M, Hinderer R, Ruchala K, Jeraj R, Olivera G, et al: Monte Carlo study of a highly efficient gas ionization detector for megavoltage imaging and image-guided radiotherapy. Med Phys 2002;29:165–175.

50 Jaffray DA: Emergent technologies for 3-dimensional image-guided radiation delivery. Semin Radiat Oncol 2005;15:208–216.

51 McBain CA, Henry AM, Sykes J, Amer A, Marchant T, Moore CM, et al: X-ray volumetric imaging in image-guided radiotherapy: the new standard in on-treatment imaging. Int J Radiat Oncol Biol Phys 2006;64:625–634.

52 Oldham M, Letourneau D, Watt L, Hugo G, Yan D, Lockman D, et al: Cone-beam-CT guided radiation therapy: a model for on-line application. Radiother Oncol 2005;75:271–278.

53 Pouliot J, Bani-Hashemi A, Chen J, Svatos M, Ghelmansarai F, Mitschke M, et al: Low-dose megavoltage cone-beam CT for radiation therapy. Int J Radiat Oncol Biol Phys 2005;61:552–560.

54 Groh BA, Siewerdsen JH, Drake DG, Wong JW, Jaffray DA: A performance comparison of flat-panel imager-based MV and kV cone-beam CT. Med Phys 2002;29:967–975.

55 Seppenwoolde Y, Shirato H, Kitamura K, Shimizu S, Van Herk M, Lebesque JV, et al: Precise and real-time measurement of 3D tumor motion in lung due to breathing and heartbeat, measured during radiotherapy. Int J Radiat Oncol Biol Phys 2002;53:822–834.

56 Harada T, Shirato H, Ogura S, Oizumi S, Yamazaki K, Shimizu S, et al: Real-time tumor-tracking radiation therapy for lung carcinoma by the aid of insertion of a gold marker using bronchofiberscopy. Cancer 2002;95:1720–1727.

57 Kitamura K, Shirato H, Seppenwoolde Y, Onimaru R, Oda M, Fujita K, et al: Three-dimensional intrafractional movement of prostate measured during real-time tumor-tracking radiotherapy in supine and prone treatment positions. Int J Radiat Oncol Biol Phys 2002;53:1117–1123.

58 Keall PJ, Joshi S, Vedam SS, Siebers JV, Kini VR, Mohan R: Four-dimensional radiotherapy planning for DMLC-based respiratory motion tracking. Med Phys 2005;32:942–951.

59 Stromberg JS, Sharpe MB, Kim LH, Kini VR, Jaffray DA, Martinez AA, et al: Active breathing control (ABC) for Hodgkin's disease: reduction in normal tissue irradiation with deep inspiration and implications for treatment. Int J Radiat Oncol Biol Phys 2000;48:797–806.

60 Cheung PC, Sixel KE, Tirona R, Ung YC: Reproducibility of lung tumor position and reduction of lung mass within the planning target volume using active breathing control (ABC). Int J Radiat Oncol Biol Phys 2003;57:1437–1442.

61 Dawson LA, Brock KK, Kazanjian S, Fitch D, McGinn CJ, Lawrence TS, et al: The reproducibility of organ position using active breathing control (ABC) during liver radiotherapy. Int J Radiat Oncol Biol Phys 2001;51:1410–1421.

62 Remouchamps VM, Vicini FA, Sharpe MB, Kestin LL, Martinez AA, Wong JW: Significant reductions in heart and lung doses using deep inspiration breath hold with active breathing control and intensity-modulated radiation therapy for patients treated with locoregional breast irradiation. Int J Radiat Oncol Biol Phys 2003;55:392–406.

63 Dawson LA, Eccles C, Bissonnette JP, Brock KK: Accuracy of daily image guidance for hypofractionated liver radiotherapy with active breathing control. Int J Radiat Oncol Biol Phys 2005;62:1247–1252.

64 Chen GT, Kung JH, Beaudette KP: Artifacts in computed tomography scanning of moving objects. Semin Radiat Oncol 2004;14:19–26.

65 Keall PJ, Starkschall G, Shukla H, Forster KM, Ortiz V, Stevens CW, et al: Acquiring 4D thoracic CT scans using a multislice helical method. Phys Med Biol 2004;49:2053–2067.

66 Rietzel E, Pan T, Chen GT: Four-dimensional computed tomography: image formation and clinical protocol. Med Phys 2005;32:874–889.

67 Wolthaus JW, Van Herk M, Muller SH, Belderbos JS, Lebesque JV, de Bois JA, et al: Fusion of respiration-correlated PET and CT scans: correlated lung tumour motion in anatomical and functional scans. Phys Med Biol 2005;50:1569–1583.

68 Nehmeh SA, Erdi YE, Pan T, Pevsner A, Rosenzweig KE, Yorke E, et al: Four-dimensional (4D) PET/CT imaging of the thorax. Med Phys 2004;31:3179–3186.

69 Sonke JJ, Zijp L, Remeijer P, Van Herk M: Respiratory correlated cone beam CT. Med Phys 2005;32:1176–1186.

70 Hawkins MA, Moseley D, Eccles C, Jaffray D, Dawson LA: Comparison of breath hold cone beam CT and orthogonal image-guided radiotherapy for liver cancer. Int J Radiat Oncol Biol Phys 2005;63(suppl 1):S555–S556.

71 Litzenberg DW, Balter JM, Hadley SW, Sandler HM, Willoughby TR, Kupelian PA, et al: Influence of intrafraction motion on margins for prostate radiotherapy. Int J Radiat Oncol Biol Phys 2006;65:548–553.

72 Nichol AM, Jaffray D, Catton C, Haycocks T, Lockwood G, Milosevic M, et al: A cohort study using cinematic magnetic resonance imaging of a bowel regimen to reduce intra-fraction prostate motion. Int J Radiat Oncol Biol Phys 2004;60(suppl 1):S429.

73 Balter JM, Wright JN, Newell LJ, Friemel B, Dimmer S, Cheng Y, et al: Accuracy of a wireless localization system for radiotherapy. Int J Radiat Oncol Biol Phys 2005;61:933–937.

74 Craig T, Moiseenko V, Battista J, Van Dyk J: The impact of geometric uncertainty on hypofractionated external beam radiation therapy of prostate cancer. Int J Radiat Oncol Biol Phys 2003;57:833–842.

75 Hugo G, Vargas C, Liang J, Kestin L, Wong JW, Yan D: Changes in the respiratory pattern during radiotherapy for cancer in the lung. Radiother Oncol 2006;78:326–331.

76 Yan D, Vicini FA, Wong JW, Martinez AA: Adaptive radiation therapy. Phys Med Biol 1997;42: 123–132.

77 Lof J, Lind BK, Brahme A: An adaptive control algorithm for optimization of intensity modulated radiotherapy considering uncertainties in beam profiles, patient set-up and internal organ motion. Phys Med Biol 1998;43:1605–1628.

78 Song WY, Schaly B, Bauman G, Battista JJ, Van Dyk J: Evaluation of image-guided radiation therapy (IGRT) technologies and their impact on the outcomes of hypofractionated prostate cancer treatments: a radiobiologic analysis. Int J Radiat Oncol Biol Phys 2006;64:289–300.

79 Yan D, Lockman D, Martinez A, Wong J, Brabbins D, Vicini F, et al: Computed tomography guided management of interfractional patient variation. Semin Radiat Oncol 2005;15:168–179.

80 Yan D, Ziaja E, Jaffray D, Wong J, Brabbins D, Vicini F, et al: The use of adaptive radiation therapy to reduce setup error: a prospective clinical study. Int J Radiat Oncol Biol Phys 1998;41:715–720.

81 Martinez AA, Yan D, Lockman D, Brabbins D, Kota K, Sharpe M, et al: Improvement in dose escalation using the process of adaptive radiotherapy combined with three-dimensional conformal or intensity-modulated beams for prostate cancer. Int J Radiat Oncol Biol Phys 2001;50: 1226–1234.

82 Pekar V, McNutt TR, Kaus MR: Automated model-based organ delineation for radiotherapy planning in prostatic region. Int J Radiat Oncol Biol Phys 2004;60:973–980.

83 Brock KK, McShan DL, Ten Haken RK, Hollister SJ, Dawson LA, Balter JM: Inclusion of organ deformation in dose calculations. Med Phys 2003; 30:290–295.

84 Pevsner A, Davis B, Joshi S, Hertanto A, Mechalakos J, Yorke E, et al: Evaluation of an automated deformable image matching method for quantifying lung motion in respiration-correlated CT images. Med Phys 2006;33:369–376.

85 Yan D, Jaffray DA, Wong JW: A model to accumulate fractionated dose in a deforming organ. Int J Radiat Oncol Biol Phys 1999;44:665–675.

Dr. Michael B. Sharpe
Department of Radiation Oncology
Radiation Medicine Program
UHN Princess Margaret Hospital
University of Toronto, 610 University Ave.
Toronto, Ont., M5G 2M9 (Canada)
Tel. +1 416 946 2000, ext. 5025
Fax +1 416 946 6566
E-Mail Michael.sharpe@rmp.uhn.on.ca

Meyer JL (ed): IMRT, IGRT, SBRT – Advances in the Treatment Planning and
Delivery of Radiotherapy. Front Radiat Ther Oncol. Basel, Karger, 2007, vol. 40, pp 94–115

Image Registration in Intensity-Modulated, Image-Guided and Stereotactic Body Radiation Therapy

Kristy K. Brock

Department of Radiation Oncology, University of Toronto and Radiation Medicine Program,
Princess Margaret Hospital, University Health Network, Toronto, Canada

Abstract

Many recent advances in the technology of radiotherapy have greatly increased the amount of image data that must be rapidly processed. With the increasing use of multimodality imaging for target definition in treatment planning, and daily image guidance in treatment delivery, the importance of image registration emerges as key to improving the radiotherapy planning and delivery process at every step. Both clinicians and nonclinicians are affected in their work efficiency. Image registration can improve the correspondence of information in multimodality imaging, allowing more information to be obtained for tumor and normal tissue definition. Image registration at treatment delivery can improve the accuracy of therapy by taking greater advantage of images available prior to treatment. Technical advances have enhanced the accuracy and efficiency of registration through several approaches to automation, and by beginning to address the tissue deformation that occurs during the planning and therapy period. When using an automated registration technique, the user must understand the components of the registration process and the accuracy and limitations of the algorithm involved. This review presents the fundamental components of image registration, compares the benefits and limitations of different algorithms, demonstrates methods of visualizing registration results, and identifies methods to optimize registration for image-guided radiation therapy.

Copyright © 2007 S. Karger AG, Basel

Image Registration and Fusion for Image-Guided Radiation Therapy

Image registration is central to every step of the radiotherapy planning and delivery process. It can improve the ease and accuracy with which multimodality images can be incorporated into a single model of the patient, by resolving the geometric discrepancies that exist between the images. This allows all the information gained from different imaging studies to be fully exploited for treatment definition. As image registration becomes more accurate, comparisons between images can be made on a voxel-by-voxel basis. Image registration can also improve the accuracy and precision of treatment delivery, by relating the volumetric images obtained just prior to treatment delivery with the images used for treatment planning. Registration of these images will allow the offset to be calculated, which can then be applied to the patient position to allow accurate delivery of the intended treatment.

Radiotherapy strives to deliver high doses of radiation to the treatment target, while sparing the surrounding normal tissues. To achieve this, precise delineation of the tumor and critical normal structures must be obtained. Multimodality imaging provides several different forms of information to allow differentiation of tissue through CT, MRI, and ultrasound, and functionality through MR spectroscopic imaging, PET, and functional CT [1–3]. Incorporating these images into one model of the patient can be challenging, since the images are obtained on different devices, each requiring the patient to be repositioned for its imaging process.

Accurate delivery of a precise treatment plan requires that the patient be in the same position as the model that was used to develop that plan. *Expected* deviations between the intended position and the actual position must be accounted for in a larger planning target volume (PTV), which increases the intended area of treatment to ensure target coverage. *Unexpected* deviations between the intended and actual positions result in a geographic miss of radiotherapy. Advances in imaging at the time of treatment, including portal imagers [4, 5], in-room CT scanners [6, 7], ultrasound [8, 9], tomographic imaging [10, 11], and cone beam imaging [12, 13], allow a reduction in the expected deviations and the potential to eliminate unexpected deviations, through daily corrections of the patient. These multiple sources of image data are most useful if they are accurately registered and fused during their evaluation.

Registration allows us to complete the loop in radiotherapy, potentially improving the accuracy of each step of the process, as shown in figure 1. The first is accurate target definition, through multimodality image registration [60, 61]. Target definition may be improved through deformable registration, as it will reduce the uncertainty in the correspondence of these multiple sources of information. The second is accurate motion assessment [62]. When multiple examples of geometry of the patient are obtained, such as inhale and exhale scans, a more accurate deformation map between the two may be generated. The next step is treatment delivery; accurate tumor guidance for online image registration may be improved using deformable registration. Finally, in accurate response follow-up, the response assessment of the tumor and changes in the normal tissue can be

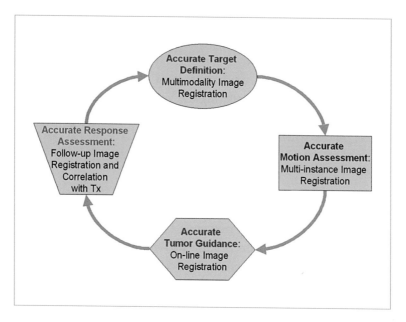

Fig. 1. The role of image registration to improve the integration of the radiotherapy process.

improved using deformable registration to compare the pretreatment images with those obtained following the completion of treatment [56].

This article reviews the methods to perform image registration, their limitations and opportunities, as well as efficient ways to view these registrations for the important tasks of treatment planning, delivery and quality assurance.

Image Registration: Basic Questions

What Is Registration?
It is simply the alignment, or calculation of the transformation, of two images to provide a more complete view of the patient by having them in the same frame of reference (fig. 2).

What Is Fusion?
Fusion is applying the transformation from the registration to the image set to view both images in the same frame of reference (fig. 3).

Why Is Registration Needed?
First, for precision treatment planning, it is often necessary to integrate multiple images, such as MR, CT, and PET scan images. Secondly, accurate correlation of

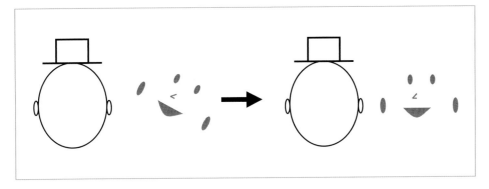

Fig. 2. Registration of the facial features image (gray) with the head image (black).

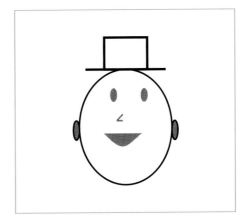

Fig. 3. Fusion of the above images.

tumor localization images at the time of treatment with high-precision treatment plans is essential. In fact, the primary focus of this section will be on the image-guided radiation therapy process of daily treatment alignment. Also, monitoring tumor response and normal tissue changes to evaluate dosimetric changes that may be occurring during the treatment course is important, and this requires image registration between the planning image and the follow-up images.

Who Performs Registration?
The *user* can perform registration by visually inspecting the image, making some adjustments manually, and deciding whether it is acceptable. A second method is the use of an *algorithm* for automated comparison and adjustment. Instead of the user inspecting the images, there is a metric of similarity calculated between the two images, and then an optimization function that seeks to maximize the similarity metric between the images by adjusting the position of the image. This is

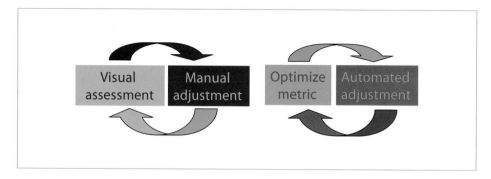

Fig. 4. Manual (left) and automated (right) registration process.

repeated, making an optimization loop that continues until a goal is achieved. Often, in the clinical setting, the two approaches are combined – user initiated and algorithm optimized. In this way, the user has the option of approving or manually adjusting further the automated result. This generally follows because soft tissue is not rigid, and the vast majority of commercially available systems rely on rigid registration, which must make a compromise to register deformed structures (fig. 4).

When Is Registration Performed?
Whenever there is more than one image! Image registration has been performed each time a radiotherapy field has been verified; methods are simply becoming more sophisticated at doing this by using more image guidance tools. The requirements to do so have enormously increased. Comparisons are now made between portal images and digitally reconstructed radiographs, between planning CT images and multimodality MR/PET/CT images, between planning CT images and volumetric images acquired prior to treatment, and between pretreatment images and follow-up images to assess tumor and normal tissue changes (fig. 5).

Why Is Image Registration a Critical Topic of Concern Now?
There are many sources of information now available to aid in creating a model of the patient, and as the number of images increases, the need for image registration increases. Analyses of patient movement, showing degrees of uncertainty that must be added into the treatment planning process, can now be obtained via four-dimensional CT or cine MRI, but these add enormously to the quantity of image data to be processed. So does the volumetric imaging that may be performed daily at the time of treatment delivery. The incorporation of this information into an efficient workflow requires a powerful, streamlined image registration process.

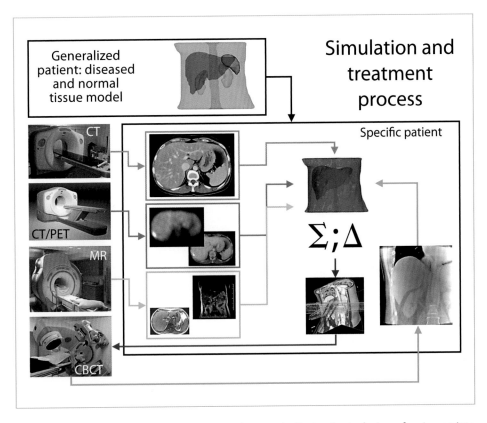

Fig. 5. Simulation and treatment process: each arrow indicates the inclusion of an image into the simulation and treatment process, therefore requiring image registration.

How Can the Burden of Registration Be Reduced?

Taking steps to set up the patient, prior to each imaging session, in a similar position will improve the starting point of registration. The most invasive method, attaching a coordinate system to the patient such as a stereotactic frame that is attached to the head, allows for a fixed reference frame to be visible in each imaging session and during treatment. This technique, although extremely accurate, is only applicable to the head and generally only for single-fraction treatments. Combining imaging modalities together, such as PET/CT, is a direct method to improve the initial registration, as the patient is set up once and images are captured sequentially. Internal anatomical motion, such as breathing, stomach or rectal filling, and small patient motions will still affect the registration and need to be accounted for in the image registration process. Reproducing the patient geometry when using more than one imaging approach, by integrating in-room lasers, treatment type couches, and stabilization devices, can also be used in the image acquisition and treatment processes.

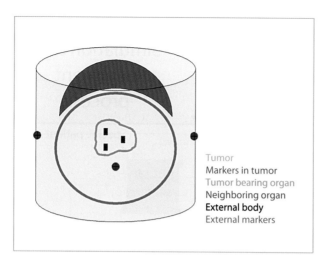

Tumor
Markers in tumor
Tumor bearing organ
Neighboring organ
External body
External markers

Fig. 6. Illustration of a patient and the various surrogates that can be used for registration.

How Is Registration Performed?
This will be the subject of the remainder of this presentation.

The Image Registration Process

Registration is a four-step process.

(1) *Determine common surrogates:* determine what is common between two images and decide how the surrogates are aligned. Options include the use of points, surfaces, and intensities.

(2) *Calculate correspondence between surrogates:* for an automatic alignment process, a quantitative metric must be identified.

(3) *Extrapolate and interpolate regions of interest (ROIs) where common surrogates are not defined:* extrapolation and/or interpolation may be simple, using translation only as for rigid registration, or may be more complicated with both translation and rotation, or modification of scale. The most sophisticated process involves deformable or nonlinear registrations, where each part of the body can move independently.

(4) *Obtain the results:* results may be a transformation map, if the goal of the registration is to determine motion; a model view, to look at how things are changing, or a fused image, to gain more information on a patient or to provide information for the treatment adjustment.

The methods involved in the first three steps are discussed further below, and the last step follows along with each of these methods.

(1) Common Surrogates

Patient imaging for treatment can be illustrated as shown in figure 6. If the position of the tumor itself is not visible on the images, as is usually the case, surrogates for that position are needed. The simplest approach, which is not image based, uses markers (i.e. tattoos) placed on the patient's skin that can be aligned to room laser coordinates. However, choosing a surrogate closer to the actual tumor will likely increase the precision. Neighboring organs, such as a bone or diaphragm that are visible in the images, can also be used as a surrogate for alignment [14, 15]. Implanting markers or fiducials into the tumor itself can create a close surrogate for the tumor [16–18], indicating the position of the tumor, but potentially not indicating deformation that is occurring in the tumor.

Guidance using the tumor-bearing organ can also increase precision; however, this still remains a surrogate, with the accuracy of its surrogacy dependent on the amount of deformation that the organ and tumor undergo, as well as on any differences in coupling between the organ motion and the tumor motion. It is sometimes possible to identify the tumor boundary on volumetric images [19, 20] obtained at the time of treatment used for guidance; however, surrogates are still used in a majority of the cases. The degree of uncertainty between the surrogate and the target for treatment must be included in the uncertainty margins in the treatment design. These uncertainties can be determined from repeat images where the tumor and the surrogate are visible.

(2) Correspondence between Surrogates

Once the surrogates are identified, the method of correspondence must be determined. This can be simple, by using points such as seed locations, or complex, by using the intensity information in the image. Three common methods for calculating correspondence of surrogates are described below: alignment by points, alignment by surfaces, and alignment by intensity pattern.

Alignment by Points

For three-dimensional alignment using points, three noncoplanar points must be identified. If no deformation exists between the position of the seeds on the initial image and the position on the secondary image, then an exact alignment of all three seeds can be performed using a rotation and translation. However, this does not happen for soft tissue anatomy, so the residual error of all the seeds must be minimized. The residual error indicates the error remaining after the correction is carried out. Equation 1 shows the formula for the minimization of three markers, α, β, and γ, where each is a three-dimensional position of a point in image 1 and image 2.

$$\sum\left[\left(\vec{\alpha}_1 - \vec{\alpha}_2\right)^2 + \left(\vec{\beta}_1 - \vec{\beta}_2\right)^2 + \left(\vec{\gamma}_1 - \vec{\gamma}_2\right)^2\right] \qquad (1)$$

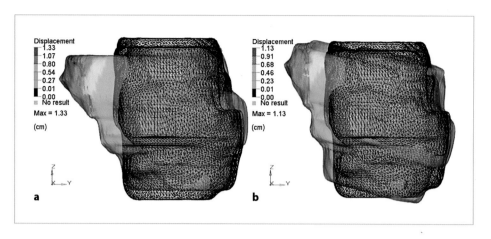

Fig. 7. Residual error of the prostate surface, due to deformation, following registration of the seeds using translation only (**a**) and translation and rotation (**b**).

An example of a common point surrogate is implanted gold fiducials in the prostate seed, which are well seen on megavoltage and kilovoltage (kV) portal images and cone beam images. With seeds, a digitally reconstructed radiograph or reference CT is obtained from planning with the seed location, and this is compared with a megavoltage, kV or volumetric image during treatment. A least-squares difference can determine the difference between these seed positions, and this displacement can provide a transformation to align the patient to the intended position. Marker implants have been shown to be a very effective method of registering the prostate prior to treatment. It is important to note, however, that these seeds are only surrogates. A study performed at Princess Margaret Hospital, where repeat MR images were obtained of the prostate and seeds, indicated the potential for substantial deformation to exist following registration of the prostate using translation only and translation and rotation [21]. Ten percent of the patients had greater than 50% of the prostate surface deformed by more than 3 mm after alignment of the seeds, with the worst case exhibiting 1.3 cm of deformation following translation and 1.1 cm of deformation following translation and rotation. Figure 7 shows the worst case of the 29 patients examined; the mesh represents the prostate position on the first MR image and the color wash represents the prostate on the second MR image, where the color wash indicates the difference, as a vector magnitude, in surface position between the prostate on the second MR image and the prostate on the first MR image.

Alignment by Surfaces
Surfaces can be used for alignment, either in two dimensions or in three dimensions, of the tumor, the tumor-bearing organ, or a neighboring organ. Surface

alignment is performed by dividing the surface into a series of points and minimizing the difference between these points, defined on both surfaces. This is commonly referred to as chamfer matching [22]. The surfaces can be defined manually or by setting a threshold in the image to define the surface.

Pretreatment alignment of the liver provides an example of surface registration for neighboring organs and the tumor-bearing organ. In two dimensions, registration is often performed using the spine to determine the left-right and anterior-posterior position and the dome of the diaphragm for the superior-inferior position. Dawson et al. [23] have shown that there can be a substantial difference in the superior-inferior motion of the tumor defined by the diaphragm on fluoroscopy and the tumor on cine MRI; differences of over 2 cm were observed in some cases. It is important to understand these uncertainties when calculating a PTV margin as well as when performing registration when images are obtained at breath hold.

With volumetric imaging, registration of the surface of the organ can be performed, increasing the precision of registration by improving the relationship between the surrogate, the tumor-bearing organ, and the tumor. The tumor-bearing organ will provide a closer surrogate for the tumor position than neighboring organs, such as bone. Registration can be performed manually, by registering the contours from the planning scan onto the pretreatment images, or by identification of the entire organ surface, either through manual contouring or autosegmentation.

Again, referring to the liver registration example, the liver, contoured on the planning CT, can then be registered to the liver contoured on the kV cone beam CT (CBCT) to match the entire organ volume. Even with good alignment, it is important to remember that this still remains only a surrogate. The organ may deform, prohibiting a rigid registration, even with rotation, to perfectly align these contours [24]. Thirteen patients treated under a liver cancer protocol with rigid registration to align the contours previously generated during treatment planning on the CT scan onto the kV CBCT images obtained prior to treatment were subsequently analyzed with deformable registration. Results showed that 4 of these patients (31%) exhibited residual, regional deformation of the liver, with more than 5% of the liver volume deformed by more than 5 mm. This could potentially have an impact on the positioning of the tumor in the field. Therefore, it is critical to know what part of the anatomy offers greatest accuracy for alignment and the degree of this uncertainty must be reflected in PTV margins, even with on-line image guidance every day.

In lung cancer therapy, registration benefits from the contrast between the lung and the tumor, allowing the tumor to be visualized on pretreatment volumetric images. In this case, alignment of the tumor itself to the planning scan volumes at the time of treatment can be performed. In addition, some tumors encompass the entire organ, such as the prostate [25]. Registration is therefore dependent on the tumor itself and residual errors, due to deformation and changes in anatomy over the course of treatment, can be visualized after registration.

Alignment by Intensity

The information inherent in the image, i.e. the intensity of each voxel, can be used to drive the registration using automated registration methods. Rather than using anatomic or contour surface details, this approach simply uses the 'raw data' of the image itself. Alignment by intensity is performed by identifying a metric that describes the similarity of the voxel intensities between the two images. A transformation is then applied to the secondary image and the similarity metric is recalculated. This is repeated several times, through an optimization algorithm, to find the optimal transformation that leads to the best similarity between the images. The similarity can be calculated using several different techniques. Three of the most common, i.e. sum of the squared difference (SSD), cross-correlation, and mutual information (MI), are described below.

Sum of the Squared Difference. The SSD between the two images is a simple and easy-to-apply metric. The optimization is driven to minimize the difference by transforming the secondary image, B, with respect to the primary image, A, as shown below in equation 2.

$$SSD(A, B) = \Sigma(A - B)^2 \tag{2}$$

The difference is calculated for each voxel in the images and the secondary image is transformed and the metric recalculated. This method is limited to images of the same modality, i.e. 2 CT images but not a CT and MR image [26, 27].

Cross-Correlation Coefficient. Cross-correlation is one of the several methods commonly available in commercial systems. It can be normalized, scaling the differences in images by the differences in local variations between the two images, for registration of images from different modalities. This metric, similar to the SSD, compares the two images on a voxel-by-voxel basis, then transforms the second image, and computes the metric again. The equation for the normalized cross-correlation (NCC) is shown in equation 3, for a comparison of images A and B. $\bar{A}$ and $\bar{B}$ are the averages or local averages of the voxels in images A and B, respectively. Essentially, this method is looking at the difference between two images as a function of the intensities in that image. For example, if image A has a white ROI on a black background and image B shows the same ROI as a light-gray ROI on a dark-gray background, the NCC would recognize that the ROIs correspond in the two images by examining the relationship between the ROI and the background in each image.

$$NCC(A,B) = \frac{\sum(A - \bar{A})(B - \bar{B})}{\sqrt{\sum(A - \bar{A})^2}\sqrt{\sum(B - \bar{B})^2}} \tag{3}$$

This technique is more complex, but offers greater flexibility, as it can be applied to images of different modalities, i.e. CT and MRI [28, 29].

Mutual Information. Another method, MI, is borrowed from information theory and uses the entropy, or information, contained in the two images [30]. The method examines the correspondence of information that is contained in each image. If the two images are completely independent, the MI is 0. MI can be used when there is a difference in the contrast or images obtained from different modalities. Equation 4 shows a common equation for MI, where the joint entropy, or combined information content in a pair of images is equal to the entropy of image A, plus the entropy of image B, minus the MI contained in images A and B.

$$H(A, B) = H(A) + H(B) - MI(A, B) \tag{4}$$

Equation 4 can be solved for MI, resulting in equation 5. This can be used as a metric for automated registration by computing the MI between two images, transforming the secondary image and recomputing the MI until the MI is maximized.

$$MI(A, B) = H(A) + H(B) - H(A, B) \tag{5}$$

This method is more complex than either SSD or NCC, but offers even more flexibility and is often the metric of choice for images of different modalities [31–34].

(3) Automated Registration
Linear Interpolation Methods

Results from an automated registration system will depend on its flexibility and accuracy in performing the interpolation and extrapolation steps required. The majority of commercially available registration algorithms use a linear interpolation, allowing the secondary image to only translate and rotate. Unfortunately, the human body does not behave in such a simplistic manner! Examining a four-dimensional CT of the lung, different motions can be observed. The lungs may move significantly in the superior-inferior direction, but the spine typically does not move at all and the ribs may move by only a fraction of the motion of the lungs. Repeat scans of the head and neck show linear motion of the skull, but variation in the motion of the neck. Complexity increases when examining longitudinal studies, such as a pretreatment image of the anatomy in the head and neck and an image obtained during the last week of treatment, where substantial changes in the volume of the tumor and surrounding normal tissue clearly indicate changes that cannot be accounted for by rotation and translation alone. In each of these cases, deformation is occurring and must be accounted for by a more sophisticated interpolation method. A few methods are briefly described later in the article, with references provided for further information. However, some methods can be performed using rotation and translation alone to improve the accuracy of registration for the ROI of most importance. These methods are described below.

Clip Box. When an automated registration is performed using an intensity-based method described above, the registration will examine the intensity throughout the entire image. If substantial deformation occurs between the two images, the alignment results may not be satisfactory since the algorithm optimized using a linear transformation when a deformable registration was required. The particular linear optimization that the algorithm chose may not be the best one from a clinical viewpoint. For example, if a head and neck patient is imaged prior to treatment and the flexion in the neck is different than that in the CT scan, which is the reference image, the registration algorithm needs to know which area is most important for registration. The user can indicate this by using a clip box, or a box that encompasses the ROI of greatest interest. The registration algorithm then focuses only on the image intensities in this box.

An example is shown below for a head and neck case using the Synergy XVI R3.5 General Release software (Elekta Limited, Crawley, UK) with a clip box to perform image guidance at the time of treatment. The algorithm sets a threshold for the bones and then performs a surface match on the segmented bone [22]. The reference image is a CT image and the secondary image is a kV CBCT image. In figure 8a, the clip box is placed on the neck, resulting in good registration of the neck but poor registration of the skull, due to deformation resulting from neck flexion between the primary (green) and secondary (purple) images. In figure 8b, the clip box is placed on the front skull, resulting in good registration of the skull and poor registration of the neck.

Organ Limitation. A second optimization approach, similar to the clip box, is to use the contoured ROI to limit the registration region. This approach allows a more tailored ROI, but requires user intervention with contouring of the ROI. For treatment planning purposes, contouring the ROI is already required, so registration can take advantage of this more detailed type of clip box.

The example shown in figure 9 is an inhale and exhale breath hold image of the abdomen for a liver cancer patient. The primary image (fig. 9a) is at exhale breath hold. The liver has been contoured, indicated by the purple outline. Figure 9b is at inhale breath hold. The spine and ribs have not moved substantially between the two image sets and will cause problems for a rigid registration algorithm; however, if the liver contour is used to limit the registration, the results, shown in figure 9c, are very good for the liver, which is the important ROI in this case. This registration was performed using MI in Pinnacle 6.2 (Philips Medical Systems, Madison, Wisc., USA).

It is important to understand which ROI is important for the treatment planning and guidance procedure. It is also critical to understand when these tradeoffs

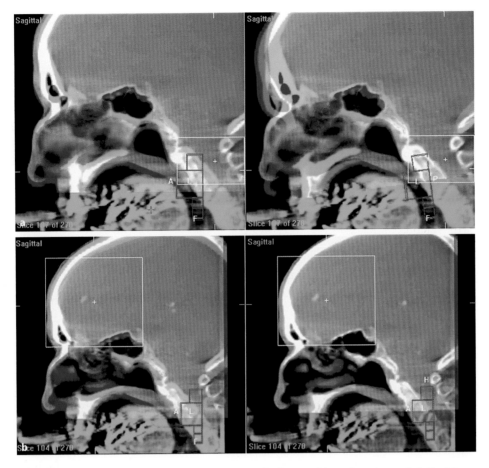

Fig. 8. a Head and neck image alignment using a clip box positioned on the neck. **b** Registration of the same head and neck, with a clip box placed on the front skull. A correct match will appear in gray by overlaying green and purple.

should not be made and an intervention, either repositioning the patient or replanning the treatment, should be performed. For example, if a clip box is used to focus the registration on a lung tumor, to overcome registration errors due to deformation, but the results of the registration places the spinal cord into the high-dose region, caution should be taken before treatment of the patient.

Deformable Registration Methods

As illustrated above, the human body does not behave in a linear fashion. Deformation exists due to internal physiological motion and external patient positioning, and the tumor and normal tissue responses to them. Accounting for this deformation in the registration process is currently the subject of much research. Several different approaches are being investigated and although it is out of

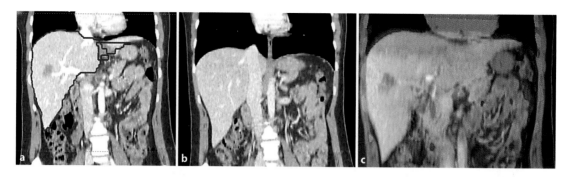

Fig. 9. Exhale breath hold CT image (**a**) with liver contour for limiting the ROI of registration, inhale breath hold CT image (**b**), and results of the registration (**c**).

the scope of this article to describe them in detail, four of the primary algorithms are briefly described: fluid flow, optical flow, spline-based, and biomechanical methods.

Fluid Flow. In a fluid flow approach, the deformations in the images are modeled as a fluid. The algorithm optimizes a similarity metric, described above, while constraining the interpolation by the laws of continuum mechanics. This method is currently being investigated by several groups for four-dimensional CT registration [3, 35, 36], intracavitary brachytherapy [37], and the brain [38, 39]. The approach can be fully automatic, invertible and has shown accuracy of less than 4 mm in the lung. Two potential limitations include accommodating noncontinuous motion, such as the stationary spine next to the moving lung, and accommodating a lack of intensity correspondence, such as an image with a full rectum being registered to an image with an empty rectum. For multimodality registration, this algorithm must be implemented with NCC or MI.

Optical Flow. Optical flow uses the differences between the images and the gradient of the image as forces to drive the registration, while maximizing a similarity metric. This approach is often referred to as the 'demon's approach', which was first implemented by Thirion [40]. Additional forces, such as an active force, based on the gradient in the moving image, can also be added to improve the outcome of the registration [41, 42]. This algorithm has been investigated in the head and neck and prostate [41]. It can also be fully automatic and has shown good efficiency. As with the fluid flow, accommodating noncontinuous motion may be a limitation in some instances as well as accommodating lack of intensity correspondence. These are only potential problems, and research is ongoing to solve these issues for this type of registration.

Brock

Thin-Plate Spline and B-Spline. A spline-based approach deforms the image using control points that are placed in specific locations (thin-plate spline) or on a regular grid (B-spline). The control points guide the deformation of the image as a similarity metric is optimized. In a thin-plate spline approach, each control point effects the deformation of the entire image; the extent depends on the distance to the control point, making this approach best for single organ registration. The control points in B-spline only affect a local area of the registration, allowing for a multiorgan registration to be performed. Spline approaches have been used in a variety of anatomical sites, including the liver [31, 43–45], lung [27, 46–48], and prostate [49–51]. The algorithm can be fully automated and efficient and an accuracy of 1.0–3.5 mm has been shown. Potential limitations are the same as for the fluid and optical flow, accommodating noncontinuous motion and lack of intensity correspondence.

Biomechanical Method. A biomechanical approach deforms the image according to the material properties of the tissue, i.e. depending on whether the material is hard or soft. The approach is typically implemented using a finite element model of the anatomy in the image, which represents each ROI as a series of connected nodes, forming tetrahedrons and solved using finite element analysis. Boundary conditions are required, which describe the motion and deformation of certain parts of the model; these are determined using a similarity metric, often by deforming the contoured ROI on one image to the contoured ROI on a secondary image. This approach has been used for several anatomical sites, including the thorax [52–54], abdomen [52, 55, 56], and pelvis [57–59]. Accuracy of 1.2–2.5 mm has been shown. Potential limitations include the dependence of contours on the registration and the uncertainty in defining the material properties of the anatomy that is modeled.

Quality Assurance

No model is perfect, and this includes the models for image registration. It is necessary to know and understand the uncertainties that may be involved. While gaining quality assurance data can be challenging, there are some techniques available such as looking at anatomic landmarks and visual assessments.

Quantitative Accuracy
Quantitative accuracy of rigid registration can be performed using a phantom and displacing the phantom by a known amount, obtaining images at both positions. The images can then be used as input to the registration algorithm and the accuracy can be computed by comparing the predicted displacement, from the

registration algorithm, with the actual displacement, from the known shift. Unfortunately, phantoms behave much better than human subjects, as they do not deform and they do not generate unique artifacts in each image! For patient data, quantitative accuracy assessments can be computed by identifying naturally or implanted fiducials in the body, such as implanted gold seeds in the prostate or bronchial bifurcations in the lung. The accuracy of identifying these fiducials will limit the confidence of the accuracy assessment, but studies have shown that the reproducibility is very good for naturally occurring fiducials in the liver and lung [47, 52, 56], as well as implanted seeds in the prostate [16–18, 63]. The predicted displacement between the fiducials from the registration can be compared with the actual displacement of the fiducials between the two images. Repeat registrations can also be performed to quantify the variability in the registration results.

Qualitative Accuracy

In the absence of quantitative accuracy, qualitative accuracy can be performed by examining the results of the registration. Image overlay is a visual method of assessing the differences. Examples of image overlay have been demonstrated throughout this discussion. Figure 7 uses a color overlay, where one image is green, the other is purple, and where they agree the image turns gray. This is a very effective way of visualizing differences, as areas that lack correspondence stand out. Figure 9 shows another color overlay, where one image is a gray scale and the other a thermal scale image, where the variation in intensity is displayed as a range of red and orange. This allows visualization of both images. In addition, both images may be shown in gray scale and a checkerboard or sliding window can be used to see the correspondence between both images. Figure 10 shows an example of a checkerboard, dividing the image into 4 quadrants, with the diagonal quadrants displaying the same image; clear misregistrations can be seen. The position of the quadrant can be moved interactively, allowing the user to see the registration at different regions of the image. The number of divisions can also be increased, allowing more comparisons of fine features to be examined.

Conclusion

Advances in image registration allow multimodality imaging and volumetric imaging at the time of treatment to be fully integrated into the radiotherapy process. The increasing use of multimodality imaging for treatment planning and the growing use of volumetric imaging for image guidance has demanded automated registration algorithms that are efficient and accurate.

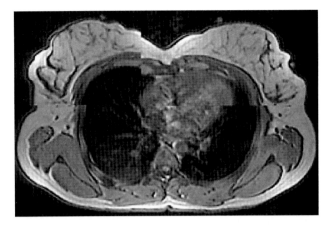

Fig. 10. A single checkerboard, dividing the image space into 4 quadrants, the upper right and lower left display one image and the upper left and lower right display the other.

The four components of registration are: (1) determining common surrogates; (2) calculating the correspondence between surrogates; (3) interpolating between surrogates, and (4) evaluating and displaying results. Several surrogates can be used depending on the application, including points, surfaces, and image intensities. Calculating the correspondence depends on the surrogate and can be as simple as minimizing the difference, for points and surfaces, or complex, such as MI for comparing image intensities. The appropriate surrogate and correspondence must be selected for each problem and the limitations of the surrogates must be understood and included in the PTV margins for the treatment delivery. Currently, most commercially available systems interpolate the image space between the surrogates using a linear translation, accounting for rotation and translation only. This is a limitation for soft tissue, which deforms due to physiological motion, flexibility in patient positioning, and anatomical changes over the course of treatment. Deformable registration algorithms, which allow for more complex interpolations, are currently being developed. Local improvements in linear registration can be achieved in the presence of deformation by optimizing the registration to focus on the ROI that is most important. The use of clip boxes or ROI delineations can restrict the algorithm to the ROI of importance; however, caution should be used to ensure that the misregistrations outside of the ROI would not significantly violate planning or treatment constraints.

Quality assurance of the registration results is very important. Quantitative approaches are possible, but are less efficient and should be performed off-line to evaluate a new registration algorithm or application to a new anatomical site. Qualitative evaluation, such as looking at image overlays, is very efficient and should be used to ensure that each registration is acceptable prior to proceeding with the treatment or planning process.

Image registration can complete integration of the radiotherapy process. As registration becomes fully integrated into the radiotherapy process, improvements may be possible in target delineation, motion assessment, image guidance, and response assessment. Research is actively pursuing deformable registration algorithms, which will further improve the registration process and reduce the need for user intervention for optimization of linear registration in the presence of deformation.

Acknowledgements

The author acknowledges the contributions of the faculty and staff of Princess Margaret Hospital, especially Laura Dawson, Douglas Moseley, Michael Sharpe, and David Jaffray for their contributions and suggestions.

References

1 Glatstein E, Lichter AS, Fraass BA, Kelly BA, van de Geijn J: The imaging revolution and radiation oncology: use of CT, ultrasound, and NMR for localization, treatment planning and treatment delivery. Int J Radiat Oncol Biol Phys 1985;11:299–314.

2 Yap JT, Carney JP, Hall NC, Townsend DW: Image-guided cancer therapy using PET/CT. Cancer J 2004;10:221–233.

3 Keall PJ, Starkschall G, Shukla H, Forster KM, Ortiz V, Stevens CW, Vedam SS, George R, Guerrero T, Mohan R: Acquiring 4D thoracic CT scans using a multislice helical method. Phys Med Biol 2004;49:2053–2067.

4 McParland BJ, Kumaradas JC: Digital portal image registration by sequential anatomical match-point and image correlations for real-time continuous field alignment verification. Med Phys 1995;22:1063–1075.

5 Michalski JM, Graham MV, Bosch WR, Wong J, Gerber RL, Cheng A, Tinger A, Valicenti RK: Prospective clinical evaluation of an electronic portal imaging device. Int J Radiat Oncol Biol Phys 1996;34:943–951.

6 Barker J, Garden A, Dong L, O'Daniel J, Wang H, Court L, Morrison W, Rosenthal D, Chao C, Mohan R, Ang K: Radiation-induced anatomic changes during fractionated head and neck radiotherapy: a pilot study using an integrated CT-LINAC system. Int J Radiat Oncol Biol Phys 2003; 57(2 suppl):S304.

7 Cheng CW, Wong J, Grimm L, Chow M, Uematsu M, Fung A: Commissioning and clinical implementation of a sliding gantry CT scanner installed in an existing treatment room and early clinical experience for precise tumor localization. Am J Clin Oncol 2003;26:e28–e36.

8 Ghanei A, Soltanian-Zadeh H, Ratkewicz A, Yin FF: A three-dimensional deformable model for segmentation of human prostate from ultrasound images. Med Phys 2001;28:2147–2153.

9 Mohan DS, Kupelian PA, Willoughby TR: Short-course intensity-modulated radiotherapy for localized prostate cancer with daily transabdominal ultrasound localization of the prostate gland. Int J Radiat Oncol Biol Phys 2000;46:575–580.

10 Mackie TR, Holmes T, Swerdloff S, Reckwerdt P, Deasy JO, Yang J, Paliwal B, Kinsella T: Tomotherapy: a new concept for the delivery of dynamic conformal radiotherapy. Med Phys 1993;20: 1709–1719.

11 Ruchala KJ, Olivera GH, Kapatoes JM, Schloesser EA, Reckwerdt PJ, Mackie TR: Megavoltage CT image reconstruction during tomotherapy treatments. Phys Med Biol 2000;45:3545–3562.

12 Jaffray DA, Siewerdsen JH: Cone-beam computed tomography with a flat-panel imager: initial performance characterization. Med Phys 2000; 27:1311–1323.

13 Ford EC, Chang J, Mueller K, Sidhu K, Todor D, Mageras G, Yorke E, Ling CC, Amols H: Cone-beam CT with megavoltage beams and an amorphous silicon electronic portal imaging device: potential for verification of radiotherapy of lung cancer. Med Phys 2002;29:2913–2924.

14 Dawson LA, Brock KK, Kazanjian S, Fitch D, McGinn CJ, Lawrence TS, Ten Haken RK, Balter J: The reproducibility of organ position using active breathing control (ABC) during liver radiotherapy. Int J Radiat Oncol Biol Phys 2001;51:1410–1421.

15 Wong JW, Sharpe MB, Jaffray DA, Kini VR, Robertson JM, Stromberg JS, Martinez AA: The use of active breathing control (ABC) to reduce margin for breathing motion. Int J Radiat Oncol Biol Phys 1999;44:911–919.

16 Dehnad H, Nederveen AJ, van der Heide UA, van Moorselaar RJ, Hofman P, Lagendijk JJ: Clinical feasibility study for the use of implanted gold seeds in the prostate as reliable positioning markers during megavoltage irradiation. Radiother Oncol 2003;67:295–302.

17 Balter JM, Lam KL, Sandler HM, Littles JF, Bree RL, Ten Haken RK: Automated localization of the prostate at the time of treatment using implanted radiopaque markers: technical feasibility. Int J Radiat Oncol Biol Phys 1995;33:1281–1286.

18 Litzenberg D, Dawson LA, Sandler H, Sanda MG, McShan DL, Ten Haken RK, Lam KL, Brock KK, Balter JM: Daily prostate targeting using implanted radiopaque markers. Int J Radiat Oncol Biol Phys 2002;52:699–703.

19 Welsh JS, Bradley K, Manon R, Lock M, Patel R, Ruchala K, Mackie TR, Mehta M: Megavoltage CT imaging for adaptive helical tomotherapy of lung cancer. Int J Radiat Oncol Biol Phys 2003;57(2 suppl):S429.

20 Letourneau D, Martinez AA, Lockman D, Yan D, Vargas C, Ivaldi G, Wong J: Assessment of residual error for online cone-beam CT-guided treatment of prostate cancer patients. Int J Radiat Oncol Biol Phys 2005;62:1239–1246.

21 Jaffray DA, Brock KK, Nichol A, Moseley DJ, Catton C, Warde P: An analysis of interfraction prostate deformation relative to implanted fiducial markers using finite element modeling. Int J Radiat Oncol Biol Phys 2004;60(suppl 1):S334–S335.

22 van Herk M, Kooy HM: Automatic three-dimensional correlation of CT-CT, CT-MRI, and CT-SPECT using chamfer matching. Med Phys 1994;21:1163–1178.

23 Dawson LA, Eccles C, Kirilova A, Brock KK: Three-dimensional motion of liver tumours using cine MRI compared to liver motion assessed at fluoroscopy. Radiother Oncol 2006;A483:S214.

24 Hawkins MA, Brock KK, Eccles C, Moseley D, Jaffray D, Dawson LA: Assessment of residual error in liver position using kV cone-beam computed tomography for liver cancer high precision radiation therapy. Int J Radiat Oncol Biol Phys 2006;66:610–619.

25 Smitsmans MH, de Bois J, Sonke JJ, Betgen A, Zijp LJ, Jaffray DA, Lebesque JV, van Herk M: Automatic prostate localization on cone-beam CT scans for high precision image-guided radiotherapy. Int J Radiat Oncol Biol Phys 2005;63:975–984.

26 Keall PJ, Joshi S, Vedam SS, Siebers JV, Kini VR, Mohan R: Four-dimensional radiotherapy planning for DMLC-based respiratory motion tracking. Med Phys 2005;32:942–951.

27 Rietzel E, Chen GT, Choi NC, Willet CG: Four-dimensional image-based treatment planning: target volume segmentation and dose calculation in the presence of respiratory motion. Int J Radiat Oncol Biol Phys 2005;61:1535–1550.

28 Dong L, Boyer AL: An image correlation procedure for digitally reconstructed radiographs and electronic portal images. Int J Radiat Oncol Biol Phys 1995;33:1053–1060.

29 Fitchard EE, Aldridge JS, Reckwerdt PJ, Mackie TR: Registration of synthetic tomographic projection data sets using cross-correlation. Phys Med Biol 1998;43:1645–1657.

30 Viola PA, Wells WM: Alignment by maximization of mutual information. Proc 5th Int Conf Comput Vision, IEEE, New York, 1995, pp 16–23.

31 Meyer CR, Boes JL, Kim B, Bland PH, Zasadny KR, Kison PV, Koral K, Frey KA, Wahl RL: Demonstration of accuracy and clinical versatility of mutual information for automatic multimodality image fusion using affine and thin-plate spline warped geometric deformations. Med Image Anal 1997;1:195–206.

32 Maes F, Vandermeulen D, Suetens P: Comparative evaluation of multiresolution optimization strategies for multimodality image registration by maximization of mutual information. Med Image Anal 1999;3:373–386.

33 Kim J, Fessler JA, Lam KL, Balter JM, Ten Haken RK: A feasibility study of mutual information based setup error estimation for radiotherapy. Med Phys 2001;28:2507–2517.

34 D'Agostino E, Maes F, Vandermeulen D, Suetens P: A viscous fluid model for multimodal non-rigid image registration using mutual information. Med Image Anal 2003;7:565–575.

35 Keall P: 4-Dimensional computed tomography imaging and treatment planning. Semin Radiat Oncol 2004;14:81–90.

36 Keall PJ, Siebers JV, Joshi S, Mohan R: Monte Carlo as a four-dimensional radiotherapy treatment-planning tool to account for respiratory motion. Phys Med Biol 2004;49:3639–3648.

37 Christensen GE, Carlson B, Chao KS, Yin P, Grigsby PW, Nguyen K, Dempsey JF, Lerma FA, Bae KT, Vannier MW, Williamson JF: Image-based dose planning of intracavitary brachytherapy: registration of serial-imaging studies using deformable anatomic templates. Int J Radiat Oncol Biol Phys 2001;51:227–243.

38 Christensen GE, Joshi SC, Miller MI: Volumetric transformation of brain anatomy. IEEE Trans Med Imaging 1997;16:864–877.

39 Haller JW, Banerjee A, Christensen GE, Gado M, Joshi S, Miller MI, Sheline Y, Vannier MW, Csernansky JG: Three-dimensional hippocampal MR morphometry with high-dimensional transformation of a neuroanatomic atlas. Radiology 1997;202:504–510.

40 Thirion JP: Image matching as a diffusion process: an analogy with Maxwell's demons. Med Image Anal 1998;2:243–260.

41 Wang H, Dong L, Lii MF, Lee AL, de Crevoisier R, Mohan R, Cox JD, Kuban DA, Cheung R: Implementation and validation of a three-dimensional deformable registration algorithm for targeted prostate cancer radiotherapy. Int J Radiat Oncol Biol Phys 2005;61:725–735.

42 Wang H, Dong L, O'Daniel J, Mohan R, Garden AS, Ang KK, Kuban DA, Bonnen M, Chang JY, Cheung R: Validation of an accelerated 'demons' algorithm for deformable image registration in radiation therapy. Phys Med Biol 2005;50:2887–2905.

43 Brock KK, McShan DL, Ten Haken RK, Hollister SJ, Dawson LA, Balter JM: Inclusion of organ deformation in dose calculations. Med Phys 2003;30:290–295.

44 Brock KM, Balter JM, Dawson LA, Kessler ML, Meyer CR: Automated generation of a four-dimensional model of the liver using warping and mutual information. Med Phys 2003;30:1128–1133.

45 Rohlfing T, Maurer CR Jr, O'Dell WG, Zhong J: Modeling liver motion and deformation during the respiratory cycle using intensity-based nonrigid registration of gated MR images. Med Phys 2004;31:427–432.

46 Rosu M, Chetty IJ, Balter JM, Kessler ML, McShan DL, Ten Haken RK: Dose reconstruction in deforming lung anatomy: dose grid size effects and clinical implications. Med Phys 2005;32:2487–2495.

47 Coselmon MM, Balter JM, McShan DL, Kessler ML: Mutual information based CT registration of the lung at exhale and inhale breathing states using thin-plate splines. Med Phys 2004;31:2942–2948.

48 Paganetti H, Jiang H, Adams JA, Chen GT, Rietzel E: Monte Carlo simulations with time-dependent geometries to investigate effects of organ motion with high temporal resolution. Int J Radiat Oncol Biol Phys 2004;60:942–950.

49 Schaly B, Bauman GS, Battista JJ, Van Dyk J: Validation of contour-driven thin-plate splines for tracking fraction-to-fraction changes in anatomy and radiation therapy dose mapping. Phys Med Biol 2005;50:459–475.

50 Venugopal N, McCurdy B, Hnatov A, Dubey A: A feasibility study to investigate the use of thin-plate splines to account for prostate deformation. Phys Med Biol 2005;50:2871–2885.

51 Schaly B, Kempe JA, Bauman GS, Battista JJ, Van Dyk J: Tracking the dose distribution in radiation therapy by accounting for variable anatomy. Phys Med Biol 2004;49:791–805.

52 Brock KK, Sharpe MB, Dawson LA, Kim SM, Jaffray DA: Accuracy of finite element model-based multi-organ deformable image registration. Med Phys 2005;32:1647–1659.

53 Schnabel JA, Tanner C, Castellano-Smith AD, Degenhard A, Leach MO, Hose DR, Hill DL, Hawkes DJ: Validation of nonrigid image registration using finite-element methods: application to breast MR images. IEEE Trans Med Imaging 2003;22:238–247.

54 Zhang T, Orton NP, Mackie TR, Paliwal BR: Technical note: a novel boundary condition using contact elements for finite element-based deformable image registration. Med Phys 2004;31:2412–2415.

55 Brock KK, Hollister SJ, Dawson LA, Balter JM: Technical note: creating a four-dimensional model of the liver using finite element analysis. Med Phys 2002;29:1403–1405.

56 Brock KK, Dawson LA, Sharpe MB, Moseley DJ, Jaffray DA: Feasibility of a novel deformable image registration technique to facilitate classification, targeting, and monitoring of tumor and normal tissue. Int J Radiat Oncol Biol Phys 2006;64:1245–1254.

57 Liang J, Yana D: Reducing uncertainties in volumetric image-based deformable organ registration. Med Phys 2003;30:2116–2122.

58 Yan D, Jaffray DA, Wong JW: A model to accumulate fractionated dose in a deforming organ. Int J Radiat Oncol Biol Phys 1999;44:665–675.

59 Bharatha A, Hirose M, Hata N, Warfield SK, Ferrant M, Zou KH, Suarez-Santana E, Ruiz-Alzola J, D'Amico A, Cormack RA, Kikinis R, Jolesz FA, Tempany CM: Evaluation of three-dimensional finite element-based deformable registration of pre- and intraoperative prostate imaging. Med Phys 2001;28:2551–2560.

60 Sailer SL, Rosenman JG, Soltys M, Cullip TJ, Chen J: Improving treatment planning accuracy through multimodality imaging. Int J Radiat Oncol Biol Phys 1996;35:117–124.

61 Schad LR, Boesecke R, Schlegel W, Hartmann GH, Sturm V, Strauss LG, Lorenz WJ: Three dimensional image correlation of CT, MR, and PET studies in radiotherapy treatment planning of brain tumors. J Comput Assist Tomogr 1987;11:948–954.

62 Langen KM, Jones DT: Organ motion and its management. Int J Radiat Oncol Biol Phys 2001;50:265–278.

63 Parker CC, Damyanovich A, Haycocks T, Haider M, Bayley A, Catton CN: Magnetic resonance imaging in the radiation treatment planning of localized prostate cancer using intra-prostatic fiducial markers for computed tomography co-registration. Radiother Oncol 2003;66:217–224.

Dr. Kristy K. Brock
Department of Radiation Oncology
University of Toronto and Radiation Medicine Program
Princess Margaret Hospital
University Health Network, 610 University Ave.
Toronto, Ont., M5G 2M9 (Canada)
Tel. +1 416 946 4501, ext. 6565
Fax +1 416 946 6566
E-Mail kristy.brock@rmp.uhn.on.ca

Meyer JL (ed): IMRT, IGRT, SBRT – Advances in the Treatment Planning and
Delivery of Radiotherapy. Front Radiat Ther Oncol. Basel, Karger, 2007, vol. 40, pp 116–131

Kilovoltage Volumetric Imaging in the Treatment Room

D.A. Jaffray

Radiation Medicine Program, Princess Margaret Hospital/Ontario Cancer Institute, Departments
of Radiation Oncology and Medical Biophysics, University of Toronto, Toronto, Canada

Abstract

Flat-panel cone beam CT is maturing to a stable imaging modality. Applications are being developed for radiotherapy, volumetric diagnostic scanning, rotational angiography and mobile C-arm
technologies with soft tissue imaging capabilities. Volumetric image-guided radiotherapy is tech-
nologically feasible, and has been proven clinically useful with cone beam CT, CT on rails and tomotherapy design configurations. Soft-tissue-based guidance of field placement is now possible for
many sites. Evaluation of the relative merits of these technologies requires that the objective of imaging be well defined. Relevant questions include: Can the target or normal structure of interest be
localized with the desired precision and accuracy? Can the patient's position be adjusted based on
this information within the time constraints of the clinical workload? We must be prepared to compromise diverse clinical objectives and technical features in order to achieve systems with defined
and useful functionality. These imaging technologies will lead to a better understanding of the weaknesses, and provide opportunity to reduce errors and improve technical execution of radiotherapy
delivery.   Copyright © 2007 S. Karger AG, Basel

Volumetric Imaging in Radiotherapy

The development of volumetric imaging in the treatment room and the opportunity for on-line guidance of radiotherapy offer strategies to increase the precision
and accuracy of dose placement in the body. The enhanced accuracy of targeting
can permit reduced exposure of normal tissues for equivalent target coverage,
since smaller planning target margins may be employed. There is a related benefit

that is of equal importance, if not greater. It is simply the assurance that the treatment will be executed as it was planned. There is a growing body of evidence regarding the inconsistency in anatomy between what is planned upon and what is actually being treated [1, 2]. On-line information will allow us to identify this inconsistency and to act to correct it.

There are three general approaches that are providing volumetric imaging as a solution throughout the body. First, there are conventional CT approaches using adjacent kilovoltage (kV) CT scanners ('in-line' or 'on-rails') [3] or integrated megavoltage (MV) scanning as developed with tomotherapy [4]. Second, there are cone beam CT approaches at both MV and kV X-ray energies [5–8]. Third, there are MR approaches being developed. In this volume, the MV cone beam CT approach is discussed by Pouliot [this vol., pp. 132–144], and tomotherapy is discussed by Tomé et al. [this vol., pp. 162–178]; see also the article by Kupelian and Meyer [this vol., pp. 289–314] for a discussion of the MR approach. This section will primarily discuss the kV cone beam CT approach, with some reference to the other approaches to provide a basis for intercomparison.

Kilovoltage Cone Beam CT

Technology
Cone beam CT is a simple process using a point X-ray source and a robust two-dimensional X-ray sensor such as a current generation flat-panel X-ray detector, both rotated about an object of interest to generate high-quality projection data. From those data, an estimate of the attenuation coefficients of the object of interest can be generated using a filtered back-projection process [9, 10]. Several vendors are now providing or developing such systems. The Elekta Synergy™ platform is an integrated imaging and delivery system that includes the source and the flat-panel detector rotating about the axis at 90° to the therapy beam. Imaging doses typically range from 0.5 to 4 cGy [11], though one can use higher or lower levels depending on the quality of the image required. In some systems, saturation of the detector can limit higher doses from being applied. The total number of projections depends upon the scan time and the frame rate of the flat-panel detector employed. Imaging acquisition typically requires 0.5–2.0 min of scan time. From that, a volumetric data set of arbitrary size can be reconstructed up to the limit of the detector field of view. Factors limiting the data set size include processing time, available memory, and limiting resolution of the system. Data sets up to $1,024^3$ have been reported [9]. This quantity of data represents a dramatic change in the amount of information that is available compared with conventional electronic portal imaging. Remarkably, this is achieved with comparable imaging doses and imaging times to those of localization port films.

The cone beam CT systems provide large fields of view (FOVs), with a z (superior-inferior) dimension of up to 25 cm and axial dimensions of 26, 40 and 50 cm. Spatial resolution on the order of 500 μm can be reconstructed, giving more than sufficient detail for precise patient positioning. The resulting volumetric images are referenced to the treatment isocenter through a calibration procedure [12]. Treatment planning data can be registered to the resulting images to determine the current patient position relative to the planned isocenter location. It is anticipated that displays of planned dose distributions will be available for online review as the technology matures.

The driving concerns for the development of this technology have been its applications in the clinic, and clinical observations made to date illustrate the performance and potential uses of kV cone beam CT.

Applications

At Princess Margaret Hospital (PMH), cone beam CT has been investigated in a wide variety of applications. It has been evaluated in guiding target positioning of radiotherapy to the breast – in many cases, breast internal soft tissue detail can be observed. It has been studied for preoperative radiotherapy for sarcoma patients, where the soft tissue tumors may be directly identified, giving distinct advantage for this guidance approach. Imaging in the thorax demonstrates its potential for use in stereotactic body radiotherapy of spine, liver, and lung lesions. For the prostate, there has been a comparison of cone beam CT and conventional markers for optimizing radiotherapy accuracy [13]. Other investigators have explored its use for bladder neoplasms and those of the head and neck [14]. The imaging objectives of these initiatives vary depending on their clinical objectives.

Soft Tissue Detail

Cone beam CT is an option for guiding radiation therapy when soft tissue targets are of interest, as in prostate cancer where it permits the localization of the gland and surrounding normal structures in most cases. This emphasizes the ability of cone beam CT to image soft tissue detail sufficiently for clinical use. However, when imaging the thoracic area, there may be substantial breathing motion that can induce artifacts, and these may require management of the motion by a variety of techniques (gating, breath hold, retrospective sorting). Fortunately, the high contrasts in the lung allow images of more than sufficient quality to be obtained [15]. Figure 1 shows the detail that can be achieved for soft tissue sarcomas during preoperative treatment. Excellent imaging is seen of the tumor itself, as well as of the skin, muscle and even vasculature. Since positioning of patients can sometimes be troublesome with extremity soft tissue tumors, direct visualization of the tumor offers significant advantage for target alignment before treatment, and allows monitoring of therapy-induced changes during a treatment course.

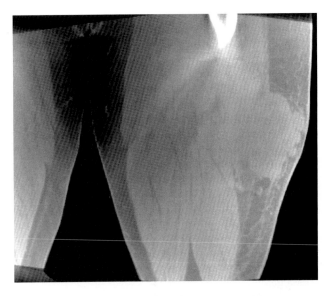

Fig. 1. kV cone beam CT image of a patient receiving preoperative radiation therapy for a sarcoma. The image is generated on the Elekta Synergy Research Platform and corresponds to an imaging dose of approx. 3 cGy. The image demonstrates the soft tissue and spatial resolution performance of these systems. Courtesy of Princess Margaret Hospital, Toronto, Canada.

Bone Detail

One can also obtain very-high-resolution imaging of bone structures. Figure 2 illustrates free-breathing reconstructions of the spine in a lung cancer patient using kV cone beam CT. Reconstruction at a pitch of 120 μm exceeds the limiting resolution of the imaging system and allows visualization of the limits of resolution of the system in the region of the spine. The trabecular bone structure is visible in this reconstruction, consistent with the 0.6-mm full width at half maximum point spread function reported upon previously [16]. The ability to localize with this level of precision and accuracy would make retreatment of targets near the cord feasible. In the context of palliation, incremental treatment of targets along the spinal column can be greatly facilitated.

Organ Movement

Unlike the detectors employed in conventional CT, flat-panel detectors were developed for fluoroscopy and radiography. Their continued application in this manner is useful for assessing internal organ movement on the treatment unit. This approach is being used at PMH for monitoring moving structures during respiration for high-precision radiotherapy of liver and lung cancers [17]. A more complete review of this is given by Taremi et al. [this vol., pp. 272–288]. Active breathing control [18] is employed if appropriate in this patient population, and

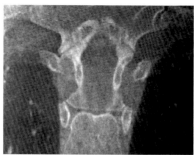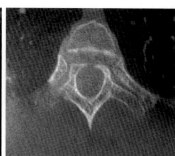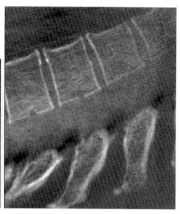

Fig. 2. A high-resolution reconstruction of the spine (120 μm voxel pitch) demonstrates the limiting resolution of the imaging system. Previous reports suggest that a spread function in the order of 0.6 mm can be achieved for the detector, focal spot, and geometry used in the Elekta system. Courtesy of Princess Margaret Hospital, Toronto, Canada.

radiographic and fluoroscopic imaging is used to confirm the anatomic position during the breath hold. During treatment of liver cancers, patients are maintained under active breathing control for treatment periods of about 10 s. Using two orthogonal kV fluoroscopic image sets, each for 10 s, one can evaluate how stable the diaphragm is over time.

Cone beam CT can be used for a form of four-dimensional target localization and phase determination through the respiratory cycle [15, 19, 20]. Operationally, the cone beam CT provides continuous monitoring of all points in the FOV through time as it rotates through the 360°. For example, a full rotation may yield a set of >600 projections containing a few minutes of periodic breathing motion (approx. 30+ breathing cycles). The problem is that there is no single, consistent object to be reconstructed. However, for periodic motions, the image sets can be sorted retrospectively to provide reconstruction at a number of phases of a periodic set of objects. The content of the projection images can be analyzed and used directly to sort the projection sets according to the phases of the breathing cycle. For instance, one could evaluate only the expiration phase projections, the longest phase of respiration. Alternatively, one could sort into multiple phase or amplitude bins over the entire respiratory cycle, thereby creating a four-dimensional cone beam CT data set just prior to treatment. This clearly has application in an on-line process in the delivery of stereotactic body radiation therapy for lung tumors. At PMH, the cone beam CT system is used to perform an on-line adjustment based on the blurred-out image with motion present. The images of the planning and on-treatment scans are registered, an adjustment is made, the couch shift determined and the patient treated. Those data sets are then reviewed off-line using

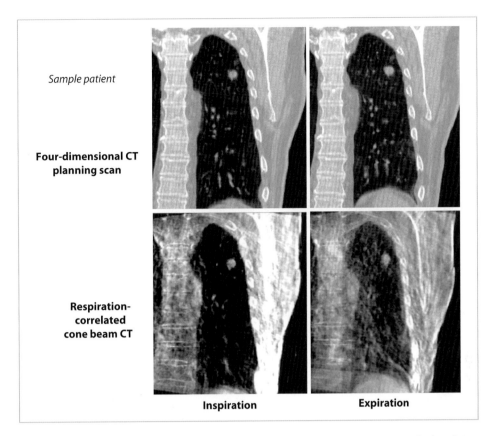

Fig. 3. Demonstration of four-dimensional respiration-correlated cone beam CT for localizing the target at two extremes of the respiratory cycle. The method used to achieve this sorting employs the projection images directly and does not rely on a secondary surrogate [19]. The limited number of projections used in each phase results in a decrease in the image quality. Fortunately, the high contrast of the structures in the lung allows visualization. Courtesy of Princess Margaret Hospital, Toronto, Canada.

retrospective four-dimensional sorting, to evaluate whether the range of motion at the time of treatment was consistent with the range of motion observed on four-dimensional CT that was used in the planning process (fig. 3, 4) [15]. Additional information on four-dimensional image analysis for lung intensity-modulated radiation therapy is reported in the article by Lagerwaard and Senan [this vol., pp. 239–252].

Fiducial Markers
High-precision radiotherapy of prostate cancer was the original focus for much of the work with cone beam CT. At PMH, a study involving 16 patients was performed to compare prostate (or marker) localization using cone beam CT and MV

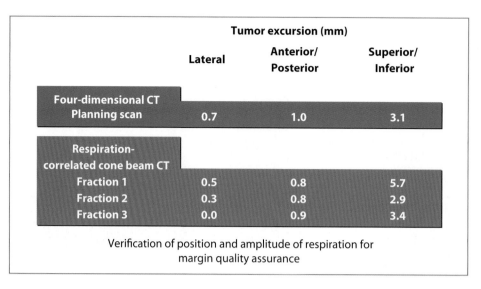

	Tumor excursion (mm)		
	Lateral	Anterior/ Posterior	Superior/ Inferior
Four-dimensional CT Planning scan	0.7	1.0	3.1
Respiration- correlated cone beam CT			
Fraction 1	0.5	0.8	5.7
Fraction 2	0.3	0.8	2.9
Fraction 3	0.0	0.9	3.4

Verification of position and amplitude of respiration for margin quality assurance

Fig. 4. Sample data from the use of four-dimensional cone beam CT for verification of the range of tumor motion during respiration. This approach can be used to assure that appropriate margins are being applied. For stereotactic body radiation therapy applications, the need for assurance of coverage is heightened by the small number of fractions typically used to deliver the therapy courses. Courtesy of T. Purdie, Princess Margaret Hospital, Toronto, Canada.

portal imaging [paper submitted]. The markers are quite visible on both cone beam CT and MV portal images. Their three-dimensional position each day can be easily extracted and the appropriate couch shift plotted according to each of these modalities. Correlation coefficients between cone beam CT and portal image-based results were well over 0.8, with 1.0 being perfect correlation. This high level of correlation emphasizes the stability of the image guidance device and procedures (both MV portal imaging and kV cone beam CT) over the 6-month-long course of the investigation. There was a lower correlation between markers and alignments based on soft tissue alignment. While there was an increased dispersion correlation for markers and soft tissue, it is important to note that the mean position in the correlation plots remained quite close to zero (fig. 5). That is, on average these corrections kept the prostate near what was estimated based on MV markers. Overall, the study shows that kV marker-based guidance has a high correlation with MV guidance, and that there was a lower correlation using soft tissue image guidance. However, systematic error was very small in both cases. This is key, because it is the dominant factor in determining the planning margins [21]. Based on the results of this study, a number of patients who have not been able to have markers implanted have now gone through daily soft tissue imaging based on cone beam CT.

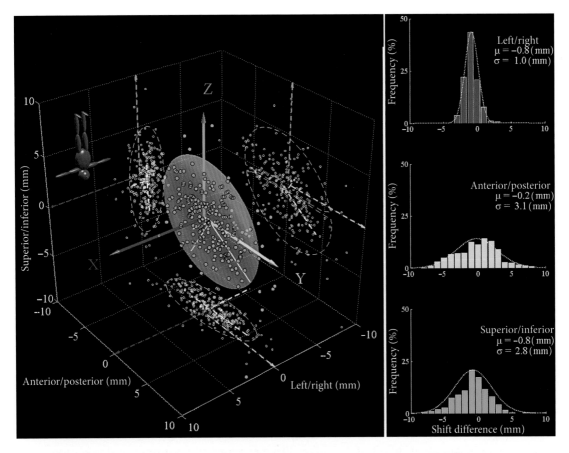

Fig. 5. Differences between MV marker-based positioning and kV cone beam CT soft tissue targeting in radiation therapy of the prostate. Marker-marker-based comparisons show excellent correlation (see text). The reduced correlation between marker- and soft-tissue-based methods is attributed to both image quality (observer detection) and deformation of the gland relative to the markers [22]. From these investigations, the level of performance of the soft tissue guidance has been deemed sufficient for on-line image-guided radiation therapy for those patients that decline or cannot participate in the marker program at PMH. See [13] for a complete analysis of these results.

Contrast Agents

The use of high-atomic-number contrast agents in patients is another consideration for imaging with kV cone beam CT devices. For instance, in the therapy of liver tumors some patients may have received transarterial chemoembolization, including iodine content that can be imaged on treatment and used as a tumor surrogate for targeting. Similar use of other contrast agents could reasonably be considered for other tumor sites, and the development of agents specifically for image guidance applications has been an area of investigation. For instance, Zheng et al. [23] reported on a liposomally encapsulated mixture of conventional gadolinium and iodine contrast agents for long-lasting contrast enhancements. This agent is maintained in the vasculature for up to 7 days and would be a useful tool for increasing contrast in the context of image-guided radiation therapy without the deleterious effects of having fiducials present in follow-up exams.

Kilovoltage Cone Beam CT and Other Image Guidance Technologies

Strengths of kV Cone Beam CT
As a technology, kV cone beam CT has a number of strengths. Some of these advantages are shared with other image guidance technologies, while others are unique to the kV imaging energies used or the technical platforms that have been developed to date. kV cone beam CT achieves the basic goal of providing geometrically robust imaging at the time of radiation delivery that is clinically useful for its guidance and correction. Typically, it can accomplish this without change in the patient's position between imaging and treatment. As important, it provides a fully three-dimensional characterization of the target position, so that it can reduce or eliminate ambiguity in the interpretation of radiographs. The kV cone beam may actually accelerate the interpretation of positioning especially of complex three-dimensional structures.

In practice, kV cone beam CT can provide a large FOV that is up to 50 cm in diameter × 25 cm in length in a single rotation. The image acquisition time is rapid, in the range of 32–100 s. Submillimeter geometric accuracy and precision in three dimensions relative to the treatment machine isocenter is expected, since the system has been demonstrated to be mechanically robust over time. It provides higher contrast radiographs as compared with MV portal imaging. Further enhancement of image quality using flat panels can be expected, since there are ongoing efforts to improve detector performance, including lower additive noise, faster readout speed and multigain acquisition modes [24].

With kV approaches, there is potential for the utilization of contrast agents for increasing the visibility of low-contrast structures. Contrast enhancement at MV energies can also be achieved to some degree using low-density agents (e.g. air pockets). For instance, the insertion of rectal balloons has been seen in clinical practice.

The low imaging dose of the kV cone beam CT approach is a strength [11]. For high-contrast structures such as bone, images of value can be generated with doses at the level of 0.05 cGy. For low-contrast objects such as soft tissue targets including the prostate, the dose remains reasonable at 2–3 cGy, which is not greatly different from that being reported for MV cone beam CT [7] or tomotherapy [25].

Current developments with kV cone beam CT allow independent imaging and delivery systems for detection during delivery, which could be a strength in certain applications, although this is not currently in routine use. The radiographic and fluoroscopic modes permit flexible rates of image monitoring, from greater than 7 frames per second to less than 1 frame every 10 s. kV cone beam CT provides for on-line and off-line guidance, as well as a basis for evaluating the overall progression of the therapy. The four-dimensional retrospective cone beam CT for phase and amplitude determination in radiotherapy has proven to be of great importance in regions influenced by respiratory motion, especially for thoracic targets.

Finally, the logistics of integrating new kV cone beam CT technologies into existing radiotherapy clinics are manageable. The approach leverages the existing investment in C-arm type linear accelerator systems, including their quality assurance programs and positioning devices. Equally important, it continues and enhances the existing staff experience with current linear accelerator equipment and their standards of care. In the experience at PMH, the system 'uptime' is comparable with those of a conventional linear accelerator. Currently, it appears that the cost is limited to capital increases, at roughly a 25–30% increase over conventional linear accelerators. These prices may be further reduced by lowering the performance requirements for the portal imaging devices currently employed on the systems.

Limitations of kV Cone Beam CT

What are some of the weaknesses of the kV cone beam CT approach? In general, the image quality is not as good as that generated by the conventional CT scanners employed in the planning process. This is due to a number of factors. To date, the detectors have been selected as the higher-grade product from the flat-panel production process and have not been specifically designed for use with CT, though there is an effort in that direction now. Current flat-panel detectors do not have the dynamic range of conventional CT detectors, and suffer to a varying degree from memory effects – referred to as lag and ghosting [26]. These can introduce subtle artifacts under conditions of high contrast or elevated levels of consistent exposure at the detector.

A fundamental challenge with the cone beam CT approach is the large acceptance angle of the detector and the large volume of tissue irradiated during imaging. These result in a significant quantity of X-ray scatter reaching the detector and being accumulated with the primary image. For larger FOVs, very high percentages of the total fluence are attributed to the scatter fluence [27]. This fluence results in errors in estimating the CT numbers within the object of interest. Furthermore, the errors vary over the FOV, resulting in distracting shading artifacts that confound the visibility of low-contrast structures of interest.

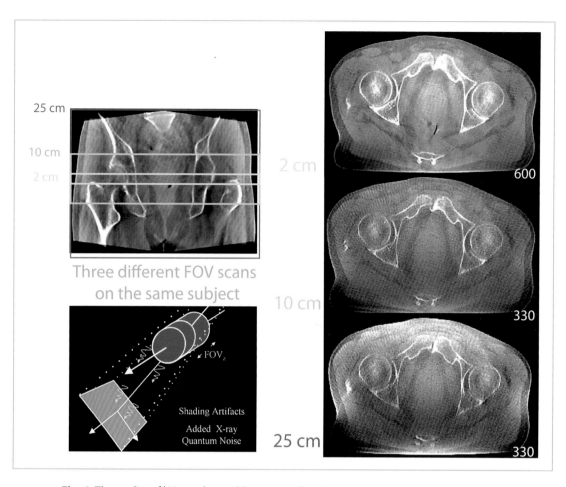

25 cm

10 cm

2 cm

Three different FOV scans on the same subject

2 cm

10 cm

25 cm

FOV$_z$

Shading Artifacts
Added X-ray
Quantum Noise

600

330

330

Fig. 6. The quality of kV cone beam CT images suffers from the presence of X-ray scatter reaching the detector. Generating images over a range of longitudinal extent by varying the superior-inferior collimator aperture illustrates the effect. The lower cone angle data set (2 cm FOV) has lower scatter at the detector and results in reduced shading artifacts. Also note the influence of doubling the number of projections (shown in the bottom right corner of each image) on the quality of the image.

As an example, the cone beam CT images of the pelvis for a 25-cm FOV are shown in figure 6. If the same region is imaged instead with a smaller superior-inferior FOV (2 or 10 cm achieved by collimating the X-ray exposure in the superior-inferior direction), one can see that the image quality deteriorates with increasing FOV, as X-ray scatter becomes more problematic. In the 2-cm scan there is very little scatter to the detector and the image is much more uniform. This image set also shows the advantages of using more projections (600 in the 2-cm FOV vs. 330 with larger FOVs); the number of projections obtained is largely limited by the detector readout rates at this point. At the 25-cm FOV, there is more shading and X-ray noise, because the X-ray scatter that interacts in the detector adds noise without adding additional contrast. This is a significant problem, and the solution is not clear. Important developments such as autosegmentation will not be easy with this level of definition. This physical effect also limits the system's ability to obtain accurate CT numbers.

Other weaknesses include the presence of clipping artifacts from dental fillings and other metal implants, which are also seen on diagnostic CT as voids of signal loss or dramatic streaks. In addition, the retraction and extension of the imager supports could be an issue with respect to access to the patient for couch rotations and the like, and should be considered.

The acquisition period, which is greater than a few seconds, can prevent the generation of high-quality images in the abdomen where there is nonperiodic motion from peristalsis. As previously discussed, if (and only if) the movement is periodic, one can exploit this periodicity to create a four-dimensional-like image. However, movement from peristalsis in abdominal structures is not periodic, sorting cannot be applied, and troublesome artifacts inevitably result. This can be a significant problem, and is reminiscent of the limitation in the use of early diagnostic CT outside of fixed structures like the head. In addition, there can be subtle cone beam CT artifacts arising from the simple circular trajectory of the source and detector about the patient. In clinical practice, these are not significant for the geometries employed in radiation therapy.

While the issues of image quality need to be addressed, the existing level of quality is highly functional for many guidance tasks and the imaging and guidance process is a technically robust system.

Other Image Guidance Technologies

Other approaches to image guidance are discussed in several articles in this volume, and are highlighted in the paper by Sharpe et al. [this vol., pp. 72–93]. Technical comparisons of these approaches are outlined in table 1. In comparison to kV cone beam CT approaches, several points can be discussed.

Image Quality

All of these guidance approaches will image soft tissues, though with varying spatial resolution and contrast resolution. At present, MV imaging will not approach the resolution and soft tissue performance found at kV energies without significant increases in dose; Pouliot [this vol., pp. 132–142] discusses aspects of MV imaging and strategies to optimize it in this volume. Beam-hardening artifacts and clipping artifacts, as around metal implants, will invariably be more prominent with kV approaches. Accurate electron density estimates are achieved with tomotherapy but are not as robust with current kV cone beam CT approaches, for the reasons discussed earlier.

Table 1. Comparison of tomographic guidance systems

Specification	In-room CT	MV CT (tomo-therapy)	MV cone beam CT	kV cone beam CT
Energy	80–140 kV	approx. 3.5 MV	2–6 MV	80–140 kVp
Resolution (min., aperture based) mm^3	0.5	1 × 1 × 2	<0.5	<0.5
Soft tissue imaging	Y	Y	Y	Y
Dose	no minimum	no minimum	no minimum	no minimum
Typical dose, cGy	5–10	1–3	4–8	1–3
Physical aperture, cm	70	85	90	90
Maximum FOV, cm	XY: 50 Z: 2 × N	XY: 40 Z: 0.2-5 × N	XY: 30 Z: 30	XY: 50 Z: 26
Scan time for Z: 15 cm, sec	<10	15 × 10/rot: 150	60	60
General functionality				
Registered to isocenter (<mm)	Y	Y	Y	Y
Repeat imaging (verification)	N	Y	Y	Y
Time delay relative to PI, min	+5	N/A	+2	+2
Verification of noncoplanar fields	Y with PI	N/A	Y with PI	Y
Special features				
Accurate CT numbers (1–5+)	+5	+5	+2	+1
Beam-hardening artifacts	Y	N	N	Y
Clipping artifacts (metal)	Y	N	N	Y
Independent operation during radiotherapy	N	N	N	Y
Fluoroscopy	Y with PI	N	Y with PI	Y
Real-time tracking	Y with PI	N	Y with PI	Y
Contrast agents	Hi-Z	Air	Air	Hi-Z
Demonstrated four-dimensional capability	Y	N	Y	Y
Logistics				
Incremental cost, USD	0.5–1.0 M	N/A	<0.5 M	0.5–1.0 M
Integration with existing systems	Y	N	Y	Y
Integration with existing image review	N	N	N	N
Fits in conventional treatment room	Possibly	Y	Y	Y
Multivendor	Y	N	N	Y

Dimensions for the comparison between the various volumetric imaging technologies currently available for image-guided radiation therapy. The intent is to provide the community with a range of metrics that may be pertinent in a selection process. The particular assignments and values may vary as the technology advances and as manufacturers implement novel approaches. Please seek updated values from the literature and manufacturers when comparing technologies.
PI = Portal imaging; M = million.

Dose for Imaging
It should be recognized that imaging deteriorates even on a conventional CT scanner as the imaging dose decreases. While there are no minimum doses for guidance devices, the necessary dose will depend in part on what one would like to see. If it is to identify bone structures, then very low doses can be used, well under 0.1 cGy for kV cone beam, and well under 1 cGy for MV cone beam technologies. Since soft tissue anatomy is the more usual objective, larger doses are required, and typically reported doses for tomotherapy and kV CT are in the range of 1–3 cGy.

Field of View
The FOV can be quite large, 50 cm, on a conventional CT scanner. Supplemented with spiral technology, the longitudinal FOV can be as large as desired. This is also true of MV tomotherapy, which carries a nominal aperture of 40 cm but is functionally limited only by the length of couch travel. The FOV for MV cone beam CT is limited by the primary jaws in the delivery unit. This gives a 40-cm CT reconstruction aperture, the same as the treatment beam width. The effective reconstruction FOV for the kV cone beam CT systems is as large as 50 × 26 cm, depending on the detector size and imaging geometry.

Scan Times and Time Delay Relative to Portal Imaging
The scan times vary somewhat between the basic design approaches. For tomotherapy, scan time may be longer than for other approaches; a scan of 15 cm that is assuming a 1-cm pitch might require 150 s. On MV or kV cone beam CT, scan times will range between 30 and 200 s. In another light, the time for all of these approaches is becoming competitive to the acquisition time for a pair of orthogonal portal images.

Fluoroscopy and Independent Operation during Radiation Therapy
The kV system is unique in permitting one to monitor the patient with imaging while MV therapy is being delivered. For the existing cone-beam CT systems, this still needs to be demonstrated as functional in the clinical context but conceptually it is attainable, and could be very important for tracking targets over time. The magnitude of MV-induced X-ray scatter at the kV detector and the potential for interference due to MV beam pulsation will need to be overcome if low-dose fluoroscopic monitoring is to be achieved with the kV systems.

   Evaluation of the various approaches to image guidance is challenging. Overall, there is a lack of quantitative assessment of *imaging performance* for the currently available commercial systems; hopefully this will be addressed in the near future as these systems mature. Quantitative assessment of *guidance performance* for clinical processes that use these technologies needs to be reported as well.

Depending on the objective, a robust process for guidance (alignment, registration, remote couch correction) may be of greater value than further improvements in image quality. These processes should also extend to support on-line and off-line image guidance approaches. In summary, there are numerous valid options for generating images for localizing the patient anatomy with respect to the treatment isocenter. Continued efforts are required to assure that these systems are provided with appropriate tools such that this valuable information can be readily employed to improve the quality of radiation therapy in all sites.

References

1 de Crevoisier R, Tucker S, Dong L, Mohan R, Cheung R, Cox J, Kuban D: Increased risk of biochemical and local failure in patients with distended rectum on the planning CT for prostate cancer radiotherapy. Int J Radiat Oncol Biol Phys 2005;62:965–973.

2 Yan D, Lockman D, Martinez A, Wong J, Brabbins D, Vicini F, Liang J, Kestin L: Computed tomography guided management of interfractional patient variation. Semin Radiat Oncol 2005;15: 168–179.

3 Uematsu M, Shioda A, Tahara K, Fukui T, Yamamoto F, Tsumatori G, Ozeki Y, Aoki T, Watanabe M, Kusano S: Focal, high dose, and fractionated modified stereotactic radiation therapy for lung carcinoma patients: a preliminary experience. Cancer 1998;82:1062–1070.

4 Mackie TR, Balog J, Ruchala K, Shepard D, Aldridge S, Fitchard E, Reckwerdt P, Olivera G, McNutt T, Mehta M: Tomotherapy. Semin Radiat Oncol 1999;9:108–117.

5 Jaffray DA, Drake DG, Moreau M, Martinez AA, Wong JW: A radiographic and tomographic imaging system integrated into a medical linear accelerator for localization of bone and soft-tissue targets. Int J Radiat Oncol Biol Phys 1999;45:773–789.

6 Ford EC, Chang J, Mueller K, Sidhu K, Todor D, Mageras G, Yorke E, Ling CC, Amols H: Cone-beam CT with megavoltage beams and an amorphous silicon electronic portal imaging device: potential for verification of radiotherapy of lung cancer. Med Phys 2002;29:2913–2924.

7 Pouliot J, Bani-Hashemi A, Chen J, Svatos M, Ghelmansarai F, Mitschke M, Aubin M, Xia P, Morin O, Bucci K, Roach M, Hernandez P, Zheng Z, Hristov D, Verkey L: Low-dose megavoltage cone-beam CT for radiation therapy. Int J Radiat Oncol Biol Phys 2005;61:552–560.

8 Seppi EJ, Munro P, Johnsen SW, Shapiro EG, Tognina C, Jones C, Pavkovich JM, Webb C, Mollov I, Partain LD, Colbeth RE: Megavoltage cone-beam computed tomography using a high-efficiency image receptor. Int J Radiat Oncol Biol Phys 2003;55:793–803.

9 Jaffray DA, Siewerdsen JH, Wong JW, Martinez AA: Flat-panel cone-beam computed tomography for image-guided radiation therapy. Int J Radiat Oncol Biol Phys 2002;53:1337–1349.

10 Feldkamp LA, Davis LC, Kress JW: Practical cone-beam algorithm. J Opt Soc Am 1984;1:612–619.

11 Islam MK, Purdie TG, Norrlinger BD, Alasti H, Moseley DJ, Sharpe MB, Siewerdsen JH, Jaffray DA: Patient dose from kilovoltage cone beam computed tomography imaging in radiation therapy. Med Phys 2006;33:1573–1582.

12 Sharpe MB, Moseley DJ, Purdie TG, Islam M, Siewerdsen JH, Jaffray DA: The stability of mechanical calibration for a kV cone beam computed tomography system integrated with linear accelerator. Med Phys 2006;33:136–144.

13 Moseley DJ, White EA, Wiltshire KL, Rosewall T, Sharpe MB, Siewerdsen JH, Bissonnette J-P, Gospodarowicz M, Warde P, Catton CN, Jaffray DA: Comparison of localization performance with implanted fiducial markers and cone-beam computed tomography for on-line image-guided radiotherapy of the prostate. Int J Radiat Oncol Biol Phys 2007;67:942–953.

14 McBain CA, Henry AM, Sykes J, Amer A, Marchant T, Moore CM, Davies J, Stratford J, McCarthy C, Porritt B, Williams P, Khoo VS, Price P: X-ray volumetric imaging in image-guided radiotherapy: the new standard in on-treatment imaging. Int J Radiat Oncol Biol Phys 2006;64: 625–634.

15 Purdie TG, Moseley DJ, Bissonnette JP, Sharpe MB, Franks K, Bezjak A, Jaffray DA: Respiration-correlated cone-beam computed tomography and 4DCT for evaluating target motion in stereotactic lung radiation therapy. Acta Oncol 2006;45:915–922.

16 Jaffray DA, Siewerdsen JH: Cone-beam computed tomography with a flat-panel imager: initial performance characterization. Med Phys 2000; 27:1311–1323.

17 Eccles C, Brock KK, Bissonnette JP, Hawkins M, Dawson LA: Reproducibility of liver position using active breathing coordinator for liver cancer radiotherapy. Int J Radiat Oncol Biol Phys 2006; 64:751–759.

18 Wong JW, Sharpe MB, Jaffray DA, Kini V, Robertson JM, Stromberg JS, Martinez AA: The use of active breathing control (ABC) to reduce margin for breathing motion. Int J Radiat Oncol Biol Phys 1999;44:911–919.

19 Moseley DJ, Keller H, et al: Framework for respiration-correlated cone-beam computed tomography. Med Phys 2004;31:1778.

20 Sonke JJ, Zijp L, Remeijer P, van Herk M: Respiratory correlated cone beam CT. Med Phys 2005;32: 1176–1186.

21 van Herk M: Errors and margins in radiotherapy. Semin Radiat Oncol 2004;14:52–64.

22 Nichol A, Brock KK, et al: A magnetic resonance imaging study of prostate deformation relative to implanted gold fiducial markers. Int J Radiat Oncol Biol Phys 2007;67:48–56.

23 Zheng J, Perkins G, Kirilova A, Allen C, Jaffray DA: Multimodal contrast agent for combined computed tomography and magnetic resonance imaging applications. Invest Radiol 2006;41: 339–348.

24 Roos PG, Colbeth R: Multiple-gain-ranging readout method to extend the dynamic range of amorphous silicon flat-panel imagers. Proc SPIE 2004;5368:139–149.

25 Mackie TR, Kapatoes J, Ruchala K, Lu W, Wu C, Olivera G, Forrest L, Tome W, Welsh J, Jeraj R, Harari P, Reckwerdt P, Paliwal B, Ritter M, Keller H, Fowler J, Mehta M: Image guidance for precise conformal radiotherapy. Int J Radiat Oncol Biol Phys 2003;56:89–105.

26 Siewerdsen JH, Jaffray D: A ghost story: spatiotemporal response characteristics of an indirect-detection flat-panel imager. Med Phys 1999;26: 1624–1641.

27 Siewerdsen JH, Moseley DJ, Bakhtiar B, Richard S, Jaffray DA: The influence of antiscatter grids on soft-tissue detectability in cone-beam computed tomography with flat-panel detectors. Med Phys 2004;31:3506–3520.

Dr. David A. Jaffray
Princess Margaret Hospital
610 University Avenue
Toronto, Ont., M5G 2M9 (Canada)
Tel. +1 416 946 4501, ext. 5384
Fax +1 416 946 6566
E-Mail david.jaffray@rmp.uhn.on.ca

Meyer JL (ed): IMRT, IGRT, SBRT – Advances in the Treatment Planning and
Delivery of Radiotherapy. Front Radiat Ther Oncol. Basel, Karger, 2007, vol. 40, pp 132–142

Megavoltage Imaging, Megavoltage Cone Beam CT and Dose-Guided Radiation Therapy

Jean Pouliot

University of California at San Francisco Comprehensive Cancer Center, San Francico, Calif., USA

Abstract

Elaborate methods of patient imaging for diagnostics, dose calculation, and radiation delivery are currently used to develop treatment plans with highly conformal patient dose distributions. However, the true delivered dose likely deviates from the planned distribution due to differences in patient position, anatomic changes due to weight loss or tumor shrinkage or variations of linear accelerator output during treatment. All the steps in a radiation treatment from diagnostics to the planning process are based on three-dimensional imaging, with the exception of treatment verification performed with electronic portal imaging devices (EPIDs) and two-dimensional images. Megavoltage cone beam CT (MV CBCT) generates an accurate three-dimensional representation of the patient anatomy, moments before the same X-ray beam is used for treatment. The three-dimensional images will provide additional information on the patient's treatment position and offer a wide range of opportunities to improve the delivery of radiation. The MV CBCT image can be registered with the planning CT for patient setup verification and correction. The periodic acquisition of three-dimensional images will allow the monitoring of anatomical changes over the treatment course due to tumor response or weight loss. The MV CBCT image can also be imported into the planning system to complement the regular CT in the presence of metallic objects or to measure the dosimetric impact of patient misalignment and anatomy modification on dose distribution. By combining exit dosimetry with the EPID and MV CBCT, this technology may play a key role in tracking the dose delivered to the patient, taking us into an era of dose-guided radiation therapy.

The first electronic portal imaging devices (EPIDs) became available about 15 years ago. At that time, it was difficult to foresee that an EPID and the linear accelerator treatment beam would eventually provide all the tools required to obtain a three-dimensional image of the patient in treatment position immediately before dose delivery. This is what megavoltage cone beam CT (MV CBCT) offers. In this review, we will present the general characteristics of MV CBCT and discuss a range of clinical applications for adaptive radiation therapy and dose-guided radiation therapy.

Megavoltage Cone Beam CT: General Characteristics and Performance

The MV CBCT system consists of a new amorphous silicon flat panel adapted for MV imaging attached to a Siemens linear accelerator and an integrated workflow application. This allows for the automatic acquisition of projection images, CBCT image reconstruction, automatic CT to CBCT image registration and remote couch position adjustment. It also provides a three-dimensional patient anatomy volume in the actual treatment position that can be tightly aligned to the planning CT moments before the dose delivery, allowing verification and correction of the patient position. For a typical case, 200 projection portal images are acquired with the 6-MV beam in 45 s. The MV CBCT image is then reconstructed in less than 2 min after the start of the acquisition. The image acquisition system performs very reliably and offers the possibility of performing an unlimited number of successive acquisitions. The dose used for MV CBCT depends on the clinical application but typically ranges from 2 to 10 cGy. The lower end is used when daily acquisitions are performed on a patient, while 6–10 cGy are used for tumor evolution studies or for planning purposes. The MV CBCT system demonstrates submillimeter localization precision and sufficient soft tissue resolution to visualize structures such as the prostate.

Perhaps one of the most appealing characteristics of MV CBCT is its simplicity. There is only one source, the beam itself, and one detector, the EPID. This provides easy access to the patient by the therapists. The imaging system and the treatment unit share the same isocenter, by definition. The image is directly referenced to the beam and the quality control required is kept to a minimum.

The development of MV CBCT as a clinical imaging tool in radiation oncology has been rapidly progressing. In October 2003, low-dose MV CBCT of a head and neck patient was acquired [1]. To the authors' knowledge, this was the first MV CBCT of a human subject in a clinical setting. In August 2004, MV CBCT was performed with sufficient soft tissue contrast to visualize organs such as the prostate, bladder, and rectum in the pelvic area and the eye globe in the head. In spring 2005, institutional-review-board-approved (H11386-18538-05) MV CBCT systems were installed onto two Siemens linear accelerators located in the University of California San Francisco Comprehensive Cancer Center [2], and studies begun to determine the clinical applications [3].

Since then, about 250 MV CBCT clinical scans have been acquired. The MV CBCT system is used to align patients, detect nonrigid spinal cord distortions,

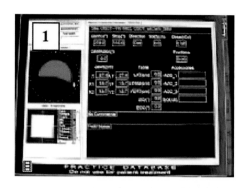

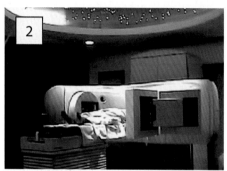

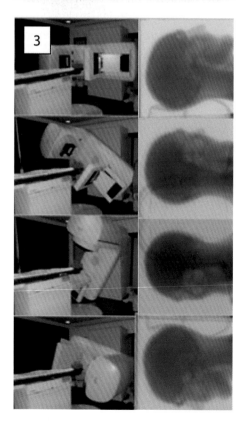

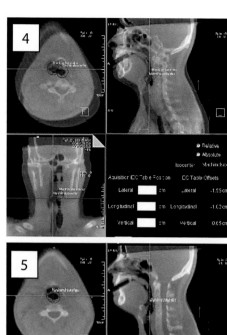

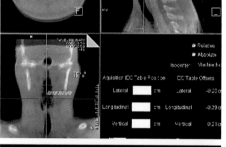

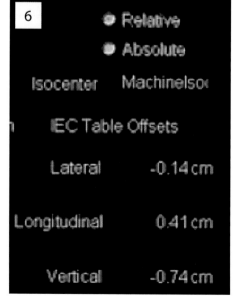

monitor tumor growth and shrinkage, position stationary tumors in the lung as well as assess the dosimetric impact of weight loss. MV CBCT has also greatly improved the delineation of structures in CT images that suffer from metal artifacts [4].

Image Acquisition and Reconstruction Steps

The steps to position a patient using MV CBCT are illustrated in figure 1 (steps 1–6). (1) The patient is first placed in the treatment position on the couch, and the cone beam acquisition mode is selected at the treatment console. (2) The linear accelerator gantry is placed in starting position, namely 270°. The reference planning CT and the reference isocenter, sent previously via DICOM from the planning system, are automatically loaded in the system when the cone beam acquisition mode is selected. This insures that CT is available for registration immediately when the cone beam image is reconstructed. (3) During the acquisition, the gantry rotates 200° until it reaches its final position, i.e. 210°. During the rotation, a portal image is acquired at each degree. The reconstruction of the cone beam image starts immediately after the first portal image has been acquired. (4) Upon completion of the reconstruction image, the cone beam image is automatically loaded in the Adaptive Targeting Software™, and the CBCT to CT image registration is performed automatically in a few seconds using a mutual information algorithm. (5) Proper alignment is validated, and manual alignment can be performed when fine-tuning is required. (6) The couch translation offset values required to obtain the best alignment of the patient at the isocenter are displayed. The couch is moved remotely from the treatment console according to these values and the patient is ready for treatment.

Clinical Applications

The clinical applications of MV CBCT can be sorted in four main categories: (1) patient setup, (2) monitoring of anatomical changes, (3) planning with non-compatible CT objects, and (4) dose calculation from MV CBCT to assess dosimetric impact.

Fig. 1. Acquisition and reconstruction steps: (1) patient setup on couch; (2) gantry is set at starting angle; (3) gantry rotates 200° and images are acquired and reconstructed; (4) CBCT image is superimposed on CT and automatic registration process starts; (5) proper alignment is validated and manual alignment can be performed when fine-tuning is required; (6) the couch translation offset values are displayed.

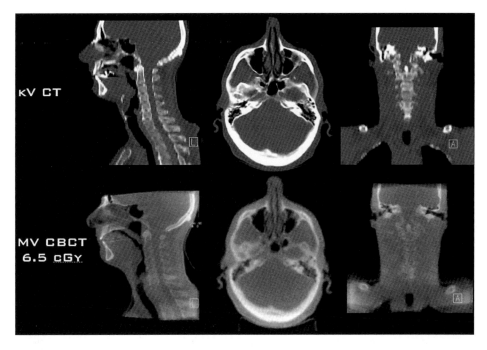

Fig. 2. Image comparison between planning CT (top) and MV CBCT (bottom) for a head and neck patient.

Patient Setup

The validity of the geometric calibration of the cone beam imaging system for absolute positioning was verified by reconstructing a gold seed placed at the isocenter with the room lasers. As expected, the center of the seed was located at the central voxel of the reconstruction (0.1, –0.2, 0.0) [5]. The mean and standard deviation of the differences between 37 arbitrary applied shifts and the measured shifts (using the phantom with gold seeds) were 0.0 and 0.3 mm, respectively. These measurements performed on phantoms indicate that MV CBCT used with the adaptive targeting tool has the potential to verify patient shifts with submillimeter precision.

Steps 4 and 5 in figure 1 depict the alignment process. Three orthogonal views of the reference CT are displayed in three distinct windows. The respective MV CBCT views are superimposed on the CT views (step 4). Using either the automatic registration tool based on a mutual information algorithm, or a manual approach, the two sets of images are registered. By adjusting the transparency level of the MV CBCT images, the user can visualize both sets of images and validate the proper alignment (fig. 1, step 5).

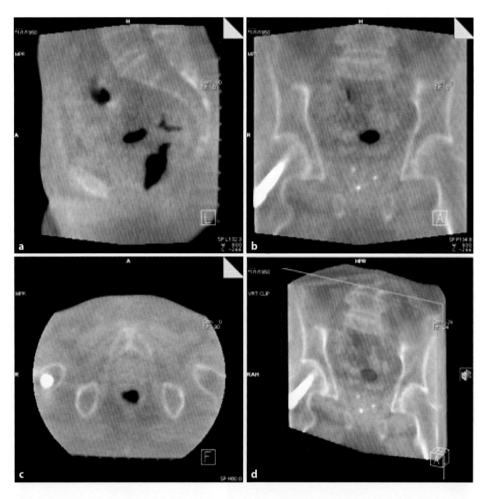

Fig. 3. Orthogonal [lateral (**a**), coronal (**b**), axial (**c**)] and three-dimensional views (**d**) of an MV CBCT (5 cGy) for a patient treated for prostate cancer. Prostate, rectum and the 3 gold markers can be seen, as well as the metallic hip rod.

In the last year, the MV CBCT system was used at the University of California San Francisco to verify and correct patient setup for different anatomical sites including head and neck (fig. 2), prostate (fig. 3), thorax, spine and lung. Several protocols are under way to determine the acquisition frequency, ranging from daily to once a week, required for optimal patient setup verification.

Monitoring of Anatomical Changes
Intensity-modulated radiation therapy for head and neck cancer permits high doses of radiation to be delivered to defined treatment volumes with sharp dose gradients to protect adjacent critical structures. Changes in patient anatomy due

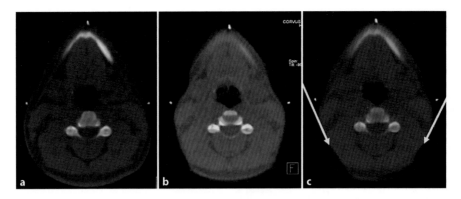

Fig. 4. Monitoring weight loss. Planning CT (red in background) with MV CBCT images overlaid (in grey levels) on first treatment day (**a**), day 24 (**b**) and day 37 (**c**). Arrows (**c**) indicate anatomical area where tissue loss was most significant.

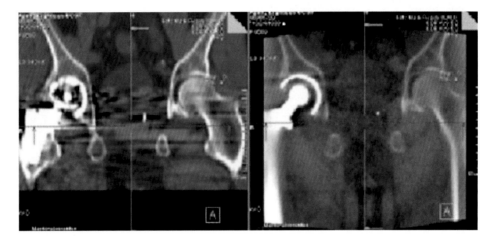

Fig. 5. Comparison of a conventional CT (left) and MV CBCT (right) for a patient with single hip replacement.

to tumor shrinkage and/or weight loss may significantly alter the dose distribution during a course of treatment. Figure 4 illustrates the feasibility of using MV CBCT to monitor changes in patient anatomy during treatment. MV CBCT images acquired on three occasions during the course of dose delivery [on the first treatment day (fig. 4a), on day 24 (fig. 4b) and on day 37 (fig. 4c)] are overlaid (in grey levels) on the planning CT (red in background). The arrows (fig. 4c) indicate the anatomical areas where tissue loss was most significant. Therefore, the periodic acquisition of MV CBCT images to verify patient alignment simultaneously provides the ability to monitor anatomical changes.

Complementing Planning CT in the Presence of Metallic Objects

A distinct advantage of MV imaging is that image quality is maintained even when high-atomic-number materials such as tooth fillings, dental implants, surgical clips, fiducial markers, or hip replacements are present. This has become of escalating importance as an increasing number of patients with hip replacements, for example, are seeking pelvic radiotherapy. According to the US Academy of Orthopedic Surgeons [6], in Europe and in the USA combined, over half a million people had a hip joint replaced in 2005. The fact that 1 out of 6 men will develop prostate cancer in their lifetime shows that this problem of hip prostheses in prostate cancer treatment by external beam radiotherapy will become increasingly significant.

For kilovoltage (kV) imaging, metallic objects create strong artifacts, as seen on the kV CT images of a patient with a hip replacement (fig. 5, on the left). In contrast, the MV CBCT images of this patient (fig. 5, on the right) clearly show the hip prosthesis, the bony anatomy, as well as soft tissues. For this reason, MV CBCT images can be used to assist in segmenting kV CT with metal artifacts for treatment planning purposes.

For 7 patients considered in a preliminary study performed at the University of California San Francisco, the prostate volumes contoured with the help of MV CBCT were generally smaller than what could be guessed from the kV CT alone in the presence of the artifacts, and this potentially prevented overdosage of the rectum. The MV CBCT image quality in the presence of large metallic objects is slightly degraded compared with the image of a regular prostate patient. However, compared with kV CT, the presence of high-Z material has relatively little impact on image quality of MV CBCT.

The next step after using MV CBCT for image segmentation is to use MV CBCT for dose calculation. Tests performed on phantoms [4] showed that the presence of a metallic object strongly impacts the Hounsfield units (up to 70% error) of a kV CT image even far away from the object, making CT inaccurate for dose calculation. Similar tests performed with MV CBCT demonstrated that Hounsfield units remain unchanged (within 3%) in the presence of metallic objects, allowing for significantly more accurate dose calculation.

Currently, the treatment plan based on kV CT is produced assuming the patient, including the metal implant, is water equivalent. Calibrating MV CBCT for density will allow the inclusion of the proper inhomogeneity corrections by directly using the calibrated MV CBCT in the treatment plan calculations. This has the potential to greatly improve the dosimetric accuracy of treatment for these patients.

Dose Calculation from MV CBCT to Assess Dosimetric Impact

MV CBCT images can be calibrated to provide accurate electron density [7] and are therefore used to assess the dosimetric impact of patient misalignment or anat-

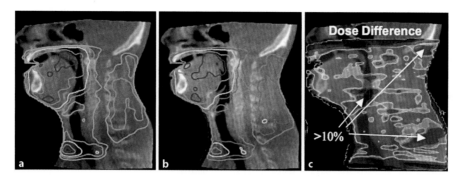

Fig. 6. Dosimetric impact of weight loss. Dose distribution during the first (**a**) and third treatment week (**b**). Dose increase (%) due to weight loss (**c**).

omy changes, enabling us to modify the treatment plan to improve the delivered dose. In the example presented in figure 6, MV CBCT images were acquired a few weeks apart (fig. 4a, c). In each case, MV CBCT was sent to the planning system (Pinnacle™) and the initial beam arrangement, used originally for planning on the diagnostic CT, was applied for dose calculation on the MV CBCT images. The dose distributions of the original CT and the first MV CBCT were within 3% or 3 mm everywhere. Comparison of the two dose distributions obtained on the MV CBCT images (fig. 6a, b) showed dose increases of more than 10% at several locations due to weight loss. Hence, in addition to providing the ability to monitor anatomical changes, one can import periodically acquired MV CBCT images into the planning system and assess the dosimetric impact of these changes.

Dose-Guided Radiation Therapy

We have recently proposed a dose-guided radiation therapy strategy in which future treatments are modified based on knowledge of the delivered dose from previous treatment fractions [8]. The main component in dose-guided therapy is the reconstruction of the delivered dose to the patient. Dose reconstruction requires two pieces of information: a three-dimensional image of the patient anatomy during or immediately before treatment and the measured energy fluence delivered by the treatment unit. The proposed dose reconstruction method uses an MV CBCT image acquired on the treatment table prior to treatment, two-dimensional portal images taken with an amorphous silicon EPID during treatment, and an independent validated dose calculation engine. The MV CBCT image should provide a more accurate depiction of the patient in the true treatment-time position as well as the necessary photon attenuation coefficients for dose calculations.

To infer the delivered energy fluence, the flat panel is used to collect portal images during treatment. The images are corrected for inhomogeneous pixel sensitivity, detector scatter, and the panel's energy response [9]. The signal is converted to energy fluence by calibrating the detector using ion chamber measurements. The energy fluence is then back-projected through the attenuation-coefficient-calibrated CBCT volume. The energy fluence is corrected for the $1/r^2$ falloff as well as for patient attenuation using the MV CBCT data. Finally, a superposition/convolution energy deposition method is used to calculate the dose.

Dose reconstruction combined with low-exposure MV CBCT has great potential to provide verification and possible improvement of dose delivery in patients with virtually no additional hardware. Knowing the true delivered dose distribution will enhance our understanding of treatment outcomes. Moreover, adaptive methods such as dose-guided radiation therapy will be developed to adjust treatment plans midcourse to compensate for differences in delivered and planned doses and improve treatment accuracy. Details of the procedure and first clinical results of dose reconstruction have been published recently [10].

Acknowledgments

This work includes the contributions from many people. The most significant efforts came from Michèle Aubin, Kara Bucci, Josephine Chen, Cynthia Chuang, Amy Gillis, Mike Lometti, Olivier Morin, Mack Roach 3rd, Lynn Verhey and Ping Xia. I would also like to thank the Siemens team, led by Ali Bani-Hashemi, for their constant participation. This work is supported by Siemens Oncology Care Systems.

References

1 Pouliot J, Xia P, Aubin M, Verhey L, Bani-Hashemi A, Ghelmansarai F, Mitschke M, Svatos M: Low-dose megavoltage cone-beam CT for dose-guided radiation therapy. 45th Annu Meet Am Soc Ther Radiol Oncol, Salt Lake City, 2003.

2 Pouliot J, Bani-Hashemi A, Chen J, Svatos M, Ghelmansarai F, Mitschke M, Aubin M, Xia P, Morin O, Bucci K, Roach M 3rd, Hernandez P, Zheng Z, Hristov D, Verhey L: Low-dose megavoltage cone-beam CT for radiation therapy. Int J Radiat Oncol Biol Phys 2005;61:552–560.

3 Morin O, Gillis A, Chen J, Aubin M, Bucci MK, Pouliot J: Megavoltage cone-beam CT: system description and IGRT clinical applications. Med Dosim 2006;31:51–61.

4 Aubin M, Morin O, Chen J, Gillis A, Aubry JF, Akazawa C, Speight J, Roach M 3rd, Pouliot J: The use of megavoltage cone-beam CT to complement CT for target definition in pelvic radiotherapy in the presence of hip replacement (abstract). 8th Biennial Eur Soc Ther Radiol Oncol Meet, Lisbon, September 2005.

5 Morin O, Gillis A, Bucci MK, Aubin M, Chen J, Pouliot J: Comparison of megavoltage cone-beam CT with electronic portal imaging for patient alignment. Proc 9th Int Workshop Electronic Portal Imaging, Melbourne, April 2006.

6 American Academy of Orthopaedic Surgeons, 2005: www.aaos.org/Research/stats/Knee%20 Facts.pdf.

7   Pouliot J, MK, Chen J, Chen H, Chuang C, Geffen M, Gillis A, Kelly K, Morin O, Roach M 3rd, Simpson L, Verhey L, Xia P: Megavoltage cone-beam CT: clinical applications for adaptive radiation therapy. Proc 9th Int Workshop Electronic Portal Imaging, Melbourne, April 2006.

8   Pouliot J, Xia P, Aubin M, Langen K, Verhey L, Bani-Hashemi A, Ghelmansarai F, Svatos M, Mitschke M: Dose-guided radiation therapy using low-dose megavoltage cone-beam CT. In 44th AAPM Annual Meeting, San Diego, Calif (abstract). Med Phys 2003;30:1337.

9   Chen J, Chuang CF, Morin O, Aubin M, Pouliot J: Calibration of an amorphous-silicon flat panel portal imager for exit-beam dosimetry. Med Phys 2006;33:584–594.

10 Chen J, Morin O, Aubin M, Bucci MK, Chuang CF, Pouliot J: Dose-guided radiation therapy with megavoltage cone-beam CT. Br J Radiol 2007; 79(suppl 1):S87–S98.

Dr. Jean Pouliot
UCSF Comprehensive Cancer Center
Suite H1031, 1600 Divisadero Street
San Francisco, CA 94143-1708 (USA)
Tel. +1 415 353 7190, Fax +1 415 353 9883
E-Mail pouliot@radonc17.ucsf.edu

Meyer JL (ed): IMRT, IGRT, SBRT – Advances in the Treatment Planning and
Delivery of Radiotherapy. Front Radiat Ther Oncol. Basel, Karger, 2007, vol. 40, pp 143–161

The Cyberknife: Practical Experience with Treatment Planning and Delivery

Vernon Smith · Cynthia F. Chuang

Department of Radiation Oncology, University of California, San Francisco, Calif., USA

Abstract

The Cyberknife® Robotic Radiosurgery System is used at the University of California at San Francisco to provide stereotactic treatments to a range of lesions throughout the body. Image guidance is an integral part of this system and is used in every treatment to provide adaptive control during the treatment. Clinical examples are given for various types of lesions using the different image guidance techniques that are available with this technology.

This discussion provides a description of the technology of the Cyberknife, how the University of California at San Francisco applies that technology to stereotactic body treatments, and why it shows promise in solving many of the problems associated with this developing treatment approach.

The Cyberknife is emerging as an important tool among radiation oncology treatment devices; approximately 18,000 patients have been treated in 39 Cyberknife facilities in the USA and 24 facilities outside of this country. On the subject of reimbursement it is important to note that the existing stereotactic radiosurgery codes apply to the Cyberknife in the USA.

Cyberknife Hardware Components

The major components of the Cyberknife (fig. 1) include a compact linear accelerator that is mounted on a robotic arm, a treatment couch that has motions not possible with conventional treatment couches, and a pair of diagnostic X-ray

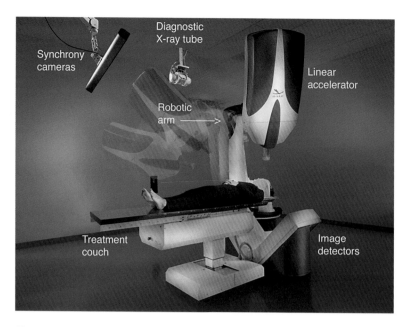

Fig. 1. Components of the Cyberknife.

sources directed at corresponding amorphous silicon image detectors for image guidance [1–3]. In addition, there are infrared cameras for the Synchrony® system.

The robot (fig. 2) has been developed from the type of robotic arm used in the automobile industry and other assembly line work, and is capable of submillimeter accuracy of movement. Each installation requires custom calibration of the robot to establish that accuracy. In theory, the robotic arm would be capable of delivering an arbitrary number of beams around the patient. In practice, the robot is programmed with a range of a hundred or so different positions in space that it can place the linear accelerator. At each position, the accelerator can then point in up to 12 different directions toward the patient, which gives a possibility of 1,200 beams. At this institute, between 50 and 250 beams are typically used for a given patient's treatment – probably more than are used at most other Cyberknife installations.

The linear accelerator (fig. 3) operates in the X-band of radiofrequencies, as opposed to the S-band used in most other medical linear accelerators. The X-band is higher in frequency by a factor of 3, which means that the components can be much smaller. This makes it possible to have a comparatively lightweight linear accelerator that can be mounted on the robotic arm. The accelerator provides approximately 400 monitor units per minute at the target site and is provided with

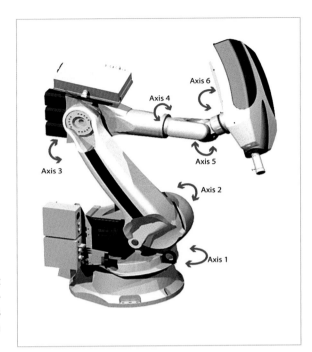

Fig. 2. Schematic of the robotic arm, with 6 axes of rotation, providing a large range of locations around the patient from which the X-ray beam can be directed.

Axis 6

Axis 4

Axis 3

Axis 5

Axis 2

Axis 1

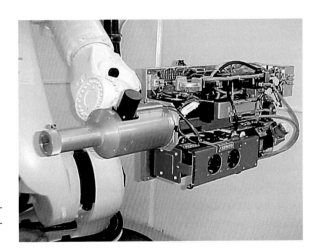

Fig. 3. Compact 6-MV linear accelerator operating in the X-band of frequencies.

a range of circular collimators having diameters at the target of 5 to 60 mm. We have never used the 60-mm, and only rarely the 5-mm collimator.

The couch (fig. 4) has unusual features. It is motorized, under software control. It has x, y and z motions as normal, but it also rotates in pitch and roll. It does not rotate in the horizontal plane, to avoid possible collision with the camera stands.

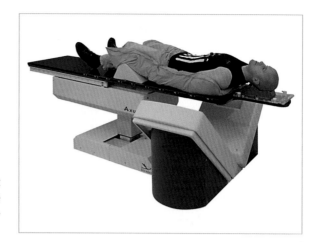

Fig. 4. Motorized treatment couch operating under software control with 5 degrees of freedom.

The Image Tracking System

The image tracking system consists of 2 diagnostic X-ray sources placed above the patient that fire down at 45° angles orthogonal to each other (fig. 1). They obtain real-time images using amorphous silicon detectors. This imaging information is used during the treatment to adjust the robot position [4]. Both skull-based and fiducial-based imaging algorithms are employed depending on the site, which provide 6-dimensional translation and rotation adjustments. The accuracy, if everything is calibrated properly, can be within 1 mm [5, 6]. A fiducial-less tracking system for spine lesions has been developed, but has only very recently been used at the University of California San Francisco.

The image tracking system allows one to calculate the deviations from the planned position, which is used for initial patient alignment. The patient is placed on the couch with immobilization devices as needed, and may be aligned with laser marks to obtain a rough alignment. Then the imaging system is used to make manual adjustments. We tend to make the adjustments until we are within 1–2 mm in translation and 1–2 degrees of rotation, with the understanding that these residual deviations are resolved during treatment by the robot.

There are 3 different tracking modalities. The skull-based tracking uses the skeletal structure of the patient as a reference (fig. 5). Basic fiducial tracking is used for extracranial lesions that do not move with respiratory motion. The Synchrony system, which also employs fiducials, allows treatment of soft tissue lesions that move with respiration [7]. During treatment, the robot compensates for motion within the range of ± 10 mm in x, y, z, plus $\pm 1°$ in pitch and roll, and $\pm 3°$ in yaw if the Axum couch is used.

Smith · Chuang

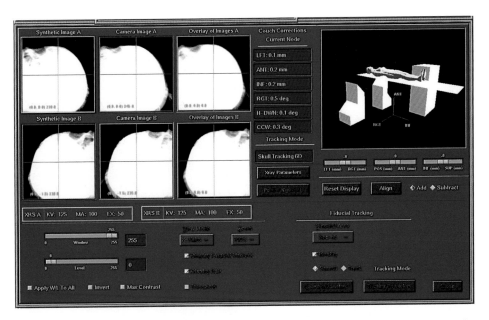

Fig. 5. Screen display of the skull-based image tracking system for cranial lesions. DRRs obtained from CT images are compared against real-time images from the detectors. Corrections in terms of 3 translations and 3 rotations are calculated that enable the robot to compensate for deviations between the plan and the actual patient position.

The fiducial tracking system employs automatic algorithms for extraction of the fiducials from the X-ray images. If at least 1 fiducial has been identified, the x, y and z adjustments can be made, and if at least 3 fiducials have been identified, rotational adjustments can be made as well. There are 2 different types of fiducials. Stainless steel screws (fig. 6) are used for spine lesions [8] and are inserted into the spinal processes, and gold fiducials (fig. 7) are used for soft tissue lesions [9].

In the screen used for fiducial tracking (fig. 8), the top row of images is for imager A, and the bottom row for imager B. The first column shows the synthetic images [digitally reconstructed radiographs (DRRs)] that are produced from the CT scan information. The fiducials are identified on the CT scans, which aids locating the fiducials at treatment. These are shown as green diamonds on the DRR images. The second column shows the images produced by the X-ray imaging system. The algorithm extracts the fiducials and identifies each with a cross. Once the fiducials have been correctly identified and have been tested to determine that they obey the laws of rigid body transformation, the corrections in x, y and z and in rotation are calculated. If the couch is moved accordingly, the crosses will line up with the diamonds and the patient will be close to alignment. As long as the residual corrections are within certain limits, treatment can be initiated and the robot will compensate accordingly.

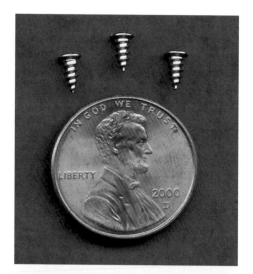

Fig. 6. Image tracking for spinal lesions is accomplished using stainless steel screws implanted in the spinal processes as fiducial markers.

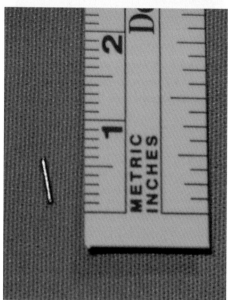

Fig. 7. Image tracking for lesions in soft tissues such as lung and liver is accomplished using gold seeds implanted in the lesion as fiducial markers.

Synchrony System

The Synchrony system (fig. 9) uses a system of 3 infrared LEDs to add respiratory motion tracking [7] to the basic fiducial tracking system. The patient wears a vest and the LEDs are placed on the vest. Three infrared cameras read the position of the fiducials and monitor the respiratory motion. During treatment, X-ray images are taken at every few nodes, resulting in a delay of a few seconds between sets of

Smith · Chuang

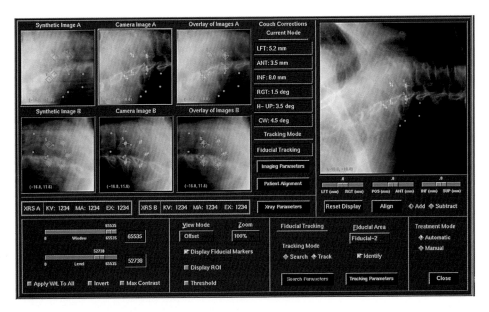

Fig. 8. Screen display of the image tracking system using fiducial markers for extracranial lesions. The predicted position of the fiducials on the DRRs based on identification on CT images is indicated by diamonds, and the position on the real-time images based on an automatic extraction algorithm is indicated by crosses. A check is made to ensure that there has been no movement of the fiducials relative to each other. If the fiducials have been located correctly, translation and rotation corrections can be calculated to enable adjustments to be made that bring the patient close to alignment. Residual corrections can be compensated for by the robot.

X-ray images. This is not fast enough to track respiratory motion, so instead the infrared diodes are used to perform the respiratory tracking. The X-ray data in conjunction with the infrared data are used to establish a correspondence model between the internal and external motion. After the initial patient setup, a recording of the LED positions is started which establishes the pattern of respiratory motion. Several sets of X-ray images are then taken. Each time a pair of X-ray images is taken, the phase of the respiratory cycle is known from the infrared data. If enough sets of images are obtained, a correspondence model can be established. As long as the patient reproduces this same breathing pattern, the model will be able to predict where the fiducials are, and provide confidence that the lesion is being treated correctly. The respiratory motion is monitored continuously throughout the treatment, and the X-ray images are taken at every 1–5 nodes. Each time a pair of X-ray images is taken, there is another check on whether the model remains accurate. If the X-ray images show that the fiducials are in the position that the model predicts, treatment proceeds. If they have deviated, as might occur when the patient coughs, then treatment stops. If the patient returns to the original position, one can proceed by using the same model after establishing its validity

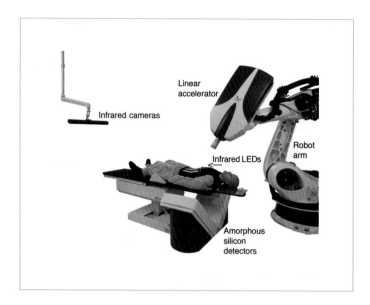

Fig. 9. Respiratory motion is continuously monitored in the Synchrony system using a set of infrared diodes placed on a vest worn on the chest and tracked by 3 infrared cameras. This is used in conjunction with internal fiducials, which are tracked with real-time images obtained every few seconds using the X-ray imaging system.

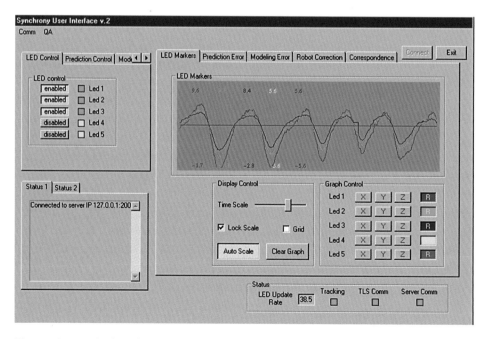

Fig. 10. Screen display of the Synchrony tracking system using infrared LEDs to track respiratory motion. Tracking can be achieved if the motion is approximately regular.

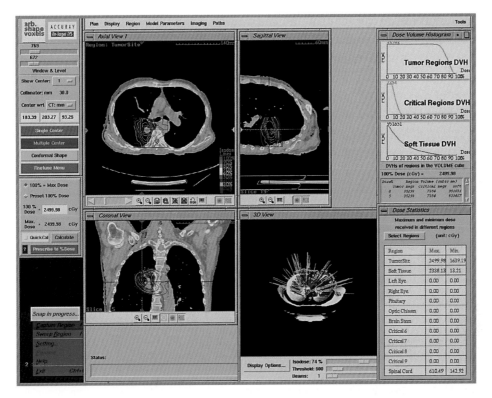

Fig. 11. Screen display of the treatment planning system. Three modes of planning are available but the conformal mode is used most often. Inverse planning requires the specification of maximum and minimum doses for the target, and maximum doses for critical structures. Variation of the degree of aggression of the constraint allows optimal plans to be obtained. The optimization routine is based on a linear programming algorithm.

by taking several pairs of X-ray images. If the model is no longer valid then it is necessary to establish a new model.

The respiratory motion tracking does not show (fig. 10) a pure sinusoidal motion. The trace is more irregular, but as long as there is periodicity about it, the system works well. It would be difficult to use this system for a patient who has compromised lung function and cannot breathe in a regular fashion.

Treatment Planning System

There are 3 modes of operation of the treatment planning system (fig. 11). Single-center planning can be used for a single small lesion. Multicenter planning can be used for multiple spherical lesions. Our cases have predominantly used conformal

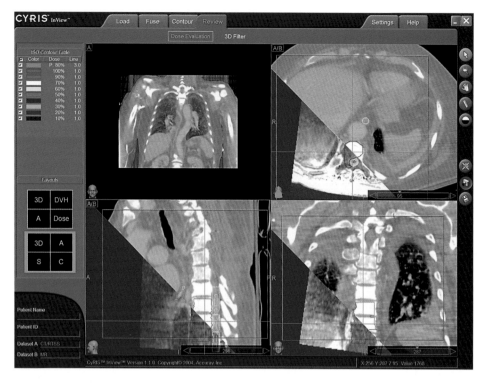

Fig. 12. The CyRIS InView package provides image registration and fusion based on mutual information theory, and tools for drawing targets and critical structures.

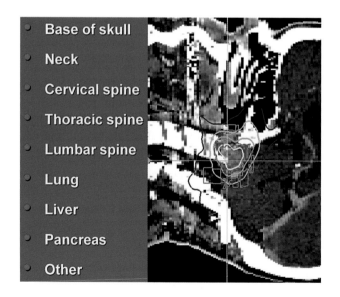

Fig. 13. A variety of extracranial tumors and lesions can be treated.

Smith · Chuang

planning, where multiple independent target points have been used. The inverse planning program requires the specification of maximum and minimum dose limits for the target, and maximum doses for critical structures. In addition, the maximum monitor unit per beam and the aggression of the constraint (in terms of exact, strict or loose) as well as other parameters, can be chosen to produce the result desired. The optimization program, unlike many others, can use gradient search or linear programming methods. After initiation of the inverse planning process, the optimization proceeds and eventually returns either with a solution that satisfies the constraints specified or, in the case of the linear programming method, possibly with no solution. If no solution has been found, then the constraints need to be modified.

Many of the lesions treated at our institution are difficult to visualize on CT scans, thus it is important that good tools are available for image registration and fusion. A relatively new package from Accuray, called CyRIS InView (fig. 12), offers tools for contouring structures, and for image registration and fusion, based on mutual information theory.

Extracranial Tumors and Lesions

A wide variety of extracranial lesions can be treated with this technology [9–12] (fig. 13). At this institution, most cases have been spine and lung lesions. Other sites such as liver and prostate have been treated as well.

The first example (fig. 14) shows a single axial image of a spine case, a rhabdomyosarcoma. The treatment plan was used to deliver 21 Gy in 3 fractions to the 78% isodose. Figure 15 is an axial view and figure 16 a sagittal view of this plan.

Figure 17 shows an MR image of a second spine case, a neurofibroma, and figure 18 the axial treatment plan on a CT image, which was used to deliver 24 Gy in 3 fractions to the 84% isodose. Figure 19 shows the sagittal view of that treatment plan.

In figure 20, a liver case is shown, as treated with the Synchrony technology to compensate for respiratory motion. The prior spine cases did not require Synchrony. Here, fiducials were implanted into the liver to track target motion. Two targets were treated as can be seen in the coronal view. They were both treated using the same treatment plan giving 30 Gy in 3 fractions to the 68% isodose. The doses to the spinal cord and other organs were kept within predefined constraints.

Figure 21 shows a lung case that was also treated with the Synchrony system. Again there were 2 targets, but only a small portion of the second one can be seen in this particular view. The isodose lines bulge out around what can be seen of the second target. This plan was treated with 36 Gy in 3 fractions to the 72% isodose, and doses to the spinal cord and esophagus were minimized.

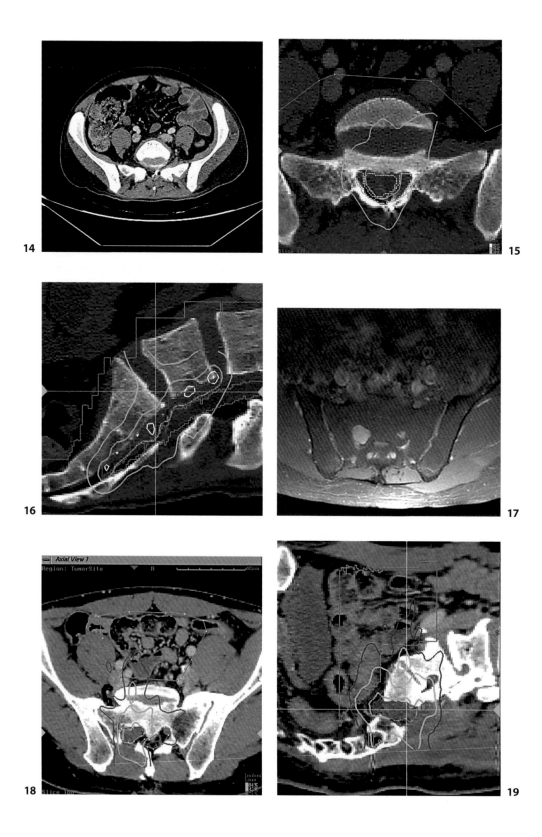

14

15

16

17

18

19

Smith · Chuang

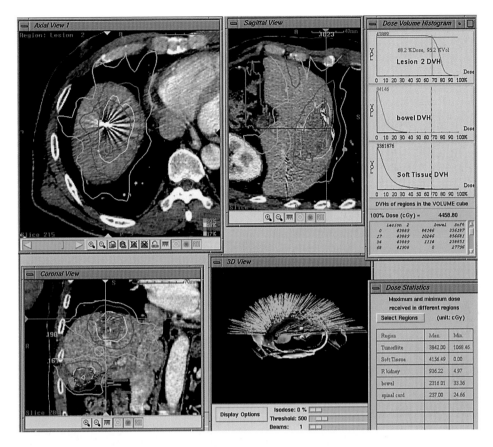

Fig. 20. Treatment plan for a patient with metastatic colon cancer to the liver with 2 targets. This was treated with the Synchrony system with fiducials implanted in the liver. The 68% isodose was chosen to deliver 30 Gy in 3 fractions to the target.

Fig. 14. Pretreatment axial CT image of a patient with metastatic rhabdomyosarcoma to the L_5-S_1 region of the spine.

Fig. 15. Treatment plan of the same patient showing isodose curves on an axial image. The prescription was chosen to deliver 21 Gy in 3 fractions to the 78% isodose.

Fig. 16. Treatment plan of the same patient showing isodose curves on a sagittal image.

Fig. 17. Pretreatment axial MR image of a patient with neurofibroma to the L_5-S_2 region of the spine.

Fig. 18. Axial image of the treatment plan. The 84% isodose was chosen to deliver 24 Gy in 3 fractions to the target.

Fig. 19. Sagittal view of the treatment plan.

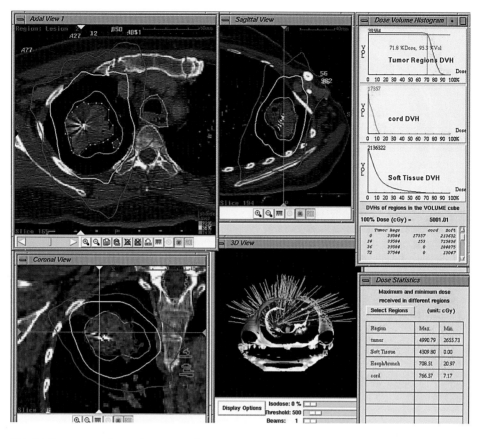

Fig. 21. Treatment plan with 2 targets for a patient with a recurrent lung adenocarcinoma. This was treated with the Synchrony system with fiducials implanted in the lung tumor. The 72% isodose was chosen to deliver 36 Gy in 3 fractions to the target.

Alternative Techniques for Lung Lesions

In using the Synchrony system for lung lesions, one of the issues that must be faced is the possibility of pneumothorax caused by implanting fiducials. In certain cases, our physicians have elected not to place fiducials in the lesion itself. Two techniques have been developed that make it possible to treat these lesions, but without the danger of pneumothorax. When the decision is made not to place fiducials in the lesion, we instead insert 2 sets of fiducials subcutaneously, one in the anterior and one in the posterior chest wall. One of two techniques is then selected. The first technique employs the anterior chest wall fiducials and uses Synchrony, so that respiratory motion is still being tracked. The second technique uses the posterior chest wall fiducials and is a non-Synchrony treatment. The constraints on these 2 techniques are as follows: Synchrony treatment with fiducials placed in the

Smith · Chuang

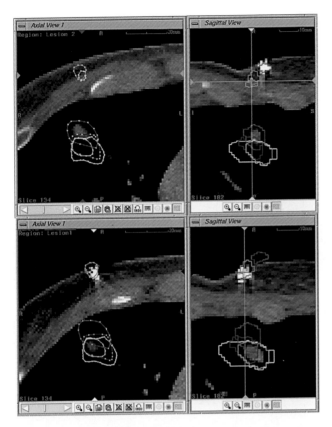

Fig. 22. Lung lesion patient that was a good candidate for tracking with fiducials implanted in the anterior chest wall to track respiratory motion using the Synchrony system. The fiducials tracked the lesion to within 1–2 mm in x and y, and to within 5 mm in z. The deviation in z motion was compensated for by extending the target volume in the z direction.

anterior chest wall is only appropriate if the fiducial motion actually approximates the lesion motion, which needs to be validated. The second technique, which does not use Synchrony, requires knowledge of how the lesion, as well as a target volume that encompasses the lesion, are moving at all phases of respiration. Fiducials in the posterior chest wall do not move with respiration, so they are only appropriate for a non-Synchrony treatment. For all of our lung lesions, we perform CT imaging consisting of 3 sets of CT scans at full inspiration, full expiration and mid inspiration. Each set has 300 slices, 1.25 mm thick, and each set is obtained during one breath hold of approximately 16 s with a GE Lightspeed multislice scanner. We have access to both an 8-slice and a 16-slice CT scanner.

Figure 22 shows an example that we considered a good candidate for the anterior chest wall technique. The lesion and the fiducial have been contoured on all 3 scans. We analyzed the relative motion between the fiducial and the lesion on all

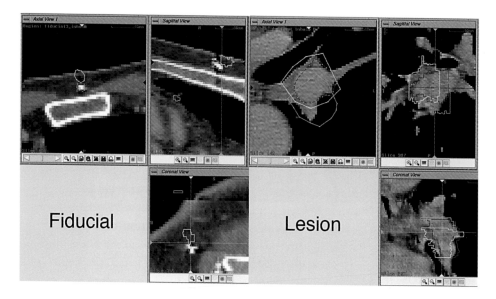

Fig. 23. Lung lesion patient that was a poor candidate for tracking with fiducials implanted in the anterior chest wall. The relative motion between the fiducials and the lesion was of the order of 2 cm. Non-Synchrony tracking was performed using fiducials implanted in the posterior chest wall.

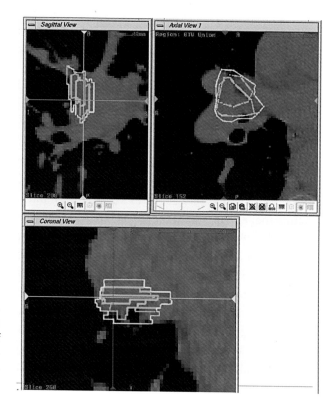

Fig. 24. A lung tumor case. The target volume was drawn to encompass the position of the target as seen on expiration, inspiration and mid-breath CT images.

relevant scan slices. In this case, the relative motion in x and y was about 1–2 mm, and in z about 5 mm. The relatively larger amount of z motion was compensated for by extending the target volume in the z direction by that amount. The white contour is the extended target volume.

Figure 23 shows a second example that was found to be a poor candidate for anterior chest wall fiducials. In this case, the relative motion between the fiducials and the lesion was large, in the order of a couple of centimeters. We were forced to use the posterior chest wall fiducials and an enlarged target volume. Figure 24 shows another lung case that required posterior chest wall fiducials and an enlarged target volume. The target was drawn on all 3 sets of CT slices and then an overall target volume was drawn to include all excursions of the target during respiration; this volume was used to plan the treatment. Figure 25 shows the treatment plan without Synchrony and figure 26 presents the plan we could have used if Synchrony had been an option (that is, if we could have placed fiducials in the lesion). The volume for the non-Synchrony treatment is some 65% larger than the Synchrony volume.

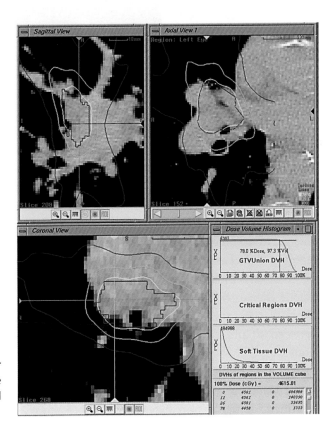

Fig. 25. Treatment plan for the enlarged target volume seen in figure 24 as treated without Synchrony.

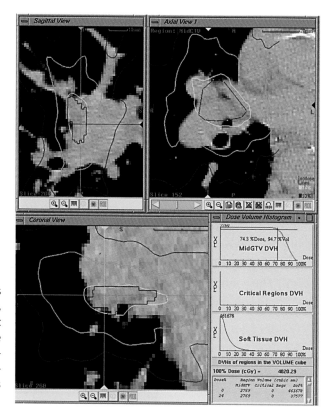

Fig. 26. The same patient as shown in the prior figure, now showing the treatment plan for the smaller volume that could have been treated with Synchrony. The volume as treated (fig. 25) was 65% larger than this volume.

Conclusions

We conclude that the Cyberknife system provides a powerful means of performing stereotactic body treatments but requires substantial resources including a linear accelerator vault and machine room, good physics support, and access to a multislice CT scanner. A primary advantage of this technique is that it provides the potential of treating all parts of the body with the accuracy and high-dose gradients previously obtained only with radiosurgery. Secondly, image guidance is integral to the treatment, and motion monitoring and tracking including respiratory motion are also fully integrated, rather than being an adjunct. The disadvantage is that difficult cases may need long planning and treatment times. The planning time can be from 30 min to many hours. The treatment time is usually between 40 and 120 min, with the longer times necessary only for complex lesions.

For all technologies used to deliver SBRT, a fundamental goal is to minimize target inaccuracy at the time of treatment. It has been suggested that a goal of treatment should be to reduce inaccuracy to about 2 mm, and that this would be

Smith · Chuang

difficult to achieve without many quality assurance measures including adjusting beam delivery during treatment. The Cyberknife provides an integrated technology to perform these targeting measures, and to achieve this level of accuracy for radiation treatment delivery.

References

1 Adler JR Jr, Murphy MJ, Chang SD, Hancock SL: Image-guided robotic radiosurgery. Neurosurgery 1999;44:1299–1307.

2 Chang SD, Murphy MJ, Doty JR, Hancock SL, Adler JR: Image-guided robotic radiosurgery: clinical and radiographic results with the CyberKnife; in Kondziolka D (ed): Radiosurgery. New York, Karger, 1999.

3 Coste-Maniere E, Olender D, Kilby W, Schultz RA: Robotic whole body stereotactic radiosurgery: clinical advantages of the CyberKnife integrated system. Int J Med Robotics Comput Assist Surg 2005;1:28–39.

4 Murphy MJ: Tracking moving organs in real time. Semin Radiat Oncol 2004;14:91–100.

5 Chang SD, Main W, Martin DP, Gibbs IC, Heilbrun MP: An analysis of the accuracy of the CyberKnife: a robotic frameless stereotactic radiosurgical system. Neurosurgery 2003;52:140–146.

6 Yu C, Main W, Taylor D, Kuduvalli G, Apuzzo ML, Adler JR Jr: An anthropomorphic phantom study of the accuracy of Cyberknife spinal radiosurgery. Neurosurgery 2004;55:1138–1149.

7 Schweikard A, Shiomi H, Adler J: Respiration tracking in radiosurgery. Med Phys 2004;31:2738–2741.

8 Gerszten PC, Ozhasoglu C, Burton SA, Vogel WJ, Atkins BA, Kalnicki S, Welch WC: CyberKnife frameless stereotactic radiosurgery for spinal lesions: clinical experience in 125 cases. Neurosurgery 2004;55:89–98.

9 Murphy MJ, Chang SD, Gibbs IC, Le QT, Hai J, Kim D, Martin DP, Adler JR Jr: Patterns of patient movement during frameless image-guided radiosurgery. Int J Radiat Oncol Biol Phys 2003;55:1400–1408.

10 Ponsky LE, Crownover RL, Rosen MJ, Rodebaugh RF, Castilla EA, Brainard J, Cherullo EE, Novick AC: Initial evaluation of Cyberknife technology for extracorporeal renal tissue ablation. Urology 2003;61:498–501.

11 Whyte RI, Crownover R, Murphy MJ, Martin DP, Rice TW, DeCamp MM Jr, Rodebaugh R, Weinhous MS, Le QT: Stereotactic radiosurgery for lung tumors: preliminary report of a phase I trial. Ann Thorac Surg 2003;75:1097–1101.

12 Koong AC, Le QT, Ho A, Fong B, Fisher G, Cho C, Ford J, Poen J, Gibbs IC, Mehta VK, Kee S, Trueblood W, Yang G, Bastidas JA: Phase I study of stereotactic radiosurgery in patients with locally advanced pancreatic cancer. Int J Radiat Oncol Biol Phys 2004;58:1017–1021.

Dr. Vernon Smith
Department of Radiation Oncology
University of California San Francisco
Box 0226, 505 Parnassus Ave., Long 75
San Francisco, CA 94143-0226 (USA)
Tel. +1 415 353 8900, Fax +1 415 353 8679
E-Mail smith@radonc17.ucsf.edu

Meyer JL (ed): IMRT, IGRT, SBRT – Advances in the Treatment Planning and
Delivery of Radiotherapy. Front Radiat Ther Oncol. Basel, Karger, 2007, vol. 40, pp 162–178

Helical Tomotherapy: Image Guidance and Adaptive Dose Guidance

Wolfgang A. Tomé · Hazim A. Jaradat · Ian A. Nelson ·
Mark A. Ritter · Minesh P. Mehta

Department of Human Oncology, University of Wisconsin School of Medicine and
Public Health, Madison, Wisc., USA

Abstract

Helical tomotherapy is a volumetric image-guided, fully dynamic, intensity-modulated radiation therapy (IMRT) delivery system. The daily use of its pretreatment megavoltage (MV) CT imaging for patient setup verification allows one to correct for interfraction setup error. This is a primary requirement for the accurate delivery of complex IMRT treatment plans, which give differential radiation doses to various target volumes while conformally avoiding normal critical structures. In particular, image guidance using MV CT allows for direct target position verification with the patient in the actual treatment position just prior to therapy delivery. Moreover, since helical MV CT imaging is a slow CT imaging technique, it allows for the encoding of target motion in the resulting MV CT data set, and therefore the pretreatment verification of a motion envelope defined from four-dimensional CT.

Copyright © 2007 S. Karger AG, Basel

Helical tomotherapy is a volumetric image-guided, fully dynamic, intensity-modulated radiation therapy (IMRT) delivery system. It has been developed at the University of Wisconsin and is now commercially manufactured as the Tomotherapy Hi·Art System [1]. At the core of this system lies a short gantry-mounted linear accelerator that is used both for treatment and pretreatment megavoltage (MV) CT imaging. Helical tomotherapy offers the potential for image-guided IMRT at most tumor sites and a broad range of applications in the cancer clinic.

The daily use of its pretreatment MV CT imaging for patient setup verification allows one to correct for interfraction setup error. This is a primary requirement for the accurate delivery of complex IMRT treatment plans giving differential radiation doses to various target volumes while conformally avoiding normal critical structures. In particular, image guidance using MV CT allows for direct target position verification with the patient in the actual treatment position just prior to therapy delivery.

Using a commercially available CT quality assurance phantom, the work presented here shows that helical MV CT images have good density resolution, spatial linearity, spatial resolution, and image uniformity. For a typical 30-fraction treatment schedule, daily imaging delivers a total exposure dose to the imaged volume of less than 1 Gy. A possible disadvantage of helical MV CT images is that the soft tissue contrast can be less than with kilovoltage (kV) CT. Nonetheless, MV CT images are far superior to planar images (either kV or MV) for the verification of correct patient setup. Moreover, helical MV CT imaging is a slow CT imaging technique that allows for the encoding of target motion in the resulting MV CT data set (see fig. 10, 11), and therefore the pretreatment verification of a motion envelope defined from four-dimensional CT.

Several reports give additional information on the design, dosimetry and quality assurance of helical tomotherapy machines [2–10]. In this discussion, the focus will be on the characterization of MV CT images and their use for pretreatment image guidance, and on two demonstrations of major clinical applications in radiotherapy, for prostate and lung tumors.

Helical Tomotherapy

The device is shown in figure 1. The primary collimator and the jaws set the beam width, the superior-inferior extent of the beam. The beam is also collimated by a binary multileaf collimator generating a fan beam of intensity-modulated radiation.

Intensity-Modulated Radiation Therapy

The jaw width is held constant (typically 2.5 or 5 cm) during treatment delivery. Laterally the beam is modulated using a binary multileaf collimator, which consists of 64 leaves each of a width of 0.625 cm (projected to the isocenter) for a total possible lateral beam dimension at an isocenter of 40 cm. Modulation is varied with the gantry angle. Individual modulation patterns are defined over rotational intervals ('projections') of just greater than 7°, corresponding to exactly 51 separate intensity-modulated projections per gantry revolution.

Image-Guided Radiation Therapy

The Hi·Art System allows for the acquisition of a helical pretreatment MV CT scan that can be used for online image guidance. Precise interfraction positioning of

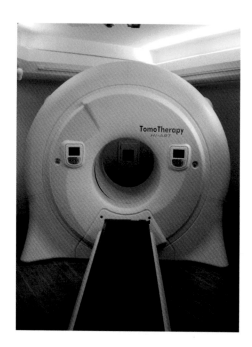

Fig. 1. Hi·Art tomotherapy machine.

the patient in the actual treatment position can be performed just prior to the start of treatment. The scanning provides soft tissue anatomic detail, especially useful when bone anatomy is not a good surrogate for target location. Daily MV CT imaging also allows assessment of changes in normal anatomy or the tumor extent during the course of therapy which may lead to repeat planning for more accurate treatment delivery.

Due to its unique design, the Hi·Art System allows highly conformal dose distributions to be delivered to patients in a helical fashion. Patients are treated lying on a couch that is translated through the bore of the machine as the gantry rotates, therefore the Hi·Art System is the therapy equivalent of helical CT [11]. Since this approach to therapy is fully dynamic, it requires synchrony of gantry rotation, couch translation, linear accelerator pulsing, and the opening and closing of the leaves of the binary multileaf collimator used for beam modulation.

Basics of Megavoltage CT Acquisition on Helical Tomotherapy

MV CT scans are acquired in a helical fashion with the patient in the treatment position just prior of treatment. One full gantry rotation takes 10 s, and therefore the total scan time is 10 s times the number of slices acquired (regardless of the slice width). The reconstruction of the MV CT image data set starts during acquisition and takes an additional 2–4 min once the scan is finished, depending upon the number of slices acquired. The resulting MV CT image data set is then fused to the treatment planning kV CT image data set to obtain the shifts necessary for precisely aligning the internal treatment target.

Integral Radiation Dose to the Patient
The radiation dose to the total imaged volume from daily MV CT pretreatment image guidance is a concern, including the theoretical possibility of induction of secondary cancers in the imaged volume outside of the high-dose target. The total dose to the imaged volume that is external to the high-dose treatment volume can be estimated as follows. Assume that we are planning to deliver a 30-fraction treatment course and that we use helical pretreatment MV CT for every fraction. The typical dose to the patient from MV CT imaging has been estimated to range from 0.015 to 0.03 Gy per image acquisition [1]. Hence, for 30 fractions this yields a dose of only 0.9 Gy to the imaged volume from the pretreatment MV CT.

MV CT Image Quality: Physical Characteristics
Image quality is a concern for all image-guided radiation therapy approaches. To objectively evaluate the MV CT images of this device, a commercially available CT quality assurance phantom was used to characterize the density resolution, spatial linearity, spatial resolution, image uniformity, and low-density contrast of MV CT images [The Catphan (CPT) 504 (Phantom Laboratory, Salem, N.Y., USA)]. The device contains various modules that allow the quantification of the tested characteristics using a single-scan acquisition. A kV CT of the CPT 504 phantom was obtained and sent to the tomotherapy planning system, and a simple plan was then generated on the phantom. The purpose of this procedure was to properly enter the phantom into the tomotherapy database, and therefore allow for proper pretreatment MV CT acquisition. The CPT 504 phantom was then centered both laterally and vertically within the tomotherapy bore, and a 256 × 256 MV CT image was acquired with a slice thickness of 2.0 mm. The MV CT images of the CPT 504 were then sent to the Pinnacle [2] treatment planning system version 7.9v via Dicom transfer and imported.

(1) Density Resolution
Procedure: To verify the density resolution of MV CT images in terms of CT numbers, a circular region of interest was drawn inside each of the regions (corresponding to different materials) shown in figure 2. The CT number and standard deviation of each material was then measured and tabulated along with the accepted mean values provided by the Phantom Laboratories (table 1).

Since the materials/expected CT numbers (shown in the middle column of table 1) are intended for use with CT images from a kV source, complete coinci-

Table 1. MV CT numbers for various materials

Material	Mean CT number	Measured CT number
Air	–1,000	–885±26
PMP	–200	–62±31
LDPE	–100	34±29
Polystyrene	–35	82±31
Delrin	340	444±35
Teflon	990	919±26

LDPE = Low-density polyethylene; PMP = polymethylpentene.

Table 2. Distances between the distance verification holes in the CPT 504 phantom

Distance between points	Nominal distance, mm	Accuracy %	Measured distance, mm
POI_1 and POI_2	50	±1	49.88
POI_2 and POI_3	50	±1	50.07
POI_3 and POI_4	50	±1	49.90
POI_4 and POI_1	50	±1	50.01

dence cannot be expected when using an MV source. However, the overall qualitative behavior is correct. Air has the lowest CT number, Teflon has the highest, and every other material falls in between according to its nominal CT number. It is interesting to note that one can resolve a contrast difference of 3–4% using MV CT images. The low-density polyethylene insert having a measured mean CT number of 82 is easily distinguished from the surrounding medium having a nominal CT number of 0.

(2) Spatial Linearity Measurement

Procedure: To determine the spatial accuracy of MV CT images, we measured the distances between the verification holes located in the CPT 504 phantom. For this purpose, we placed a point of interest in the center of each of the four verification holes and determined the distances between each of these points (fig. 3). In table 2, we show the results of this test along with the nominal distances supplied by Phantom Laboratories. Each measured distance easily falls within the 1% accuracy standard.

Tomé · Jaradat · Nelson · Ritter · Mehta

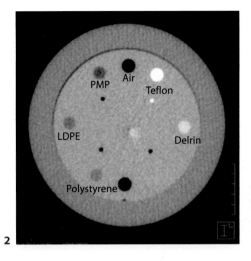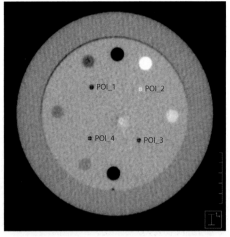

Fig. 2. MV CT image of the density resolution module of the phantom. LDPE = Low-density polyethylene; PMP = polymethylpentene.
Fig. 3. MV CT image of the density resolution module of the phantom.

(3) Image Uniformity

Procedure: To assess image uniformity, five regions of interest were placed in the image uniformity module of the CPT 504. Four of the five regions of interest were placed in the periphery at cardinal angles and one region of interest was placed in the center of the image (fig. 4; table 3).

(4) Spatial Resolution

Procedure: Spatial resolution of the MV CT images was quantified using the high-resolution module in the CPT 504 phantom. This test yields the minimal separation distance two well-defined objects must have in order to be resolved. Figure 5 shows the resulting MV CT image (table 4).

The arrow in figure 5 indicates the highest line pair that could be resolved using a 256 × 256 MV CT image, corresponding to a minimum separation distance of 0.125 mm. Incidentally, our in-house CT scanner can resolve line pair 8 in figure 5, yielding a minimal distance of 0.063 cm (half the value obtained for the MV CT image). Note, however, that the kV CT image is a 512 × 512 image while the MV CT image is a 256 × 256 image. Hence for the same field of view, the MV CT pixel size is twice that of the kV CT, and therefore its high spatial resolution is theoretically half that of the kV CT image, exactly what was found in this test.

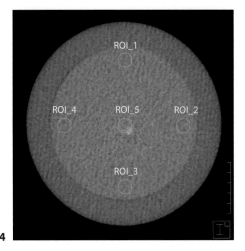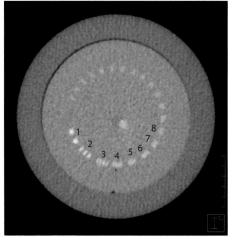

Fig. 4. MV CT image of the uniformity module of the phantom. The five regions of interest that are used to assess the image uniformity are shown in green. The central region of interest (ROI_5) contains part of a reconstruction artifact. Excluding this, table 3 demonstrates that MV CT images have good image uniformity.

Fig. 5. MV CT image of the high-resolution gauge module of the phantom.

<table>
<tr><td colspan="2">Table 3. Image uniformity of MV CT images</td></tr>
<tr><td>Region of interest</td><td>Mean CT number</td></tr>
<tr><td>ROI_1</td><td>156±26</td></tr>
<tr><td>ROI_2</td><td>159±27</td></tr>
<tr><td>ROI_3</td><td>160±29</td></tr>
<tr><td>ROI_4</td><td>152±29</td></tr>
<tr><td>ROI_5</td><td>196±49</td></tr>
</table>

Table 4. Line pair per centimeter and associated gap size

Line pair/cm	Gap size, cm
1	0.500
2	0.250
3	0.167
4	0.125
5	0.100
6	0.083
7	0.071
8	0.063

(5) Low-Contrast Resolution

Procedure: The CPT 504 phantom contains a low-contrast resolution module that allows one to assess the capability of an imaging system to resolve contrast difference ranging from 0.5 to 1%.

Figure 6 reveals the major limitation of MV CT images, namely their low-contrast resolution capability. Figure 6a shows a kV CT image and figure 6b presents an MV CT image. The same level and window was used for both images. In the kV CT image, contrast differences of 1% can be resolved while in the MV CT image they cannot. The use of an MV beam for imaging results in the loss of low-

Tomé · Jaradat · Nelson · Ritter · Mehta

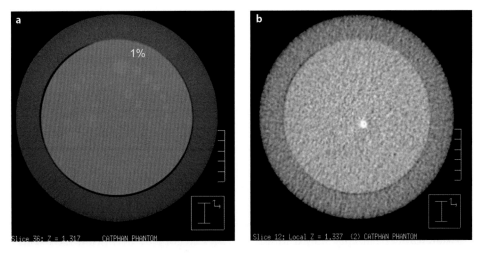

Fig. 6. kV CT (**a**) and MV CT (**b**) image of the low-density resolution module of the phantom.

contrast resolution, due to the fact that the dominant radiation interaction is Compton scattering which exhibits no dependence on the atomic number. However, we have seen in the density resolution test above that one can clearly resolve contrast differences between 3 and 4% using MV CT images, which is sufficient for high-quality pretreatment image guidance.

MV CT Image Quality: Clinical Use
Welsh et al. [12] qualitatively and quantitatively evaluated the pretreatment MV CT scans of 10 patients with lung cancer. Seven patients had lesions primarily in the lung parenchyma, 2 in the mediastinum, and 1 in both. They found that for mediastinal disease, MV CT yielded suboptimal visualization due to the loss of soft tissue contrast mentioned above. However, for lesions primarily in the lung, MV CT imaging did yield good visualization with visible detail. When the MV CT images were quantitatively compared with the treatment planning kV CT images, Welsh et al. [12] found that volumetric agreement between observers in patients with parenchymal lesions was good in 5 of 7 patients for a volume threshold of 25% between the kV CT and MV CT.

Clinical Applications of Helical Tomotherapy

In this section, two clinical applications that highlight the unique capabilities of tomotherapy and MV CT image guidance will be presented. The first example is of pelvic nodal irradiation for high-risk prostate cancer. This illustrates a large-field IMRT treatment along the cephalad-caudad axis for which tomotherapy is ideally suited, since it has no field length limitations in that direction. With tomotherapy, one can treat virtually any field length in the cephalad-caudad direction, the only limitation being the length of time needed to deliver the treatment. The second clinical example is of stereotactic body radiation therapy for peripheral T1–2 N0 M0 lung tumors. Since one can image the patient in the actual treatment position without having to move or reposition the patient prior to the treatment delivery, tomotherapy (and by the same token a linear accelerator with cone beam CT) is ideally suited for this hypofractionated high-dose, high-precision therapy.

Pelvic Nodal Dose Escalation with Prostate Hypofractionation

Prostate cancer patients staged in a high-risk category by definition have a significant risk of regional lymph node metastases, which probably represents a major cause of biochemical failure. However, even when whole-pelvis irradiation is used, treatment outcomes have not shown consistent improvement. For squamous cell carcinomas of the head and neck involving regional lymph nodes, the radiation doses necessary to sterilize small-volume disease (≤ 1 cm^3) with greater than 90% probability are in the order of 54–60 Gy, as opposed to the 45–50.4 Gy common for prostate adenocarcinoma when using whole-pelvis irradiation [13]. With tomotherapy, one can potentially safely increase the dose to the lymph nodes at risk, and therefore increase the likelihood of eradicating microscopic lymph node disease in patients with high-risk prostate cancer.

Hong et al. [14] have examined hypofractionation of the prostate with concurrent treatment of the pelvis using conformal avoidance. In this treatment technique, patients are placed prone on a bowel displacement board to reduce bowel exposure. Also, a displacement rectal balloon is used to decrease the amount of rectal wall in the high-dose volume and to effectively immobilize the prostate [15].

Figure 7 shows the resulting tomotherapy hypofractionated conformal avoidance-defined treatment plan for the treatment of high-risk prostate cancer that includes elective nodal irradiation. Seventy gray in 2.5-Gy fractions is delivered to the prostate planning target volume (PTV) and 56 Gy in 2-Gy fractions is delivered to a nodal region PTV defined using conformal avoidance. Conformal avoidance is especially useful when the target is diffuse, as in regional lymphatic volumes, and when the organs at risk are easily identified. The design of the conformal avoidance target begins with the conventional field design, which in the case of high-risk prostate cancer is a large 4-field design. From that initial field design, one then excludes the normal structures that do not contain lymph tissue. The remainder represents the intended conformal avoidance clinical target volume, which is shown as the blue region of interest in figure 7.

Tomé · Jaradat · Nelson · Ritter · Mehta

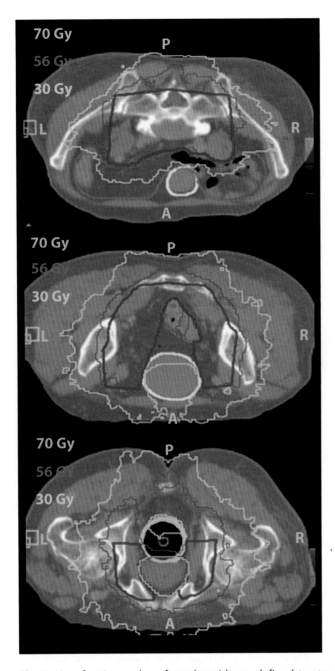

Fig. 7. Hypofractionated conformal avoidance-defined treatment plan for the treatment of high-risk prostate cancer that includes elective nodal irradiation to 56 Gy in 2-Gy fractions. The 70-Gy isodose line is shown in green, the 56-Gy isodose line is shown in red, and the 30-Gy isodose line is shown in sky blue. Other colors denote ROI.

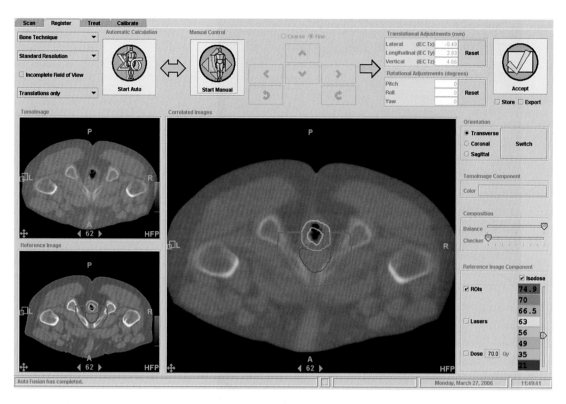

Fig. 8. Image guidance module of tomotherapy. The upper image on the left-hand side is the fused MV CT and the image below is the treatment planning kV CT. The image on the right shows the treatment planning contours for the prostate and the conformal avoidance-defined nodal region overlaid on the MV CT. The shifts necessary to align the patient are shown in the upper right-hand corner under the heading 'translational adjustments'.

For daily treatment, the patient is aligned via wall-mounted lasers and a pre-treatment MV CT scan is obtained. The resulting MV CT image is then fused to the treatment planning kV CT image. One can verify the fusion either by comparing anatomical landmarks in both image sets or by overlaying the regions of interest that have been defined during the treatment planning process onto the pretreatment MV CT scans. In figure 8, the lower image on the left-hand side shows the treatment planning kV CT and the image above shows the pretreatment MV CT. The large image on the right shows the treatment planning contours for the prostate and the conformal avoidance-defined nodal region overlaid on the pretreatment MV CT. The shifts necessary to align the treatment target are shown in the upper right-hand corner under the heading 'translational adjustments'. Once the treating physician has verified the fidelity of the image fusion, the daily translational adjustments are applied and treatment commences.

Image-Guided Stereotactic Body Radiotherapy of Non-Small-Cell Lung Cancer
In image-guided stereotactic body radiotherapy, patients are immobilized using a double vacuum whole-body mold with an abdominal pressure pillow (Bodyfix™, Medical Intelligence, Munich, Germany). A vacuum of 80 mbar together with an abdominal pressure pillow is used to reduce tumor motion associated with respiration. For treatment planning, a regular thin-slice CT is acquired for localization, and a four-dimensional CT data set is acquired to define the motion envelope of the treatment target. To define the planning target volume, a 6-mm margin is added to the motion envelope. Dosimetric margins are chosen such that the ratio of the minimum peripheral dose volume and the prescription isodose volume to the target volume is less than or equal to 1.2.

A dose fractionation schedule consisting of 5 fractions of 12 Gy each has been adopted at our institution for image-guided stereotactic body radiotherapy of peripheral lung tumors. Based on currently available clinical data, this fractionation schedule should allow one to achieve a progression-free survival at 30 months of $\geq 80\%$ if proliferation can be neglected [16]. In order to keep the incidence of clinically significant radiation pneumonitis below 20%, the mean normalized total dose to the residual healthy lung (both lungs – PTV) is determined for each treatment plan and is kept below 18 Gy_3 [17] (fig. 9).

MV CT images acquired prior to treatment are used to realign the internal target before treatment (fig. 10). Since the tomotherapy machine is a slow CT imager (one full gantry rotation takes 10 s), the motion pattern of the target is encoded into the pretreatment MV CT scan. The fusion module can then be used to align this motion-defined target to the intended position. One can check for each fraction that the motion-defined target lies within the PTV of the motion envelope (defined from the four-dimensional CT data set) by overlaying the contours onto the pretreatment MV CT. In figure 10, observe that the motion-encoded treatment target achieved this goal: it lies fully within the motion-defined PTV.

Figure 11 shows the pretreatment MV CT scans of 4 T1/2 N0 M0 non-small-cell lung cancer patients that have undergone stereotactic body radiation therapy using tomotherapy. The target definition is clear, showing the good potential of pretreatment MV CT image guidance for stereotactic body radiation therapy of peripheral lung tumors.

Adaptive or Dose-Guided Radiotherapy

Currently, pretreatment MV CT image guidance allows one to verify the correct patient setup and internal target position just prior to treatment. Corrections to the patient's position or an internal target's position can be made based on the

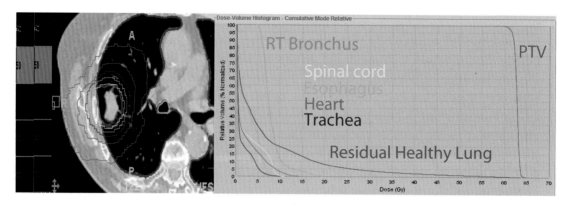

Fig. 9. The stereotactic body radiation therapy plan for the treatment of a T1/2 N0 M0 non-small-cell lung cancer. The following isodose lines are shown: 60 Gy (yellow), 50 Gy (green), 40 Gy (blue), 30 Gy (red), and 20 Gy (purple). On the right a dose-volume histogram is shown for the following structures: motion-defined PTV (red), residual healthy lung (blue), right main bronchus (aquamarine), trachea (dark purple), heart (purple), spinal cord (yellow), and esophagus (green).

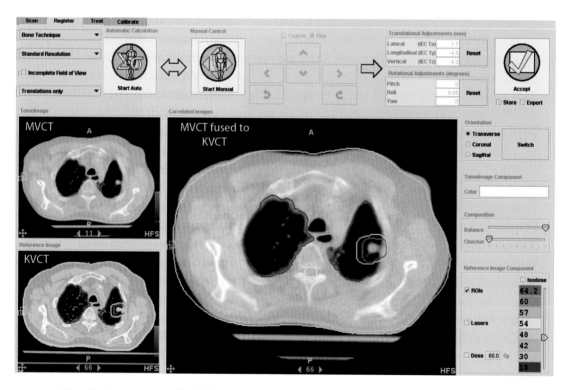

Fig. 10. Pretreatment MV CT for image-guided stereotactic body radiation therapy for T1/2 N0 M0 non-small-cell lung cancer.

Tomé · Jaradat · Nelson · Ritter · Mehta

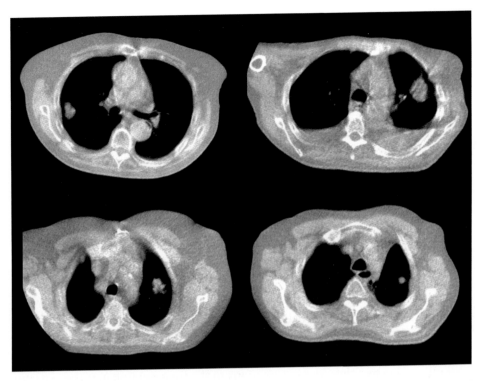

Fig. 11. Pretreatment MV CT scans for 4 lung cancer patients treated using image-guided stereotactic body radiation therapy.

results of the correlation of the pretreatment MV CT to the treatment planning kV CT. This process is graphically depicted in figure 12.

Figure 13 shows the pretreatment dose guidance that is currently possible with tomotherapy. The overlaid isodose cloud can be used to visually verify that the intended targets lie within the high-dose region and that organs at risk lie outside the high-dose region.

In figure 14, one of the possible approaches to adaptive or dose-guided radiotherapy is shown. The left-hand side of figure 14 is identical to figure 12, that is, one would still employ pretreatment MV CT image guidance to ensure correct patient setup and internal target alignment. However, instead of simply delivering the intended treatment plan, one would take an exit dose measurement during treatment and reconstruct the dose distribution that has been delivered. Using any of a number of metrics, one could then compare this actually delivered dose distribution with the intended one.

Since one aligns the treatment target accurately using MV CT image guidance, one could choose to follow an iso-normal tissue complication probability (NTCP)

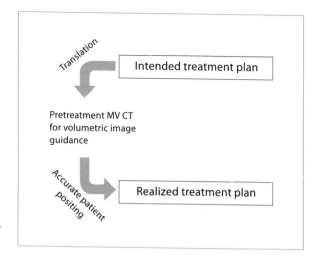

Fig. 12. Current state of pretreatment image guidance.

dose guidance strategy. In this dose guidance strategy, one accumulates dose to organs at risk up to the last delivered treatment fraction. It is well known that organs at risk can undergo interfraction motion and are not necessarily in the same position they were in at the time of treatment planning kV CT acquisition. This allows one to either make corrections to the treatment plan, if the expected NTCP for an organ at risk is predicted to exceed the planned value, or to escalate the dose to the target, if the actual NTCP is below the threshold set at the time of treatment planning.

Future Directions

What processes need to be accomplished before dose guidance can become a reality on tomotherapy? First and foremost, one needs to be able to calculate the dose actually delivered during therapy. The actually delivered dose can be calculated from collected exit dose measurements during treatment using back-projection [18, 19].

Secondly, one has to have the ability to reliably track four-dimensional target motion envelopes since tomotherapy is a fully dynamic therapy. An attempt to solve this problem has been made by Zhang et al. [20] using the breathing synchronized delivery technique. Breathing synchronized delivery can be employed to track the four-dimensional motion of a target due to breathing during therapy.

Last but not least, one needs to be able to reliably contour changes in the target and to quantify organ deformation. Target variation and organ deformation can be handled using deformable image registration and projecting the contours from the old data set onto the new data set using nonlinear transformation [21, 22].

Each of these goals is within reach, and can add adaptive, dose-guided delivery to the practical benefits of image guidance already achieved using helical tomotherapy.

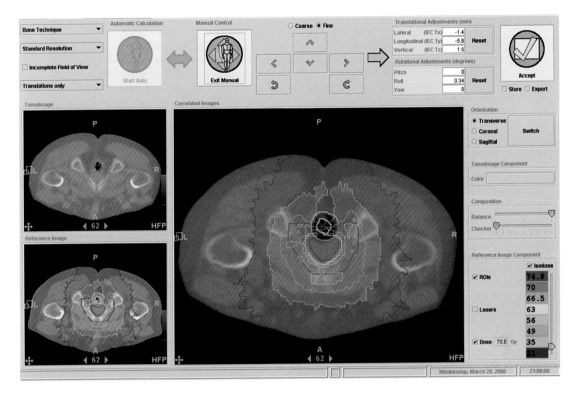

Fig. 13. Pretreatment dose guidance.

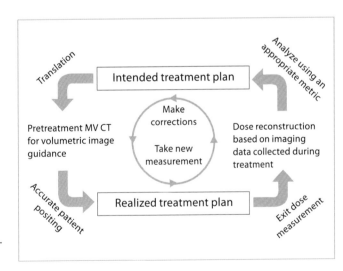

Fig. 14. Possible schema for adaptive dose-guided therapy.

References

1 Mackie TR, Olivera GH, Kapatoes JM, et al: Helical tomotherapy; in Palta JR, Mackie TR (eds): Intensity-Modulated Radiation Therapy – The State of the Art. Madison, Medical Physics Publishing, 2003, pp 247–284.

2 Mackie TR, Holmes T, Swerdloff S, et al: Tomotherapy: a new concept for the delivery of dynamic conformal radiotherapy. Med Phys 1993;20:1709–1719.

3 Mackie TR, Balog J, Ruchala K, et al: Tomotherapy. Semin Radiat Oncol 1999;9:108–117.

4 Balog JP, Mackie TR, Reckwerdt P, et al: Characterization of the output for helical delivery of intensity-modulated slit beams. Med Phys 1999;26:55–64.

5 Balog JP, Mackie TR, Wenman DL, et al: Multileaf collimator interleaf transmission. Med Phys 1999;26:176–186.

6 Balog JP, Mackie TR, Pearson D, et al: Benchmarking beam alignment for a clinical helical tomotherapy device. Med Phys 2003;30:1118–1127.

7 Balog J, Olivera G, Kapatoes J: Clinical helical tomotherapy commissioning dosimetry. Med Phys 2003;30:3097–3106.

8 Fenwick JD, Tomé WA, Jaradat HA, et al: Quality assurance of a helical tomotherapy machine. Phys Med Biol 2004;49:2933–2953.

9 Fenwick JD, Tomé WA, Kissick MW, Mackie TR: Modelling simple helically delivered dose distributions. Phys Med Biol 2005;50:1505–1517.

10 Kissick MW, Fenwick J, James JA, et al: The helical tomotherapy thread effect. Med Phys 2005;32:1414–1423.

11 Kalender WA, Polacin A: Physical performance characteristics of spiral CT scanning. Med Phys 1991;18:910–915.

12 Welsh JS, Bradley K, Ruchala KJ, Mackie TR, Manon R, Patel R, Wiederholt P, Lock M, Hui S, Mehta MP: Megavoltage computed tomography imaging: a potential tool to guide and improve the delivery of thoracic radiation therapy. Clin Lung Cancer 2004;5:303–306.

13 Mendenhall WM, Million RR, Bova FJ: Analysis of time-dose factors in clinically positive neck nodes treated with irradiation alone in squamous cell carcinoma of the head and neck. Int J Radiat Oncol Biol Phys 1984;10:639–643.

14 Hong TS, Tomé WA, Jaradat HA, Reisbeck B, Ritter MA: Pelvic nodal dose escalation with prostate hypofractionation using conformal avoidance defined (H-CAD) intensity-modulated radiation therapy. Acta Oncol 2006;45:717–727.

15 Patel RR, Orton N, Tome WA, Chappell R, Ritter MA: Rectal dose sparing with a balloon catheter and ultrasound localization in conformal radiation therapy for prostate cancer. Radiother Oncol 2003;67:285–294.

16 Tomé WA, Fenwick JD, Mehta MP: How can tumor effect and normal tissue effect be balanced in stereotactic body radiotherapy. Radiosurgery 2006;6:87–98.

17 Seppenwoolde Y, Lebesque J, de Jaeger K, et al: Comparing different NTCP models that predict the incidence of radiation pneumonitis. Int J Radiat Oncol Biol Phys 2003;55:724–735.

18 McNutt TR, Mackie TR, Paliwal BR: Analysis and convergence of the iterative convolution/superposition dose reconstruction technique for multiple treatment beams and tomotherapy. Med Phys 1997;24:1465–1476.

19 Kapatoes JM, Olivera GH, Balog JP, Keller H, Reckwerdt PJ, Mackie TR: On the accuracy and effectiveness of dose reconstruction for tomotherapy. Phys Med Biol 2001;46:943–966.

20 Zhang T, Jeraj R, Keller H, Lu WG, Olivera GH, McNutt TR, Mackie TR, Paliwal P: Treatment plan optimization incorporating respiratory motion. Med Phys 2004;31:1576–1586.

21 Lu WG, Chen ML, Olivera GH, Ruchala KJ, Mackie TR: Fast free-form deformable registration via calculus of variation. Phys Med Biol 2004;49:3067–3087.

22 Zhang T, Orton NP, Tomé WA: On the automated definition of mobile target volumes from 4D-CT images for stereotactic body radiotherapy. Med Phys 2005;32:3493–3502.

Dr. Wolfgang Tomé
University of Wisconsin School of
Medicine and Public Health
Department of Human Oncology, K4/344 CSC
600 Highland Ave.
Madison, WI 53792 (USA)
Tel. +1 608 263 8510, Fax +1 608 263 9947
E-Mail tome@humonc.wisc.edu

Tomé · Jaradat · Nelson · Ritter · Mehta

II. IMRT / IGRT Clinical Treatment Programs

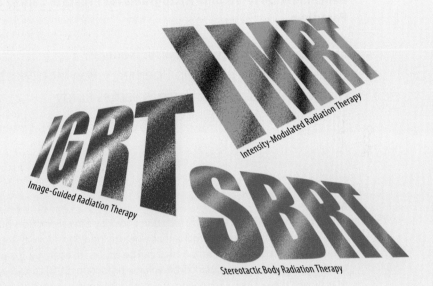

Meyer JL (ed): IMRT, IGRT, SBRT – Advances in the Treatment Planning and
Delivery of Radiotherapy. Front Radiat Ther Oncol. Basel, Karger, 2007, vol. 40, pp 180–192

Introducing New Technologies into the Clinic

Benchmark Dose-Volume Histograms for Prostate Cancer as a Paradigm

Srinivasan Vijayakumar · Samir Narayan ·
Claus Chunli Yang · Philip Boerner · Rojymon Jacob ·
Mathew Mathai · Rick Harse · James Purdy

Department of Radiation Oncology, University of California, Davis Cancer Center,
Sacramento, Calif., USA

Abstract

Introducing new technologies into radiation oncology clinical practices poses very specific logistical dilemmas. How do we determine that a new technology's dose distribution is better than the 'standard' and what are the methods that can be applied to easily compare the 'new' with the 'old'? We consider how the benchmark dose-volume histogram (DVH) can serve as a conceptual model to approach these issues. Comparing dosimetric differences using benchmark DVHs helps a 'global' comparison of the area under the curve that is intuitive, relatively efficient and easily implemented. These concepts, applied in prostate cancer in this communication, have wider applications in other disease sites and in the introduction of technologies beyond intensity-modulated radiation therapy.

The Benchmark Dose-Volume Histogram

The introduction of new technologies into our clinical practice of radiation oncology poses very specific logistical dilemmas. At what point can one say that the new technologies offer potential advances in treatment outcomes? How often can these potential outcomes be expected? In daily clinical work, these questions eventually resolve to: will a specific patient's problem be aided by the use of the new technology? New technologies are often accompanied by added technical costs, staff time in implementation, and practical concerns regarding the reliability of the new processes and their outcomes. New technologies designed for clinical use, though acquired with considerable cost and effort, will likely suffer deferment of use on a day-to-day basis unless quantitative measures permit a clear definition of their new and immediate roles in improving outcomes for specific patient groups.

Dose-volume histograms (DVHs) are generated during the treatment planning process [1–3], and assist in defining the dose distributions of rendered plans to regions of interest. In comparing rival plans, DVHs can be used for making treatment decisions in therapy by comparing the dose distributions to normal and tumor tissues. In so doing, DVHs can objectively compare the treatment technologies themselves, their role for individual patients, and ultimately their role in the technical environment of individual treatment clinics, each with its unique army of diverse technologies.

The benchmark DVH is a conceptual model to facilitate an efficient way to define the relative role of a new radiation delivery technology. A *benchmark* is a standard of measurement or evaluation, 'a point of reference for judging value, quality, change or the like; standard to which others can be compared'. By using the benchmarking of DVHs as a strategy, one can objectively define a path of progress in improving radiotherapy dose distributions, and utilizing the new technologies that provide those improved dose distributions.

A new technology may give a better dose distribution to the planning target volume (PTV), and thus to the gross tumor volume (GTV) and clinical target volume (CTV). This might be either a more uniform dose distribution or a biologically advantageous dose gradient ('hot spot') within the PTV that could potentially improve outcomes. In addition, a new technology could be instrumental in reducing doses to critical tissues. In turn, these dosimetric advantages can improve outcomes, including survival, local control, quality of life, and toxicity endpoints. The new technology might also be more efficient or cost less. Benchmarks can help assess all of these important considerations.

Important questions remain in the development of new intensity-modulated radiation therapy (IMRT) approaches for radiotherapy. For example, are IMRT plans always better than conventional or three-dimensional conformal radiation therapy (3DCRT) plans? How does one quantitatively compare IMRT with other plans? How much additional time is required for IMRT in terms of planning treatment, monitoring quality assurance, and delivering therapy? What additional resources are needed for its implementation and confirming its reliability? Which patients should receive this new technology and which will not benefit from it? How can exact guidelines for use be developed? More generally, why would one want to change to a new technology when an older technology may appear adequate? These questions are universal for the introduction of any new technology into our clinics. The differences that can be defined by benchmark DVHs can lead

Table 1. Considerations regarding the value of IMRT compared with 3DCRT

Consideration	Response
Better dose distribution?	yes
Lower doses to the critical tissues?	yes
Improved outcomes?	
Survival	unknown
Local control	yes
Quality of life	possibly
Fewer toxicities	yes
More efficient than 3DCRT?	no
Lower cost (decreased staff levels)?	no

not only to approval of new treatment plans, but also to the justification for the new planning and delivery processes themselves and their requirements for implementation. Benchmark DVHs can provide objective measures for the specific roles of new technologies in the radiotherapy clinic.

This discussion will illustrate these concepts using prostate cancer therapy as a model.

The Benchmark Dose-Volume Histogram and Prostate Cancer

In prostate cancer treatment, dose escalation beyond 70 Gy is becoming routine practice. This is made possible with the use of 3DCRT and more recently with the implementation of IMRT. Dose escalation, however, is often limited by rectal and bladder toxicity. Although accuracy in delivering high doses to the target and low doses to the surrounding structures is complicated by rectal dose/volume variation due to organ motion and daily repositioning errors, the likelihood of late rectal or bladder toxicity is initially investigated through evaluation using the DVH.

One of the questions regarding prostate cancer radiotherapy is whether IMRT always leads to a better dose distribution to the PTV, meaning a more uniform dose or higher dose within the CTV/GTV, than occurs with 3DCRT. Second, does IMRT lead to lower doses to the critical tissues such as the rectum, bladder, penile tissues, and femoral heads/hip joints? Third, has IMRT improved outcomes, including survival, local control, quality of life, and lower toxicity? Table 1 provides some of the commonly acknowledged answers to these questions.

However, are these answers applicable to every prostate cancer patient treated today? A response to this requires quantification of the potential benefit of IMRT specific to an individual case, and is aided by standards for comparison. In this

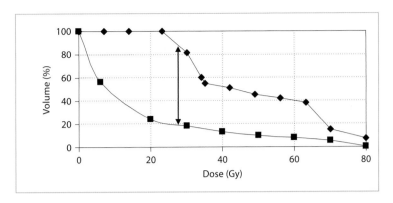

Fig. 1. Upper and lower range for bladder DVHs reported by 9 institutions in the literature.

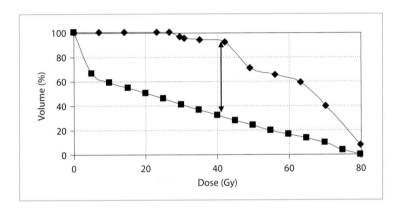

Fig. 2. Upper and lower range for rectal DVHs reported by 9 institutions in the literature.

paper, a systematic approach toward this will be presented, showing an organization of existing data on prostate therapy DVHs that should prove useful for evaluating IMRT treatment plans and expected outcomes. These concepts may be applied in other clinics for their prostate cancer therapy planning, and may be applied for other tumor sites and other technologies as well.

Benchmark Dose-Volume Histogram Data for Defining Prostate Cancer Therapy

Bladder and Rectum DVH Results in the Literature for Prostate Radiotherapy
Published DVH analyses for bladder or rectum volumes, treated using modern radiotherapy approaches for prostate cancer, are shown in figures 1 and 2. They reveal a wide range of results. These grouped data cannot be used directly to eval-

uate a single institution's DVH results. Each institution has its own set of protocols in performing simulations, positioning patients, defining targets, expanding PTV margins, and so forth. For example, some institutions use enemas to evacuate the rectum before planning treatment, and this alone could have an influence on an institution's DVH patterns for rectal volume that does not reflect any contribution of IMRT. Some institutions use intravenous contrast and some do not. Some institutions treat patients in the prone position, whereas the majority of institutions use the supine position. Therefore, the institutions must develop their own benchmark DVHs to compare their work and technologic development, and to correlate them with their outcomes once sufficient follow-up has been obtained.

There are a number of ways clinicians can analyze DVH data to optimize planning. For example, one might evaluate the mean dose to the rectum, or the rectal volume receiving more than 70 Gy, or other measures. In the experience of several groups including ours, the ideal way is to utilize the whole DVH curve, because even the lower therapy doses may significantly contribute to normal tissue complications.

At least three published studies show the importance of evaluating the area under the curve. In one, Huang et al. [4] at the MD Anderson Cancer Center examined the dosimetric, anatomical and clinical factors that may lead to late rectal toxicity after 3DCRT by retrospectively analyzing DVHs. The study was comprised of 163 patients with stage T1–T3 disease and treated from 1992 to 1999. Treatments delivered isocenter doses of 74–78 Gy, and patients were followed for a median of 62 months. To score late rectal complications, the investigators used modified Radiation Therapy Oncology Group criteria, and correlations were made at 6 years following therapy for grade 2 or higher toxicities. At 6 years, grade 2 or higher toxicities were seen in 25% of patients. Factors that correlated with late rectal toxicity included dose and volume effects: the overall percent volume of the rectum irradiated and the dose prescribed. Analyzing specific doses, there was a significant correlation of toxicity with the volume of rectum treated. Importantly, this correlation existed at several dose points, including the volume of the rectum receiving 60, 70, 75.6 and 78 Gy.

Additionally, the percentage of rectal volume treated correlated significantly with the incidence of rectal complications, as well as the absolute rectal volume, both at 70, 75.6 and 78 Gy. According to their univariate analysis, maximal dose to the CTV, maximal dose to the rectum, maximal dose to the rectum as a percentage of the prescribed dose and maximal dose delivered to 10 cm^3 of rectum were all important. The only clinical variable that was important was a history of hemorrhoids. Through DVH analysis, this study found a dose/volume correlation for developing late rectal complications, and this correlation was observed at multiple dose levels indicating that the curve itself must be considered rather than any individual dose point on the curve.

Table 2. Association of total rectal wall volume (VRW) with rectal bleeding, at the Memorial Sloan-Kettering Cancer Center

Dose and correlation with rectal bleeding	
70.2 Gy	$p = 0.06$
75.6 Gy	$p = 0.01$
Patients with similar VRWs, and volume exposed to 46 Gy	
70.2 Gy	$p = 0.02$
75.6 Gy	$p = 0.005$
Patients with volume exposed to 77 Gy	
75.6 Gy	$p < 0.005$

A second important study, from the Memorial Sloan-Kettering Cancer Center [5], looked at late rectal bleeding after 3DCRT, and specifically at the rectal wall DVHs. A total of 266 and 320 patients were treated with doses of either 70.2 or 75.6 Gy, respectively, using six-field coplanar beams. Patients were scored as having rectal bleeding or not depending on whether they showed this complication by 30 months. Within the eligible group, rectal bleeding occurred in 13 patients after 70.2 Gy and in 36 patients after 75.6 Gy. For comparison, investigators took cohorts of 39 and 83 patients from a random sample of eligible nonbleeding patients at 70.2 and 75.6 Gy, respectively. They then performed a multivariate analysis, looking at rectal wall DVH correlations, to investigate what the predictive variables might be (table 2). For patients with bleeding, the area under the rectal DVH curve (using average percent volume) was significantly greater than for patients without bleeding, for both dose groups. In both, the volume exposed to 46 Gy was very important in influencing rectal bleeding rates, indicated with significant p values. Also, the percent volume receiving 77 Gy was significant for the patients receiving 75.6 Gy. This study shows that even at 46 Gy, the absolute volume or percent volume of the rectum helps predict complications.

To guide dose escalation in prostate cancer treatment, variations in the rectal dose/volume relationship must be considered as well. In a third related study, Yan et al. [6] examined the influence of variations in rectal volume, shape, size and position between patients and in the same patient on different treatment days. This retrospective study took different PTV constructions and evaluated the effect of rectal complications on them. In 30 patients, treatment plans were generated (a four-field box beam arrangement) for each of three different PTVs: PTV with a 0.5-cm uniform margin from CTV, a 1.0-cm margin, and a patient-specific PTV constructed using treatment imaging feedback. The investigators found that sensitivity of the risk of rectal complication to rectal dose/volume variation strongly depended on both the CTV-to-PTV margin and the prescription dose (table 3) in addition to other factors.

Table 3. Factors causing rectal complications, in order of importance

1	Margin expansion, CTV to PTV
2	Prescription dose
3	Rectal volume
4	Rectal dose
5	Shape/size of rectum
6	Position of rectum

William Beaumont Hospital [6].

Using DVH Results to Strategize the Introduction of New Technologies

Clinical analyses of DVH results can be used to model improvements in our technologies and their clinical roles. Building upon these earlier studies of prostate cancer DVHs, the approach used at UC Davis to introduce IMRT for prostate cancer patients is outlined in table 4 [7, 8].

The hypothesis was that IMRT was likely to give a better dose distribution in a majority of patients but not in all patients. The percentage of patients in whom IMRT would not be different than 3DCRT was not known when examined 2–3 years ago. One way to ascertain an improved dose distribution is to compare 3DCRT with IMRT in each patient. However, this would be extremely resource intensive. By developing benchmark DVHs, one can create a more efficient method of comparing new IMRT plans with more traditional plans. This approach is equally applicable to the evaluation of other new technologies (for example, helical tomotherapy might be compared with linear accelerator-based IMRT). What follows is a description of the introduction of IMRT in a planned and phased way at UC Davis, which helped to optimize its use of resources and may be helpful for other institutions.

The strategy was to create individual 3DCRT and IMRT plans for a certain number of patients. The expectation was that patients would be treated using IMRT only if the dose distributions were better than those with 3DCRT. Benchmark DVHs were then developed after a certain number of cases and used for future comparisons. To define this benchmark standard, 97 treatment plans were used from 66 patients with prostate cancer treated at UC Davis between 2000 and 2003. Thirty-five patients, treated before routine implementation of IMRT, were treated with 3DCRT. Both 3DCRT and IMRT plans were developed for the remaining 31 patients. In order to develop baseline data, DVHs from prior work at the University of Illinois at Chicago were used to accomplish some of the average DVHs, since their outcomes were known [Vijayakumar, S., pers. commun.].

Table 4. UC Davis hypotheses, strategy and experience [8]

Hypotheses	Strategy	Experience
IMRT is likely to give better dose profiles in a majority of patients, but not all patients (the percentage in whom it may not be different than 3DCRT was unknown)	Perform 3DCRT and IMRT plans for a certain number of patients	97 treatment plans were generated on 66 patients with prostate cancer treated at our institution between April 2000 and December 2003
One way to ascertain an improved dose profile is by comparing 3DCRT vs. IMRT in each patient (however, this would be resource intense over time)	Treat those with IMRT if the dose profile is better than 3DCRT	35 patients were treated before the routine implementation of IMRT with 3DCRT
Developing benchmark DVHs will allow for a more efficient way to compare IMRT to more traditional treatment plans	Treat with 3DCRT if dose profiles are comparable (this saves resources)	Both 3DCRT and IMRT plans were developed for the remaining 31 patients
A class solution for comparing rival plans can save resources and can make the implementation of any new technology more efficient	Develop benchmark DVHs after a certain number of cases and then use the benchmark DVH for comparison	Bladder and rectum DVH data were summarized to obtain an average DVH for each technique and then compared using two-tailed paired t test analysis (fig. 3–9)

In accordance with our methods, a dose of 74 Gy in 37 fractions was prescribed to the 95% isodose surface and the dose was normalized to the isocenter. Bladder and rectum DVH data were summarized to obtain an average DVH (fig. 3, 4) for each technique, and then compared using a two-tailed paired t test. Target volumes (GTV, CTV and PTV), as well as critical tissues, were recontoured if necessary when this analysis was done, so that there was uniformity in the delineation of target volumes [7, 8].

The mean dose for 3DCRT patients was 28.8 versus 26.4 Gy for IMRT. Examining the volume receiving 70 Gy next, similar results were found. In the results for the rectum, there was an advantage for IMRT over 3DCRT both for the mean dose and volume receiving 70 Gy. For those patients who had both prostate and seminal vesicles treated, IMRT gave an advantage in terms of both the mean dose and volume receiving 70 Gy for both bladder and rectum. The mean dose to the bladder was 27.5 Gy for 3DCRT patients compared with 25.9 Gy for IMRT. Finally, in those patients receiving treatment to the prostate only, there again were advantages for IMRT for bladder and rectum [8]. For example, the mean dose to the bladder was

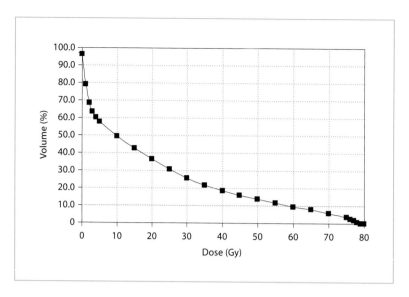

Fig. 3. UC Davis benchmark DVH for bladder, for patients receiving treatment to both prostate and seminal vesicles.

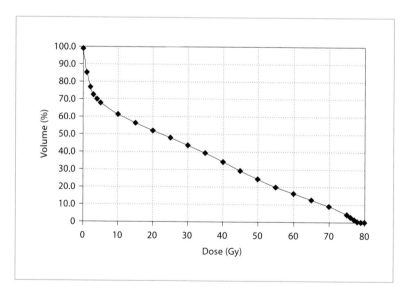

Fig. 4. UC Davis benchmark DVH for rectum, for patients receiving treatment to both prostate and seminal vesicles.

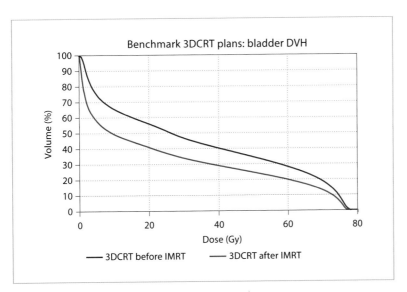

Fig. 5. Comparison of UC Davis benchmark DVHs. Shown are 3DCRT benchmarks before and after the initiation of IMRT. The upper line is the 3DCRT DVH for bladder prior to implementation of IMRT, and the lower line is the 3DCRT DVH for the next 30 patients after implementation of IMRT, which encouraged planners to achieve higher goals with 3DCRT. Note that the 3DCRT DVHs improved when a benchmark DVH was used to 'challenge' the planner.

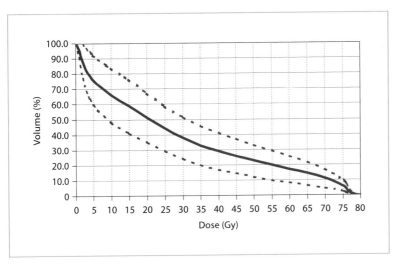

Fig. 6. Bladder IMRT DVH benchmark (bladder volume: 70–300 cm^3; average: 206 cm^3).

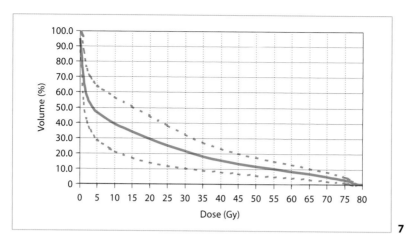

7

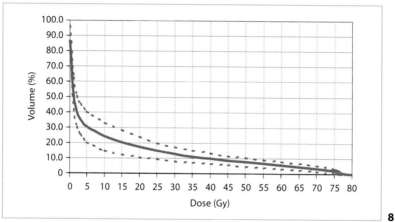

8

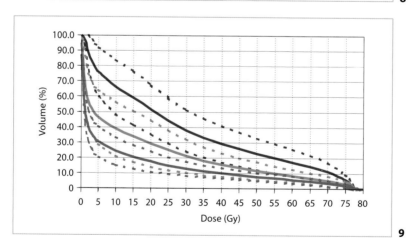

9

Fig. 7. Bladder IMRT DVH benchmark (bladder volume: 300–600 cm³; average: 449 cm³).
Fig. 8. Bladder IMRT DVH benchmark (bladder volume: 600–850 cm³; average: 722 cm³).
Fig. 9. Bladder IMRT DVH benchmark (3 categories of bladder volume: red = 70–300 cm³; green = 300–600 cm³; blue = 600–850 cm³).

31.0 Gy for 3DCRT, while it was 27.1 Gy for IMRT. For the penile tissue doses, IMRT had an advantage as well. Additional results are shown in figures 5–9. In figure 5, UC Davis benchmark DVHs are compared, showing 3DCRT benchmarks before and after the initiation of IMRT. Figures 6–9 show three categories of bladder volumes for the bladder IMRT DVH benchmarks. Since the average DVHs depended on the bladder volume, three different benchmark DVHs were developed based on bladder volumes. In figure 6, the bladder volume ranged from 70 to 300 cm³, and in figure 7 from 300 to 600 cm³. It can be seen that the average DVH has a better profile in figure 7 compared with figure 6. Similar conclusions can be drawn from figure 8, for bladder volumes >600 cm³. In figure 9, different benchmark DVHs for different bladder volumes are compared.

Summary and Conclusions

IMRT achieves better dose distributions than 3DCRT in most cases of prostate cancer. This can be documented by comparing IMRT plans with more traditional ones using benchmark DVHs. In our implementation of IMRT, bladder and rectum DVH data were summarized to obtain an average DVH for each technique, and then compared. We found that IMRT was advantageous, and showed improvement in terms of reducing both mean dose and the volume receiving 70 Gy for bladder and rectum. These advantages existed both for patients receiving treatment to the prostate plus seminal vesicles and for those receiving prostate treatment alone.

In summary, volume effects are very important at various levels of doses, not just at single levels, and the area under the curve in the DVH is important. Benchmark dose/volume data should be acquired, evaluated and used to retrospectively and prospectively assess potential new treatment programs. Such analyses should make use of the whole area under the DVH curve for optimal results. There are alternative approaches to using DVH data [9], and DVH results will likely be specific for each institution.

Comparing results from an institution's existing treatment patterns, such as their 3DCRT cases, with a new proposed technology, such as IMRT, is an important benefit of DVH data utilization. Investigators can then assure themselves that their IMRT results will be at least as good as those with 3DCRT. These same principles apply to the use of any new technology at any treatment site, to assure that improvement in dose distribution is actually achieved, how it should be clinically measured, and ultimately when a new technology should be used.

References

1 Lyman JT, Wolbarst AB: Optimization of radiation therapy. 3. A method of assessing complication probabilities from dose-volume histograms. Int J Radiat Oncol Biol Phys 1987;13:103–109.
2 Lyman JT, Wolbarst AB: Optimization of radiation therapy. 4. A dose-volume histogram reduction algorithm. Int J Radiat Oncol Biol Phys 1989; 17:433–436.
3 Kutcher GJ, Burman C, Brewster L, et al: Histogram reduction method for calculating complication probabilities for three-dimensional treatment planning evaluations. Int J Radiat Oncol Biol Phys 1991;21:137–146.
4 Huang EH, Pollack A, Levy L, et al: Late rectal toxicity: dose-volume effects of conformal radiotherapy for prostate cancer. Int J Radiat Oncol Biol Phys 2002;54:1314–1321.
5 Jackson A, Skwarchuk MW, Zelefsky MJ, et al: Late rectal bleeding after conformal radiotherapy of prostate cancer. 2. Volume effects and dose-volume histograms. Int J Radiat Oncol Biol Phys 2001;49:685–698.
6 Yan D, Xu B, Lockman D, et al: The influence of interpatient and intrapatient rectum variation on external beam treatment of prostate cancer. Int J Radiat Oncol Biol Phys 2001;51:1111–1119.
7 Narayan S, Luo CH, Yang C, Stern S, Perks J, Wang L, Mathai M, Gao MC, Goldberg Z, Chou R, Ryu J, Vijayakumar S: A competing plan methodology for optimizing the use of IMRT and 3D-CRT. Int J Radiat Oncol Biol Phys 2004; 60:S633–S634.
8 Luo CH, Yang C, Narayan S, Stern R, Perks J, Goldberg Z, Ryu J, Purdy J, Vijayakumar S: Use of benchmark DVHs in selection of optimal technique between 3D-CRT and IMRT in prostate cancer. Int J of Radiat Oncol Biol Phys, in press.
9 Miralbell R, Taussky D, Rinaldi O, et al: Influence of rectal volume changes during radiotherapy for prostate cancer: a predictive model for mild-to-moderate late rectal toxicity. Int J Radiat Oncol Biol Phys 2003;57:1280–1284.

Dr. Srinivasan Vijayakumar
Department of Radiation Oncology
University of California, Davis Cancer Center
Sacramento, CA 95817 (USA)
Tel. +1 916 734 7888, Fax +1 916 703 5069, E-Mail
srinivasan.vijayakumar@ucdmc.ucdavis.edu

Meyer JL (ed): IMRT, IGRT, SBRT – Advances in the Treatment Planning and
Delivery of Radiotherapy. Front Radiat Ther Oncol. Basel, Karger, 2007, vol. 40, pp 193–207

Delineating Neck Targets for Intensity-Modulated Radiation Therapy of Head and Neck Cancer

What Have We Learned from Marginal Recurrences?

Merav Ben David · Avraham Eisbruch

Department of Radiation Oncology, University of Michigan, Ann Arbor, Mich., USA

Abstract

Delineation of the targets for intensity-modulated radiation therapy (IMRT) of the head and neck is a crucial step in treatment planning, determining the risks of marginal or out-of-field local/regional recurrences. Delineation of the gross tumor volumes needs to take into account both radiological (CT, MRI, PET) and clinical findings, discussed in this paper. In contrast, the delineation of the clinical target volumes depends solely on the physician's judgement and knowledge of the natural history and spread pattern of head and neck cancer. While much of this information exists in older literature, new information has been gained from the pattern of recurrences observed after IMRT of head and neck cancer. This review concentrates on this information and on the lessons gained from these recurrences at our institution.

Studies in intensity-modulated radiation therapy (IMRT) of head and neck cancer have mostly concentrated on the sparing of noninvolved tissues from irradiation. Major salivary glands, minor salivary glands dispersed throughout the oral cavity, the mandible and the pharyngeal mucosa and musculature can all be partly spared, improving post-treatment quality of life compared with conventional radiotherapy (RT) [1–3]. In cases of nasopharyngeal and paranasal sinus cancers, additional critical normal tissues that may be partly spared using IMRT include the inner and middle ears, temporomandibular joints, temporal brain lobes and optic pathways [4]. In addition to sparing noninvolved tissues, IMRT offers a potential for improving tumor control by reducing the constraints on the total tumor dose imposed by adjacent critical normal tissues, especially the spinal cord and brain stem, which can be problematic with conventional RT.

The need for accurate selection and definition of the targets for IMRT is especially relevant in head and neck cancer, where a high risk of subclinical local and nodal disease exists and where adequate irradiation of the lymph nodes at risk is crucial for local-regional control and survival. For example, in standard three-field RT of oropharyngeal cancer, the first echelon and the retropharyngeal (RP) nodes are inevitably treated when the primary tumor is targeted. In contrast, these nodes will not be adequately irradiated by IMRT if they are not specified as targets on the planning CT.

Delineating Tumor and Target Volumes in the Neck

The Gross Tumor Volume in the Neck

Information for Treatment Planning

Examination, CT and MRI
In order to define the targets for head and neck cancer, the extent of the gross tumor volume (GTV) should be precisely known. The physical exam (including mirror and fiber-optic exam), in conjunction with the surgeon's report of direct endoscopy under anesthesia, are important data to define the tumor. The simulation contrast-enhanced CT is in most cases the only imaging modality required for the delineation of the targets. MRI is limited by its sensitivity to artifacts, difficulty in interpretation, long examination time and cost. However, MRI is an essential adjunct to CT for tumors close to the base of skull, i.e. nasopharyngeal and paranasal sinus cancers, where it provides better detail of the tumor extension and of the parapharyngeal and RP spaces compared with CT [5]. MRI is therefore essential for delineating the targets in these cases.

FDG-PET
FDG-PET imaging may provide additional staging information. Clinical evaluations of head and neck cancer patients, where CT, MRI and FDG-PET were all obtained and surgery was then performed to validate the primary tumor extent and lymph node involvement, have reported a small additional benefit of FDG-PET compared with CT and MRI [6, 7]. In cases of recurrent cancer, FDG-PET has demonstrated significantly higher utility compared with CT or MRI [8–10]. We utilize FDG-PET registered with CT as an adjunct to the simulation CT. The GTV may be adjusted by including the composite abnormality of both CT and PET (rather than relying on one modality). Borderline enlarged nodes noted on the CT scan, which might have been included in the subclinical target, become part of the GTV if they are PET avid. Thus, PET can alter therapy by increasing prescribed doses to sites found to be involved, compared with CT alone.

Delineating the GTV in the Neck

Based on the experience of imaging sciences and radiation oncology practice, this institution has developed some broad policies. Lymph nodes are included in the GTV if they have any of the following radiologic criteria:
  (1) diameter >1 cm (or in the case of the jugulodigastric nodes, >1.1–1.5 cm);
  (2) smaller than 1 cm with spherical rather than ellipsoidal shape;
  (3) contain inhomogeneities suggestive of necrotic centers;
  (4) cluster of 3 or more borderline nodes [11];
  (5) FDG-PET positive.

The Clinical Target Volume in the Neck

The clinical target volume (CTV) surrounding the primary tumor encompasses tissues judged to be at risk for microscopic, subclinical tumor extension. Neck CTVs consist of the neck levels at risk that do not match the radiologic criteria of node involvement. Factors used for assessing the extent of the CTV margins in each case include tumor site, size, stage, differentiation and morphology (ulcerative or exophytic, infiltrative or pushing front). Rather than simply expanding the GTV uniformly, an approach of outlining of the CTV on the planning CT on a slice-by-slice basis is recommended. Knowledge of the anatomical and clinical patterns of tumor extension, clinical judgment, and familiarity with head and neck imaging are necessary for the accurate estimation of CTV margins around the tumor. Details of CTV outlining around the primary tumor have been discussed elsewhere [12]. In this paper, we will concentrate on the delineation of the neck CTVs.

Lymphatic Drainage

Our knowledge of the pattern and risk of lymphatic drainage from different head and neck sites is based on the classic anatomical work by Rouvière [13, 14], the assessment of the location and prevalence of clinical neck metastases by Lindberg [15], and the large experience with elective neck dissections providing information about microscopic metastases reported by Byers et al. [16], Candela et al. [17] and others. These studies demonstrate that squamous cell carcinomas of the upper aerodigestive tract tend to metastasize to the neck in predictable patterns, governed by the density and drainage of the lymphatics at each site, and with increasing risk at each level if the adjoining proximal level is involved.

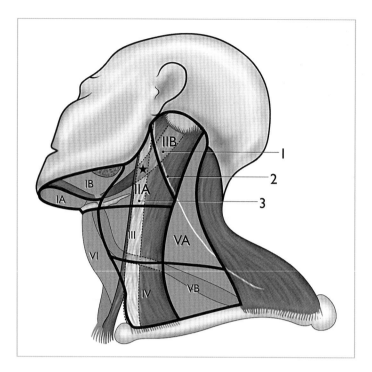

Fig. 1. Neck node levels. 1 = Posterior belly of the digastric muscle; 2 = accessory nerve; 3 = jugular vein; asterisk = jugulodigastric nodes: where jugular vein bisects the posterior belly of the digastric muscle (just below the transverse process of C1).

To create an anatomic reference system for neck nodes, surgeons from the Memorial Sloan-Kettering Hospital developed a simple division, revised by Robbins et al. [18] and Robbins [19]. Six levels were defined, each with discrete anatomic boundaries that are apparent during neck dissection. This classification allows standardized reporting of the sites of nodal involvement in the neck, as well as the sites of surgical therapy. A corresponding imaging-based nodal classification, using CT- or MRI-based criteria for these surgical anatomic landmarks, has been developed by head and neck radiologists [20]. In addition, several publications by radiation oncologists have demonstrated how to outline the lymph node neck levels as CTV on planning CT or axial MRI scans [21–23]. The above publications are highly recommended for the reader before pursuing three-dimensional conformal radiation therapy or IMRT to the head and neck for cancer treatment. An extensive review of the literature regarding the risk of metastases to each neck level has recently been published by Gregoire et al. [21]. Another tool is on the Radiation Therapy Oncology Group (RTOG) website: http://www.rtog.org/hnatlas – a detailed atlas of the head and neck with illustrations of the different neck levels [24].

Ben David · Eisbruch

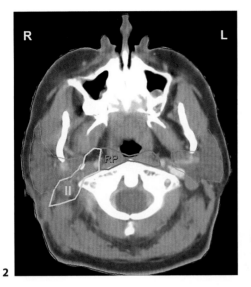 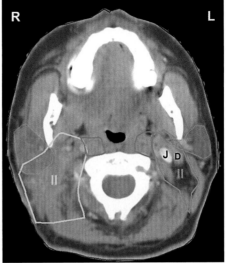

2   3

Fig. 2. A patient with oropharyngeal cancer with grossly involved lower level II nodes: targets at an axial CT image cranial to the transverse process of C1. Right level II, as well as the RP nodes, are outlined through the base of the skull, while the contralateral upper level II is not outlined.
Fig. 3. Same patient, at an axial cut below the transverse process of C1: the nodal targets are outlined in the contralateral (left) level II to ensure coverage of the jugulodigastric (subdigastric) nodes (see case study 1 for figures 2–4).

To include a neck region in the CTV, we consider that a 10% or higher risk of metastatic involvement justifies treatment. The factors affecting this risk should be taken into account for each case: tumor stage, size, thickness (3 mm or more is associated with a high metastatic risk for oral cavity tumors), differentiation, keratinization status, lymphatic vessel invasion in the tumor specimen, and whether other neck levels are involved [12].

Defining the CTV in the Neck

In defining the CTVs for head and neck cancer IMRT, the following node regions or levels (fig. 1) should be included. While these general concepts are broadly useful, specific approaches for individual tumor sites are described in detail elsewhere [23].

(1) Contralateral nodes: for cases of lateralized cancer where only the ipsilateral neck would ordinarily require therapy (small tonsillar cancers, and retromolar trigone and buccal mucosa cancers). Contralateral neck treatment is always added to the CTV when the ipsilateral neck involvement is greater than N1.

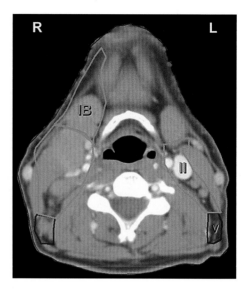

Fig. 4. Targets outlined at the mid neck. Level IB is outlined as a target in the ipsilateral (right) neck, due to the gross involvement of level II nodes, but not in the contralateral, clinically noninvolved neck.

(2) Level II nodes: level II is the most frequent nodal metastatic site for tumors in all mucosal sites. This level can be divided into the subdigastric (jugulodigastric) nodes, located below the level at which the posterior belly of the digastric muscle crosses the jugular vein, and more cranially located nodes below the base of skull ('junctional' nodes in Rouvière's [13] terminology). The subdigastric nodes are the main nodes involved when contralateral metastases occur, while the more cephalad nodes are at risk bilaterally in cases of nasopharyngeal cancer and in the neck side that contains other level II–III metastases [23] (fig. 2, 3).

(3) Level IB and IV nodes: levels IB and IV are treated in all cases in the neck side with clinical involvement of levels II or III (fig. 4).

(4) Level V nodes: level V is treated in the neck side with significant (>N1) involvement of levels II–IV, in all cases.

(5) RP nodes: the RP nodes are treated bilaterally in all cases of oropharyngeal and hypopharyngeal cancer with clinical involvement of levels II–IV (in cases of early lateralized oropharyngeal tumors with small N1 disease, treat ipsilaterally).

(6) Level VI nodes: level VI nodes are treated in all cases with clinical involvement of level IV nodes.

Target Doses

The current policy at this institute is to deliver 70 Gy to the GTV in 35 fractions (2 Gy per fraction). The high-risk CTV, which is around the GTV and the first echelon nodes, receives 63 Gy (in 1.8-Gy fractions, biologically equivalent to

60 Gy at 2.0 Gy per fraction). The lower-risk areas receive 60 Gy (1.7 Gy per fraction, biologically equivalent to 54 Gy at 2.0 Gy per fraction). These specifications are very similar to the policies at UCSF [37], Washington University [36], University of Iowa [35] and the RTOG in the nasopharyngeal protocol [38].

Lessons from Marginal Recurrences

To better understand the validity of the IMRT target delineations used at this center and others, a series of 133 patients treated for head and neck cancer were studied. If local-regional failure occurred after treatment (21 cases), the sites of failure were carefully examined (especially near the base of skull) in relation to the IMRT targets that were used for each case [25, 26]. All patients had nonnasopharyngeal head and neck squamous cell carcinomas and underwent courses of curative, parotid-sparing IMRT.

Initial Neck Treatment

For the initial treatment course, the delineation of the superiormost extent of the nodal targets was consistent, and corresponded to Rouvière's [13] observations.

Contralateral: in all patients in this study, the contralateral neck was clinically node negative but was judged to be at a high risk of subclinical disease and therefore treated. The uppermost level II nodal target was the subdigastric node group. To assure its coverage, the uppermost CTV was delineated at the axial CT image, in which the posterior belly of the digastric muscle crossed the jugular vein.

Ipsilateral: in the ipsilateral neck, which was node positive in most patients, the uppermost level II CTV was delineated through the base of the skull (fig. 2, 3). The uppermost RP nodal target was delineated at the level of the top of the C1 vertebral body, accommodating Rouvière's [13] description of the location of the lateral RP nodes.

The dose prescription was 70 Gy for the primary planning target volume, 64 and 60 Gy for the planning target volumes of the postoperative surgical beds with and without extracapsular extension, respectively, and 50–54 Gy for the planning target volumes of nonoperated subclinical disease, at 1.8–2.0 Gy per fraction.

Assessment of Tumor Recurrence

For every patient with recurrence, the volume of recurrence on CT scan was outlined and registered to the original planning CT, to evaluate the doses that were delivered to these sites of recurrence [25, 26]. Marginal recurrence was defined as occurring when only 20–95% of the recurrence volume had received >95% of the prescribed dose. In-field recurrence required that at least 95% of the recurrence volume had received >95% of the prescribed dose.

At a median follow-up period of 32 months, 21 of the 133 patients (16%) had local-regional recurrences; 17 were in-field and 4 were marginal. Details about the marginal recurrences are provided below.

Analyses of Marginal Recurrences and Conclusions for IMRT Treatment Volumes

Patient 1 and 2

Two of the marginal recurrences occurred near the base of skull, corresponding to the lateral RP nodes. Both patients had oropharyngeal cancer (one tonsillar and one base of tongue), and presented with N0 necks. In each case, the RP nodes had been defined as targets, and the cranialmost extent of the CTV was delineated at the top of C1. However, the epicenter of the recurrence volume of the two marginal RP recurrences lay cranial to the top of C1. One of these recurrences was in the ipsilateral lateral RP nodes, and the other was at the contralateral base of skull and was extensive.

Commentary: the lateral RP nodes were described by Rouvière [13] as lying medial to the carotid artery, from the top of C1 superiorly to C3 inferiorly. Details in the literature about the pattern of metastases to the RP nodes in nonnasopharyngeal cancer are scant. These nodes are not routinely dissected in surgical series, and most radiological series describing RP nodal involvement concentrate on nasopharyngeal cancer [27]. Existing surgical series assessing the incidence of RP nodal involvement in head and neck cancer report a very low rate of involvement in cases with N0 neck, apart from nasopharyngeal or pharyngeal wall cancer [27, 28]. Finally, in IMRT of nasopharyngeal cancer, these nodes are usually included in the GTV or the CTV of the primary tumor that extends cranially to the base of the skull.

In IMRT of nonnasopharyngeal cancer, there is a need for a conscientious effort to determine first, whether these nodes should be included as targets, and second, how to delineate them. Until more comprehensive information is available, and given the recurrences we have observed, we recommend the inclusion of the lateral RP nodes as targets in all cases of locally advanced oropharyngeal cancer, whether or not there is evidence of involvement of other neck levels.

How should the RP nodal targets be delineated? The findings of RP nodal recurrences whose epicenters were cranial to the top of C1 were unexpected, in view of Rouvière's [13] description that the lateral RP nodes lay in front of C1. Our results suggest that in cases that are at risk of RP nodal metastases, these targets should extend more cranially than the top of C1, from the level of the upper naso-pharynx to the base of skull. This is consistent with the recent consensus guidelines [29] (fig. 2, 3).

A literature search yielded three surgical series of RP nodal dissection in which the laterality of the RP nodal disease relative to the primary cancer was detailed. Hasegawa and Matsuura [30] reported two patients with RP recurrences contralateral to the primary tumor; one had ipsilateral RP nodal metastases at initial presentation and one did not. Ballantyne [31] reported one patient who recurred in the contralateral RP nodes following dissection of involved ipsilateral RP nodes. Amatsu et al. [32] reported 16 patients with RP nodal involvement, of whom 4 had bilateral, 9 had ipsilateral, and 3 had contralateral involvement alone. Thus, the pattern of failure reported in the surgical literature and in our series suggests that in patients with lateral primary tumors who are at a high risk of RP nodal involvement, both the ipsilateral and the contralateral nodes should be included in the RP nodal target.

Patient 3

The third recurrence in our series was in a patient with tongue cancer who had significant involvement of the low neck. After irradiation, the patient achieved complete response and later recurred in level VI.

Commentary: this recurrence highlights the risk of recurrence at any neck level when adjoining levels are involved. If lymphatic flow obstruction occurs due to metastases, retrograde lymphatic flow may result [33]. Connections from the pretracheal/prelaryngeal nodes (level VI) to the jugular nodes (levels III–IV) have been described by Rouvière [13]. These connections, in tandem with flow obstruction at level IV, explain this marginal recurrence at level VI.

Patient 4

The fourth marginal recurrence was observed in a patient who had had a neck dissection more than a year prior to recurrence of an oral cavity cancer, then treated with local excision and IMRT. He recurred again in an unpredicted anatomic site: the subcutaneous tissues of contralateral level I.

Commentary: this marginal recurrence demonstrates the effect of collateral lymphatics, which have been demonstrated to fully develop one or more years after surgery and to extend to unpredictable neck sites [13]. These collaterals develop in the submental and submandibular areas, including subdermal tissues. We currently exclude from IMRT patients who have had major neck surgery more than 1 year previously, due to the uncertainty regarding their targets.

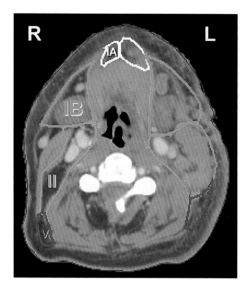

Fig. 5. Grossly involved level IA (submental) nodes on the left demonstrate the extent of the CTV (subclinical) outlining of level IA on the right (see case study 2 for this figure and next).

Additional Cases Reported in the Literature

Several head and neck cancer IMRT series have recently been published. In a series by de Arruda et al. [34], 50 patients with cancer of the oropharynx were treated with IMRT. In this series, they describe one marginal recurrence of a patient with a T4N0 base of tongue cancer. This patient had persistent disease following irradiation and therefore had right mandibulectomy and right neck dissection with 40 negative lymph nodes, 6 months after RT. One year later, he recurred in a submental node, demonstrating aberrant lymphatic drainage after neck dissection.

In a series by Yao et al. [35], the outcomes of 150 patients treated with IMRT for squamous cell carcinoma of the head and neck are detailed; no marginal failures have been observed so far, with a median follow-up of only 17 months. Chao et al. [36] reported the outcomes of 126 head and neck cancer patients treated with IMRT, which was used only in the upper neck to spare the salivary function. The lower neck was treated with a conventional AP low neck port abutted to the inferior IMRT dose distribution border. Five patients had recurrence in the supraclavicular area (28% of recurrences). This demonstrates the importance of contouring the regional lymph nodes in the low neck in cases where they are at high risk, such as cases with significant nodal involvement of the high neck, and delivering radiation to that area with appropriate dose and energy. Preferably, the low neck targets should be included in the IMRT treatment plan when they are at high risk of metastases.

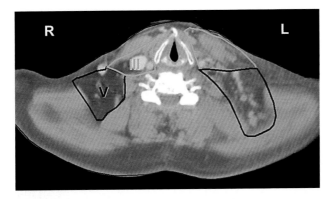

Fig. 6. Level V is involved bilaterally in a case of nasopharyngeal cancer. Note the posterior extent of the lymphadenopathy on the left. An anterior-posterior low-neck field prescribed to 3 cm depth would have underdosed the deepest nodes of level V. In cases with a high risk of low neck involvement, we prefer to include the low neck in the IMRT plan in order to avoid underdosage.

Summary Recommendations for Head and Neck IMRT Based on Marginal Recurrence Analyses

In summary, these analyses of marginal recurrences suggest the following additional recommendations for target volume delineation in IMRT, and augment those already understood.

(1) Lateral RP nodes should be included as targets in all cases of locally advanced oropharyngeal cancer, whether or not there is evidence of involvement of other neck levels.

(2) In cases that are at risk of RP nodal metastases, these targets should extend more cranially than the top of C1, from the level of the upper nasopharynx to the base of skull.

(3) In patients with lateral primary tumors that are at high risk of RP nodal involvement, both the ipsilateral and the contralateral nodes should be included in the RP nodal target.

(4) Patients who have had major neck surgery more than 1 year previously should be excluded from IMRT, due to the uncertainty regarding their targets.

(5) It is important to contour the regional lymph nodes in the low neck when they are at high risk, such as cases with significant nodal involvement of the high neck, and to deliver irradiation to the low neck with appropriate dose coverage. Preferably, the low neck targets should be included in the IMRT treatment plan in these cases.

Case Studies

Case 1

Patient. A 57-year-old male with stage T2 N2B M0 carcinoma of the right tonsil.

Treatment. IMRT concurrent with chemotherapy. Doses were 70 Gy to CTV1, 64 Gy to CTV2 and 60 Gy to CTV3. In the upper neck, CTV2 extended to the base of skull ipsilaterally and included level II and RP nodes (fig. 2). On the contralateral side of the neck (L), level II extended only to the level in which the jugular vein bisected the posterior belly of the digastric muscle (just below the transverse process of C1), to ensure coverage of the jugulodigastric nodes (fig. 3). At low level II on the right, an enlarged lymph node was observed with gross extracapsular invasion into the sternocleidomastoid muscle (fig. 4). Level II therefore was out-lined with generous margins into the surrounding tissues and the muscle. In contrast, the contralateral level was outlined to include just the fatty tissue harboring level II nodes. Also, level IB was included in the CTV on the right due to level II gross involvement, and was not included in the left CTV, the side that was node negative.

Result. This patient is currently free of disease.

Case 2

Patient. A 37-year-old female with stage T2 N2c M0 squamous cell carcinoma of the naso-pharynx.

Treatment. IMRT concurrent with chemotherapy. Doses were similar to case 1. Figure 5 shows grossly involved nodes in levels Ia, Ib, and II on the left. Note the difference in the out-lining of level II on the left compared with the clinically noninvolved level II on the right. Levels Ia–V were outlined as targets bilaterally. Figure 6 shows grossly involved levels III–IV and low level V (level VB) on the left. Note the depth in tissue in which the involved nodes are observed.

Result. This patient achieved local-regional disease control but failed with lung metas-tases.

Guidelines for Clinical Practice

For Gross Tumor Volume Delineation/Treatment
Lymph nodes are included in the gross tumor volume (GTV) if they have the following radiologic criteria:

- diameter >1 cm (or in the case of the jugulodigastric nodes, >1.1–1.5 cm);

- smaller than 1 cm with spherical rather than ellipsoidal shape;

- contain inhomogeneities suggestive of necrotic centers;

- cluster of 3 or more borderline nodes;

- FDG-PET positive.

For Clinical Target Volume Delineation/Treatment
- Contralateral nodes: for cases of lateralized cancer where only the ipsilateral neck would ordinarily require therapy (small tonsillar cancers, and retromolar trigone and buccal mucosa cancers). Contralateral neck treatment is always added to the clinical target vol-ume (CTV) when the ipsilateral neck involvement is greater than N1.

- Level II nodes: level II neck nodes are the most frequent metastatic site for tumors in all mucosal sites. These nodes can be divided into the subdigastric (jugulodigastric) nodes, located below the level at which the posterior belly of the digastric muscle crosses the jugular vein, and more cranially located nodes below the base of skull ('junctional' nodes in Rouvière's terminology). The subdigastric nodes are the main nodes involved when contralateral metastases occur, while the more cephalad nodes are at risk bilaterally in cases of nasopharyngeal cancer and in the neck side that contains other level II–III metastases.

- Level IB and IV nodes: levels IB and IV are treated in all cases in the neck side with clinical involvement of levels II or III.

- Level V nodes: level V is treated in the neck side with significant (>N1) involvement of levels II–IV, in all cases.

- Retropharyngeal nodes: the retropharyngeal nodes are treated bilaterally in all cases of oropharyngeal and hypopharyngeal cancer with clinical involvement of levels II–IV (in cases of early lateralized oropharyngeal tumors with small N1 disease, treat ipsilaterally).

- Level VI nodes: level VI nodes are treated in all cases with clinical involvement of level IV nodes.

For Dose Prescription
- GTV: the current policy at this institute is to deliver 70 Gy to the GTV in 35 fractions (2 Gy per fraction).

- High-risk CTV: the high-risk CTV, which is around the GTV and the first echelon nodes, receives 63 Gy (in 1.8-Gy fractions, biologically equivalent to 60 Gy at 2.0 Gy per fraction).

- Low-risk CTV: the lower-risk areas receive 60 Gy (1.7 Gy per fraction, biologically equivalent to 54 Gy at 2.0 Gy per fraction).

References

1 Eisbruch A, Kim HM, Terrell JE, Marsh LH, Dawson LA, Ship JA: Xerostomia and its predictors following parotid-sparing irradiation of head-and-neck cancer. Int J Radiat Oncol Biol Phys 2001;50:695–704.

2 Lin A, Kim HM, Terrell JE, Dawson LA, Ship JA, Eisbruch A: Quality of life after parotid-sparing IMRT for head-and-neck cancer: a prospective longitudinal study. Int J Radiat Oncol Biol Phys 2003;57:61–70.

3 Eisbruch A, Schwartz M, Rasch C, et al: Dysphagia and aspiration after chemoradiotherapy for head-and-neck cancer: which anatomic structures are affected and can they be spared by IMRT? Int J Radiat Oncol Biol Phys 2004;60: 1425–1439.

4 Fung K, Lyden TH, Lee J, et al: Voice and swallowing outcomes of an organ-preservation trial for advanced laryngeal cancer. Int J Radiat Oncol Biol Phys 2005;63:1395–1399.

5 Som PM: The present controversy over the imaging method of choice for evaluating the soft tissues of the neck. AJNR Am J Neuroradiol 1997; 18:1869–1872.

6 Schechter NR, Gillenwater AM, Byers RM, et al: Can positron emission tomography improve the quality of care for head-and-neck cancer patients? Int J Radiat Oncol Biol Phys 2001;51:4–9.

7 Daisne JF, Duprez T, Weynand B, et al: Tumor volume in pharyngolaryngeal squamous cell carcinoma: comparison at CT, MR imaging, and FDG PET and validation with surgical specimen. Radiology 2004;233:93–100.

8 Kubota K, Yokoyama J, Yamaguchi K, et al: FDG-PET delayed imaging for the detection of head and neck cancer recurrence after radio-chemotherapy: comparison with MRI/CT. Eur J Nucl Med Mol Imaging 2004;31:590–595.

9 Anzai Y, Minoshima S, Wolf GT, Wahl RL: Head and neck cancer: detection of recurrence with three-dimensional principal components analysis at dynamic FDG PET. Radiology 1999;212: 285–290.

10 Lapela M, Grenman R, Kurki T, et al: Head and neck cancer: detection of recurrence with PET and 2-[F-18]fluoro-2-deoxy-D-glucose. Radiology 1995;197:205–211.

11 van den Brekel MW, Stel HV, Castelijns JA, et al: Cervical lymph node metastasis: assessment of radiologic criteria. Radiology 1990;177:379–384.

12 Eisbruch A, Foote RL, O'Sullivan B, Beitler JJ, Vikram B: Intensity-modulated radiation therapy for head and neck cancer: emphasis on the selection and delineation of the targets. Semin Radiat Oncol 2002;12:238–249.

13 Rouvière H: Lymphatic System of the Head and Neck (translated by Tobias M). Ann Arbor, Edward Brothers, 1938.

14 Mukherji SK, Armao D, Joshi VM: Cervical nodal metastases in squamous cell carcinoma of the head and neck: what to expect. Head Neck 2001; 23:995–1005.

15 Lindberg R: Distribution of cervical lymph node metastases from squamous cell carcinoma of the upper respiratory and digestive tracts. Cancer 1972;29:1446–1449.

16 Byers RM, Wolf PF, Ballantyne AJ: Rationale for elective modified neck dissection. Head Neck Surg 1988;10:160–167.

17 Candela FC, Shah J, Jaques DP, Shah JP: Patterns of cervical node metastases from squamous carcinoma of the larynx. Arch Otolaryngol Head Neck Surg 1990;116:432–435.

18 Robbins KT, Medina JE, Wolfe GT, Levine PA, Sessions RB, Pruet CW: Standardizing neck dissection terminology. Official report of the Academy's Committee for Head and Neck Surgery and Oncology. Arch Otolaryngol Head Neck Surg 1991;117:601–605.

19 Robbins KT: Integrating radiological criteria into the classification of cervical lymph node disease. Arch Otolaryngol Head Neck Surg 1999;125: 385–387.

20 Som PM, Curtin HD, Mancuso AA: An imaging-based classification for the cervical nodes designed as an adjunct to recent clinically based nodal classifications. Arch Otolaryngol Head Neck Surg 1999;125:388–396.

21 Gregoire V, Coche E, Cosnard G, Hamoir M, Reychler H: Selection and delineation of lymph node target volumes in head and neck conformal radiotherapy. Proposal for standardizing terminology and procedure based on the surgical experience. Radiother Oncol 2000;56:135–150.

22 Nowak PJ, Wijers OB, Lagerwaard FJ, Levendag PC: A three-dimensional CT-based target definition for elective irradiation of the neck. Int J Radiat Oncol Biol Phys 1999;45:33–39.

23 Wijers OB, Levendag PC, Tan T, et al: A simplified CT-based definition of the lymph node levels in the node negative neck. Radiother Oncol 1999; 52:35–42.

24 Million RR CN: Management of Head and Neck Cancer: A Multidisciplinary Approach, ed 2. Philadelphia, Lippincott, 1994.

25 Eisbruch A, Marsh LH, Dawson LA, et al: Recurrences near base of skull after IMRT for head-and-neck cancer: implications for target delineation in high neck and for parotid gland sparing. Int J Radiat Oncol Biol Phys 2004;59:28–42.

26 Dawson LA, Anzai Y, Marsh L, et al: Patterns of local-regional recurrence following parotid-sparing conformal and segmental intensity-modulated radiotherapy for head and neck cancer. Int J Radiat Oncol Biol Phys 2000;46:1117–1126.

27 King AD, Ahuja AT, Leung SF, et al: Neck node metastases from nasopharyngeal carcinoma: MR imaging of patterns of disease. Head Neck 2000; 22:275–281.

28 McLaughlin MP, Mendenhall WM, Mancuso AA, et al: Retropharyngeal adenopathy as a predictor of outcome in squamous cell carcinoma of the head and neck. Head Neck 1995;17:190–198.

29 http://www.rtog.org/hnatlas/main.html.

30 Hasegawa Y, Matsuura H: Retropharyngeal node dissection in cancer of the oropharynx and hypopharynx. Head Neck 1994;16:173–180.

31 Ballantyne AJ: Significance of retropharyngeal nodes in cancer of the head and neck. Am J Surg 1964;108:500–504.

Ben David · Eisbruch

32 Amatsu M, Mohri M, Kinishi M: Significance of retropharyngeal node dissection at radical surgery for carcinoma of the hypopharynx and cervical esophagus. Laryngoscope 2001;111:1099–1103.

33 Fisch U: Lymphography of the Cervical Lymphatic System, Philadelphia, Saunders, 1968.

34 de Arruda FF, Puri DR, Zhung J, et al: Intensity-modulated radiation therapy for the treatment of oropharyngeal carcinoma: the Memorial Sloan-Kettering Cancer Center experience. Int J Radiat Oncol Biol Phys 2006;64:363–373.

35 Yao M, Dornfeld KJ, Buatti JM, et al: Intensity-modulated radiation treatment for head-and-neck squamous cell carcinoma – the University of Iowa experience. Int J Radiat Oncol Biol Phys 2005;63:410–421.

36 Chao KS, Ozyigit G, Tran BN, Cengiz M, Dempsey JF, Low DA: Patterns of failure in patients receiving definitive and postoperative IMRT for head-and-neck cancer. Int J Radiat Oncol Biol Phys 2003;55:312–321.

37 Lee N, Xia P, Fischbein NJ, Akazawa P, Akazawa C, Quivey JM: Intensity-modulated radiation therapy for head-and-neck cancer: the UCSF experience focusing on target volume delineation. Int J Radiat Oncol Biol Phys 2003;57:49–60.

38 http://www.rtog.org/members/protocols/0225/0225.pdf.

Avraham Eisbruch, MD
Department of Radiation Oncology
University of Michigan
Ann Arbor, MI 48105 (USA)
Tel. +1 734 936 9337, Fax +1 734 763 7370
E-Mail eisbruch@umich.edu

Meyer JL (ed): IMRT, IGRT, SBRT – Advances in the Treatment Planning and
Delivery of Radiotherapy. Front Radiat Ther Oncol. Basel, Karger, 2007, vol. 40, pp 208–231

Nasopharyngeal and Oropharyngeal Carcinomas: Target Delineation, Therapy Delivery and Stereotactic Boost Procedures with Intensity-Modulated/Image-Guided Radiation Therapy

Quynh-Thu Le

Department of Radiation Oncology, Stanford University, Stanford, Calif., USA

Abstract

Radiation therapy is a key component of the multidisciplinary treatment of nasopharyngeal and oropharyngeal carcinomas, which are ideal tumors for intensity-modulated radiation therapy (IMRT) because of their location and intimate relationship to the surrounding critical structures. Several studies have suggested that IMRT is superior to conventional radiation therapy in salivary preservation and holds promise for improved locoregional control of these tumors. Target delineation for IMRT in these tumors is complex and requires detailed knowledge of head and neck anatomy and pathways of tumor spread. This article focuses on target delineation for IMRT for oropharyngeal and nasopharyngeal carcinomas. In addition, we also present data on the use of stereotactic radiotherapy as a boost to improve local control of nasopharyngeal carcinomas.

This paper focuses on target delineation for nasopharynx (NP) and oropharynx (OP) cancers and the use of stereotactic radiotherapy boost for locally advanced NP carcinomas. The first half will be devoted to the use of intensity-modulated radiation therapy (IMRT) and stereotactic radiotherapy boost in the management of patients with newly diagnosed NP cancer, and the second half will concentrate on the use of IMRT as a definitive treatment for OP carcinomas.

Parotid tolerance

- University of Michigan (parotid flow)
  Mean dose   26 Gy
  45% gland   30 Gy
- University of Hong Kong (parotid flow)
  Mean dose   38.8 Gy
  >70% patients recovered 25% parotid flow at 2 years
- Mallinckrodt Institute (whole saliva)
  16 Gy – 50% saliva flow reduction
  32 Gy – 75% saliva flow reduction
- Baylor (questionnaires ≥grade 2 xerostomia)
  21–26 Gy for ipsilateral parotid
  16–21 Gy for contralateral parotid

Fig. 1. A partial summary of the literature on parotid tolerance using different approaches of assessment.

Intensity-Modulated Radiation Therapy/Image-Guided Radiation Therapy for Head and Neck Cancers

Rationale

The rationale for using innovative radiotherapy approaches such as IMRT and image-guided radiation therapy for head and neck (HN) cancers is simply to enhance locoregional control by improving target delineation. These approaches allow us to deliver higher doses to the tumor while sparing normal tissues, thereby reducing late radiation-related complications such as xerostomia and its dental consequences. In addition, for tumors located near the skull base such as NP cancer, these approaches offer means to reduce the risk of long-term neural complications and pituitary dysfunction in treated patients.

The University of Michigan group, under the leadership of Dr. Eisbruch, has performed extensive analyses on parotid tolerance after treatment with either parotid-sparing three-dimensional conformal radiotherapy or IMRT [1–3]. Figure 1 lists a partial summary of the literature on parotid tolerance that was assessed by different functional endpoints at different institutions [3–6]. The endpoints included measured parotid and whole saliva flow, and xerostomia assessed by questionnaires. These data all suggest that above a certain threshold (approximately 25–30 Gy for the mean parotid dose or 30 Gy for the dose received by ≥50% of the parotid volume), xerostomia will become permanent. We have therefore adopted a policy at our institution of maintaining the mean dose <26 Gy to the contralateral parotids.

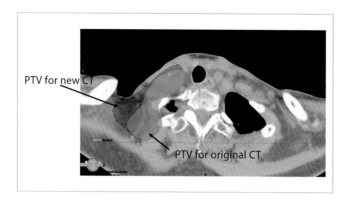

PTV for new CT

PTV for original CT

Fig. 2. The effect on nodal PTV from inadequate shoulder immobilization. The light-blue area denotes the PTV from the original treatment planning CT and the dark-blue area denotes the PTV from the new treatment planning CT.

Patient Setup

The standard thermoplastic mask provides adequate immobilization of the head; however, it does not provide sufficient immobilization of the shoulders, an important requirement when IMRT is used for comprehensive nodal irradiation. There are several home-fabricated and commercially available systems for shoulder immobilization. These include extended head and shoulder thermoplastic masks, various shoulder fixators, arm pullers, or pegboards with shoulder straps and 3-point tattoos.

Shown in figure 2 is an illustration of a significant change in the nodal planning target volume (PTV) due to poor shoulder immobilization. This particular NP cancer patient was initially set up with a slightly crooked body position for her initial treatment planning CT. On pretreatment verification, she was straightened and rescanned. When the 2 CT scans were superimposed at the isocenter level, a significant change in the PTV (light blue for the 1st scan and dark blue for the 2nd scan) was observed. The original PTV in light blue would have missed most of the inferior level V nodes, which are at risk for involvement in NP cancer. This illustrates the importance of adequate shoulder immobilization. In addition, the superior-inferior position of the shoulders can shift significantly from day to day without adequate immobilization and result in dose attenuation of the tangential fields, thereby compromising target coverage. Please see the article by Ben David and Eisbruch on neck node delineation [this vol., pp. 193–207] for an illustration of the neck node levels.

Daily setup variability has been quantified, primarily for treatment isocenters. Hong et al. [7] from the University of Wisconsin used an optically guided patient localization system to evaluate setup accuracy in 10 patients immobilized with thermoplastic masks and a baseplate fixation to the treatment couch. The details

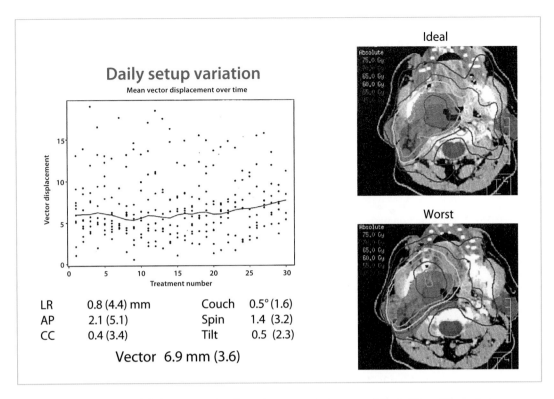

Daily setup variation

Mean vector displacement over time

LR	0.8 (4.4) mm	Couch	0.5° (1.6)
AP	2.1 (5.1)	Spin	1.4 (3.2)
CC	0.4 (3.4)	Tilt	0.5 (2.3)

Vector 6.9 mm (3.6)

Fig. 3. Quantitation of daily setup variability using an optical system. Adapted from Hong et al. [7].

of their findings are shown in figure 3. The mean setup error in any single dimension averaged 3.33 mm and the mean composite vector offset was 6.97 mm (standard deviation: 3.63 mm) when all 6 degrees of freedom were accounted for. These setup errors resulted in a decrease in the equivalent uniform dose of up to 21%. Several approaches are available to adjust interfraction patient setup variability. These include setup correction based on daily kilovoltage orthogonal or CT images.

Therapy Replanning

Another issue that needs to be addressed during fractionated IMRT for HN cancers is the observed changes in the tumor volume and the patient's anatomy over the 6–7 weeks of treatment. Often, there is rapid shrinkage in tumor and nodal volume, requiring IMRT replanning. In addition, patients can lose a significant amount of weight, causing poor fit of the initial immobilization system. Normal tissues such as parotid and submandibular glands also shrink during radiotherapy. Figure 4 shows the interfractional clinical target volume (CTV) and parotid volumes obtained from an HN cancer patient treated with IMRT at the

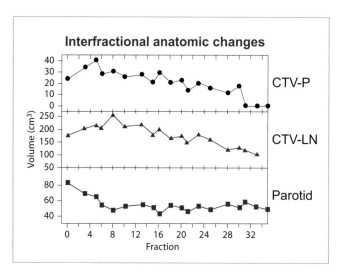

Fig. 4. Quantitation of interfractional anatomic changes, assessed by imaging at treatment using CT-on-rails. Adapted from Mohan et al. [8]. CTV-LN = Nodal clinical target volume; CTV-P = primary clinical target volume.

MD Anderson Cancer Center [8]. These volumetric changes can result in inadequate dose delivery when compared with the intended dose distribution generated from the initial treatment planning CT.

Several approaches have been proposed for on-line adaptive radiotherapy. These include:

(1) on-line near real-time IMRT replanning at daily to weekly intervals,

(2) deforming radiation intensities based on anatomic deformation seen on CT images acquired at daily to weekly intervals,

(3) generating a patient-specific confidence-limited PTV based on several initial CT scans, and correcting the planning only when the actual dose distribution is significantly different from the anticipated one.

Most of these approaches are time consuming, and it is unclear which approach will result in clinically superior treatment outcomes.

Intensity-Modulated Radiation Therapy for Nasopharyngeal Carcinomas

Target Volume Delineation
Figure 5 shows the recommended definitions for the different target volumes in NP cancer. HN MRI scans, specifically gadolinium-enhanced, fat-saturated T_1-weighted series with axial and coronal views, are critical for gross tumor volume (GTV) delineation. MRI is superior to CT scanning in defining tumor involve-

Target volume definition

- GTV: Gross tumor on CT/MRI and PET
- CTV: GTV + margin including
  nasopharynx, retropharyngeal nodes,
  clivus, skull base,
  inferior sphenoid sinus,
  pterygoid fossae,
  parapharyngeal space,
  posterior nasal cavity and maxillary sinuses
- PTV: CTV + 3–5 mm

Fig. 5. Recommended target volume definition for NP cancer.

ment of the parapharyngeal space, skull base, cavernous sinus and retropharyngeal nodes. For nodal volume delineation, treatment planning FDG-PET/CT scans can often be helpful. In rare occasions, one can see parotid nodal involvement in patients with locally advanced NP cancer (fig. 6); therefore, we do not recommend routine sparing of the ipsilateral parotids. In addition, as shown in figure 6, involvement of level V nodes is very common in NP cancer, and adequate coverage of level V in the nodal CTV is critical for NP cancer IMRT planning.

Although useful, FDG-PET scans can sometimes present false-positive findings. One of them is uptake in normal 'brown fat' in the low neck of young patients ($\leq$40 years of age). Figure 7 shows an example of a 35-year-old NP cancer patient with a large volume of brown fat. It shows a high level of FDG uptake on an initial PET scan, but pretreatment with Ativan reduced FDG uptake in the brown fat without compromising tumor uptake on a subsequent scan.

Figure 8a shows an example of a patient with a small T2A lesion with anterior extension into the nasal cavity. The GTV was delineated using merged images from the CT, MRI and PET. The CTV includes the posterior aspects of the nasal cavity, the maxillary sinuses, the pterygoid fossa with the pterygoid plates and the anterior half of the clivus. In patients who have more parapharyngeal space involvement as in T2B disease (fig. 8b), the CTV should include all of the pterygoid fossa and the lateral pterygoid muscle on the side of parapharyngeal space extension.

In patients with tumor involvement of the cavernous sinus and the prepontine cistern, as shown in figure 9a, the GTV needs to extend intracranially to cover all areas of gross disease. The CTV and PTV expansions can be rather small due to the close vicinity of the tumor to the temporal lobes laterally and the brainstem posteriorly. In this particular patient, we performed isocenter portal imaging daily before treatment in order to minimize the interfraction

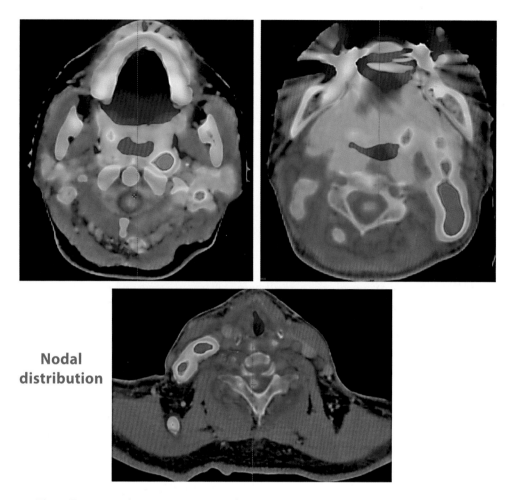

Nodal distribution

Fig. 6. Treatment planning PET-CT scan of an NP cancer patient showing different sites of nodal involvement including retropharyngeal nodes, intraparotid node and level 5 neck nodes.

setup errors. In a patient with skull base involvement (fig. 9b), the CTV should include most of the bone structures of the skull base as well as the entire clivus. The CTV dose is prescribed to ≥54 Gy. In patients without imaging evidence of the skull base or intracranial tumor involvement, the CTV generally encompasses the pterygopalatine fossae, sphenoid sinuses, part of the ethmoid and maxillary sinuses and the anterior half of the clivus (fig. 9c, d). We do not routinely cover the cavernous sinus, unless there is cranial nerve or skull base involvement, in order to achieve sparing of the temporal lobes. A 3–5-mm margin is routinely added to generate the PTV from our CTV and GTV, to account for daily setup variability. It is critical to consult your institutional radiologist for optimal target delineation.

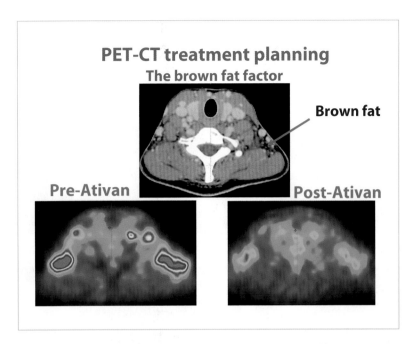

PET-CT treatment planning
The brown fat factor

Brown fat

Pre-Ativan

Post-Ativan

Fig. 7. False-positive FDG-PET findings due to the presence of brown fat in the supraclavicular fossa. Note CT did not show any obvious node. Pretreatment with Ativan resulted in decreased FDG uptake.

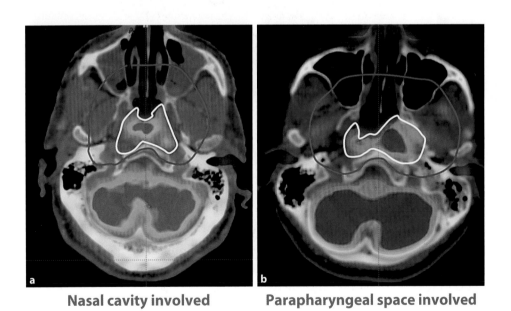

Nasal cavity involved

Parapharyngeal space involved

Fig. 8. GTV and CTV. **a** A T2a tumor with nasal cavity involvement. **b** A T2b tumor with left parapharyngeal space involvement; note more lateral extension on the left side. GTV = White line; CTV = red line.

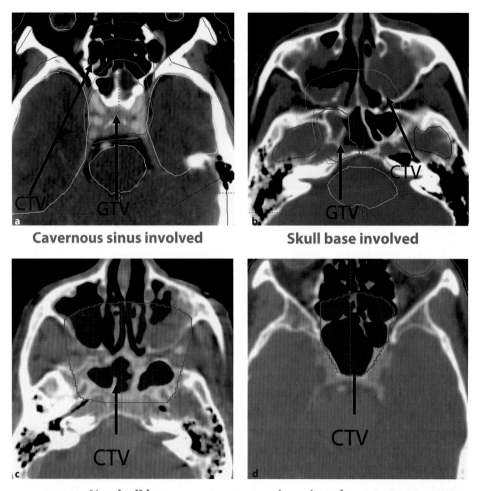

Fig. 9. Examples of GTV and CTV delineation. **a** A T4 tumor with bilateral cavernous sinus and prepontine cistern involvement. **b** A T3 tumor with skull base involvement. **c, d** A T2a tumor without either skull base or intracranial extension.

Dose Prescription

Figure 10 shows the different dose prescriptions that have been used for NP cancer. Most of these prescriptions employ a dose painting approach. For patients with large T2b–T4 tumors, the Stanford group employs a stereotactic radiotherapy boost to the area of residual disease (see below).

Bucci et al. [9] have recently updated the University of California San Francisco (UCSF) IMRT experience at the 2004 ASTRO annual meeting. Figure 11 shows an example of a treatment plan employed at the UCSF where IMRT was used to treat the tumor and upper neck nodes while a conventional anteropos-

Fig. 10. Different dose prescriptions for NP cancer. STR = Stereotactic radiotherapy. MSKCC = Memorial Sloan-Kettering Cancer Center.

UCSF IMRT technique

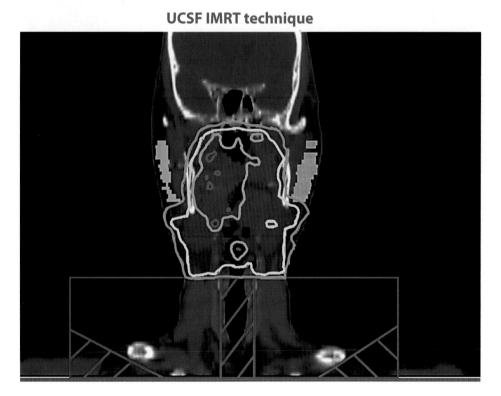

Fig. 11. Illustration of the technique used for treating NP cancer at the UCSF. IMRT is used to treat the primary tumor + upper neck nodes whereas a conventional supraclavicular field is used to treat the low neck nodes (adapted from Bucci et al. [9]).

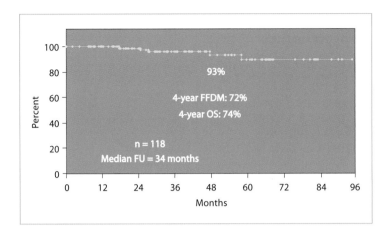

Fig. 12. Freedom from local relapse in 118 patients treated by IMRT for NP cancer at the UCSF (adapted from Bucci et al. [9]). FFDM = Freedom from distant metastases; OS = overall survival; FU = follow-up.

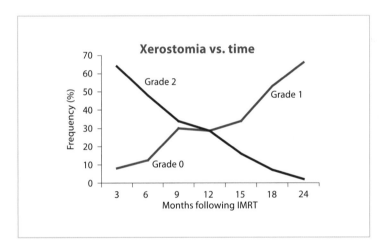

Fig. 13. Frequency of patients with grade 0–2 xerostomia over time after completion of IMRT for NP cancer (courtesy of Nancy Lee, MD).

terior supraclavicular field was used to treat the low neck nodes. The dose prescription is shown in figure 10. One hundred and eighteen patients were treated between 1995 and 2003, of which 74% had stage III/VI tumors, 90% received concomitant chemotherapy and 23% also had a high-dose-rate brachytherapy boost. The mean parotid dose was kept between 28 and 30 Gy.

Clinical Results for IMRT of NP Cancer
At a median follow-up period of 34 months, the 4-year local control rate in the UCSF experience was 93% and overall survival rate was 74% (fig. 12). The most

Le

common site of relapse was distant. Xerostomia evaluation in a subset of these patients revealed that the majority had grade 2 xerostomia at completion of radiotherapy but recovered to grade 0 or 1 at 2 years of follow-up (fig. 13) [10].

Figure 14 summarizes the IMRT experience for NP cancer from several institutions. Most of these data are preliminary and have only been reported in abstract form. Wolden et al. [11] reported on 50 NP cancer patients treated with IMRT and concurrent chemotherapy at the Memorial Sloan-Kettering Cancer Center. At a short follow-up period of less than 2 years, the local control rate was 94%. Data from the Prince of Wales Hospital are shown in figure 14b [12]. Intracavitary and conformal boosts were used routinely and 30% of the patients also received chemotherapy. At a median follow-up of 29 months, only 4 in-field failures were observed and the predominant site of relapse was distant. These results translated into a local relapse-free survival rate of 92% and an overall survival rate of 90% at 3 years. Only a quarter of the patients had grade 2 or greater xerostomia. Zhao et al. [13] (fig. 14c) presented data on 108 NP cancer patients treated with IMRT at Sun Yat-sen University at the 2004 ASTRO annual meeting. The GTV dose ranged from 64 to 70 Gy and 23% of the patients received chemotherapy. At a median follow-up of 19 months, the local control rate was 98% and the overall survival rate was 87%. Serial evaluation of parotid function with SPECT imaging in 32 patients showed that most have achieved improvement in xerostomia to grade 0–1.

Presently, there are several prospective studies evaluating the role of IMRT in NP cancer. At the Memorial Sloan-Kettering Cancer Center, patients with stage II–IV NP cancer are treated with dose painting IMRT concurrently with chemotherapy. The dose regimen is described in figure 10. The Radiation Therapy Oncology Group (RTOG) is conducting a phase II multi-institutional study (RTOG 0225) using 2.12 Gy per fraction to a total dose of 70 Gy. Patients with T-stage ≥2B or N+ node also receive concurrent and adjuvant chemotherapy.

Stereotactic Radiotherapy as a Boost for NP Cancer

The use of stereotactic radiotherapy as a boost for patients with locally advanced NP cancer at Stanford University was pioneered by Dr. D.R. Goffinet in 1992, prior to the IMRT era. It was first reported by Le et al. in 2003 [14] and recently updated by Hara et al. [15] at the 2005 American Radium Society annual meeting. The rationale for using stereotactic boost is to enhance local control, as the local recurrence rates in the prechemotherapy and IMRT eras were as high as 60%, depending on tumor stage. In addition, persistent skull base disease can result in significantly poor functional outcomes with a low salvage rate. Previous experiences using three-dimensional conformal radiotherapy and brachytherapy boost suggested that a dose-response relationship exists for NP cancer. Therefore, we performed this prospective study, evaluating the role of stereotactic radiotherapy in the management of patients with locally advanced NP tumors.

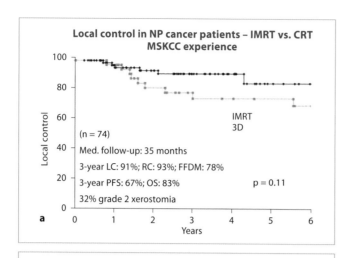

Local control in NP cancer patients – IMRT vs. CRT
MSKCC experience

(n = 74)
Med. follow-up: 35 months
3-year LC: 91%; RC: 93%; FFDM: 78%
3-year PFS: 67%; OS: 83%   p = 0.11
32% grade 2 xerostomia

a

Prince of Wales Hospital experience

- n = 63; III/IV: 57%; DMLC
- 66 GTV; 60 PTV; 54–60 for N0 neck
- Boost: IC for T1–T2a; conformal for T >2a
- 30% had chemotherapy
- Median follow-up: 29 months (8–45)
- Failure: 4 in-field, 1 regional, 13 distant
- 3-year LRFS 92%; DMFS 79%; OS 90%
- Grade 2–3 xerostomia at 2 years: 23%

b

Sun Yat-sen University experience

- n =106; III/IV: 50%
- Corvus 3.0 / MIMiC
- GTV: 64–70 Gy; CTV(I): 55–66 Gy; CTV(II): 42–54 Gy
- 23% had chemotherapy (CDDP/5FU)
- Median follow-up: 19 months
- 3-year LPF 98%; DM-free 98%; OS 87%

c

Fig. 14. Reported IMRT experience for NP cancer at the Memorial Sloan-Kettering Cancer Center (MSKCC) [11] (**a**), Prince of Wales Hospital [12] (**b**), and Sun Yat-sen University [13] (**c**). LC = Local control; RC = regional control; FFDM = freedom from distant metastases; PFS = progression-free survival; OS = overall survival; DMLC = dynamic multileaf collimator; IC = intracavitary; LRFS = local relapse-free survival; LPF = local progression-free survival; DMFS or DM-free = distant metastasis-free survival.

From September 1992 to September 2004, we treated 65 patients using this approach. Figure 15a shows the patient distribution by age, gender, ethnicity and WHO histology; figure 15b shows the treatment characteristics and figure 15c the staging distribution. The fractionated external beam dose was 66 Gy, delivered using a conventional approach in 45 patients and with IMRT in 20 patients. For the stereotaxis, two thirds were treated via a frame-based approach and one third via a frameless approach with the Cyberknife. Figure 16a shows an example of a Cyberknife boost plan for a patient with an initial T2b tumor, where a 12-Gy dose was prescribed to the 80% isodose line, covering the entire NP and area of residual tumor. Figure 16b shows another plan for a patient with T4b tumor with skull base involvement and intracranial extension. The patient received 8 Gy to the area of persistent abnormality on MRI; the prescribed dose was lowered to meet the dose constraint to the optic chiasm and the brainstem. Overall, the most commonly prescribed dose was 8–12 Gy and the median prescribed isodose line was 79%. Chemotherapy was used in 82% of the patients. Stereotactic therapy was generally delivered approximately 2–3 weeks after completion of fractionated external beam radiotherapy, before the first cycle of adjuvant chemotherapy.

With a median follow-up period of 45 months, only one local relapse has been observed and the 4-year Kaplan-Meier estimate of local control is 97.5% (fig. 17a). The predominant pattern of relapse was distant despite the frequent use of systemic chemotherapy (fig. 17b). The 4-year overall survival was 80% (fig. 17c).

In terms of late toxicity, there were 3 patients with asymptomatic temporal lobe necrosis (an example is shown in fig. 18a), 1 patient with carotid aneurysm in the face of hypertension (fig. 18b), 4 patients with transient cranial nerve paresis, 2 patients with permanent V2 and V3 numbness and 1 diabetic patient with retinopathy. Given the excellent control rates and some incidence of temporal lobe necrosis, we have decreased the stereotactic boost dose to 8 Gy.

Intensity-Modulated Radiation Therapy for Oropharyngeal Carcinomas

Target Volume Delineation
For OP carcinoma, treatment planning is routinely performed using contrast-enhanced CT scans. Whenever possible, a recent MRI or PET scan may be merged with the CT to aid target delineation. We have found that the PET scan is primarily useful for localizing the tumor and involved nodes, but not for exact volume delineation as the FDG-avid volume is highly sensitive to the window/level or threshold settings used.

Stanford experience
Patient characteristics

- n (period) — 65 patients (9/92–9/04)
- Mean age (range) — 44.6 (14–80)
- Male/female — 48/17
- Ethnicity Asian — 44 (67%)
  - Caucasian — 18 (28%)
  - Other — 3 (5%)
- WHO grade 3 — 32 (49%)
  - 2 — 25 (38%)
  - 1 — 7 (11%)
  - Mixed — 1 (2%)

a

Stanford experience
Treatment characteristics

- EBRT — 66 Gy (20 patients IMRT)
- SRS Frame based — 43 (66%)
  - Frameless — 22 (34%)
- SRS dose 7–<10 Gy — 11 (17%)
  - 10–12 Gy — 45 (69%)
  - >12 Gy — 9 (14%)
- Chemotherapy — 53 (82%)
- Median isodose line — 79% (range: 54–95%)

b

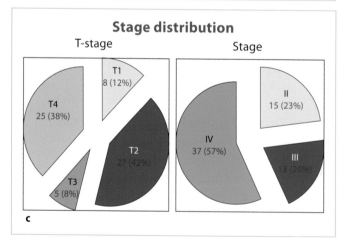

Stage distribution

T-stage — T1 8 (12%); T4 25 (38%); T3 5 (8%); T2 27 (42%)

Stage — II 15 (23%); IV 37 (57%); III 13 (20%)

c

Fig. 15. Stanford experience with stereotactic boost (SRS) for patients with locally advanced NP cancer. EBRT = External beam radiotherapy. **a** Patient characteristics. **b** Treatment characteristics. **c** Staging distribution.

Le

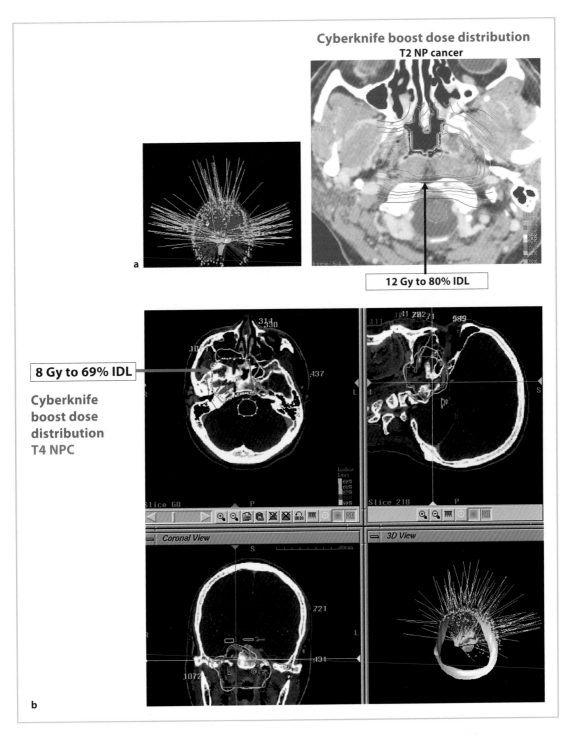

Cyberknife boost dose distribution
T2 NP cancer

12 Gy to 80% IDL

8 Gy to 69% IDL

Cyberknife
boost dose
distribution
T4 NPC

Fig. 16. Examples of stereotactic boost plans in NP cancer patients. **a** A patient with a T2b tumor receiving 12 Gy prescribed to the 80% isodose line (IDL). **b** A patient with a T4 tumor receiving 8 Gy to the 69% isodose line.

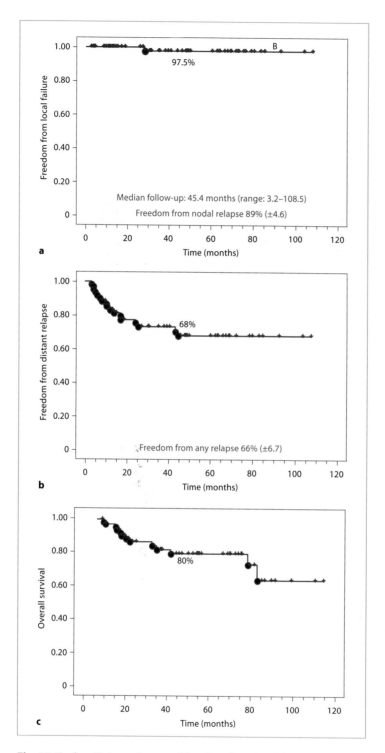

Fig. 17. Kaplan-Meier estimates of freedom from local failure (**a**), freedom from distant relapse (**b**), and overall survival in these 65 patients (**c**). The 4-year estimates are shown on the curves.

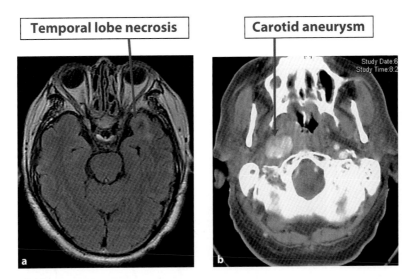

Temporal lobe necrosis **Carotid aneurysm**

Fig. 18. a Representative MRI axial image showing evidence of temporal lobe necrosis in an NP cancer patient with a previous T4 tumor. The patient is completely asymptomatic and continues to work full-time as an engineer. **b** CT scan showing a carotid aneurysm requiring coiling in a patient with T2b tumor previously treated with stereotactic boost.

Dose Prescription

The prescription schemes for OP cancer are similar to those used for NP cancer. To account for organ motion and patient setup errors, we routinely add a 3- to 5-mm margin to the GTV to generate a PTV66 (66 Gy at 2.2 Gy/fraction). In addition, for base of tongue and vallecular tumors, the entire base of tongue and vallecula are contoured in the PTV60, to ensure that these structures receive at least 60 Gy delivered at 2 Gy/fraction. Similarly, for tonsil and soft palate tumors, the entire tonsillar fossa (from the pterygoid plate insertion to the pharyngoepiglottic fold) or the entire soft palate is contoured in the PTV60. The PTV54 encompasses the clinically negative neck, which includes bilateral retropharyngeal nodes and level II–V nodes. In cases where there is level II nodal involvement, level IB nodes are also included in PTV54.

Figure 19 shows a patient with vallecular carcinoma. Note that the bilateral retropharyngeal nodes were included for treatment in this patient with bilateral nodal involvement and a history of neck surgery from an endarterectomy. In order to generate a more homogenous dose distribution for the PTV54, which is usually rather large in NP and OP carcinomas (from the skull base to the clavicle), we routinely split it into 2 different PTVs as shown in figure 20 (PTV54-1 in orange and PTV54-2 in green). Treatment plans are optimized such that >95% of PTV54-1 receives at least 54 Gy and >95% of PTV54-2 receives at least 52 Gy.

Contouring example: vallecular carcinoma

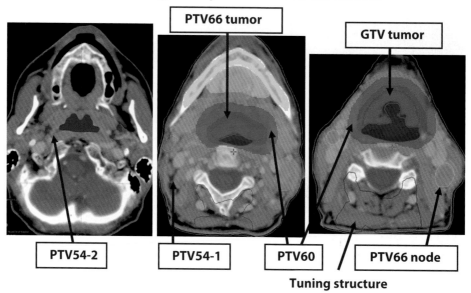

PTV66 tumor

GTV tumor

PTV54-2

PTV54-1

PTV60

PTV66 node

Tuning structure

Fig. 19. Axial images showing contour for PTV54-1, PTV54-2, PTV66 tumor, PTV66 node, PTV60 and the tuning structure. Note PTV54 was broken up in to 2 smaller volumes for treatment optimization.

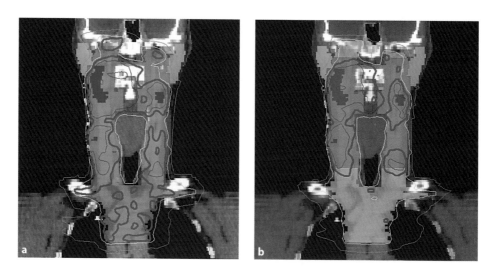

Fig. 20. Coronal slice showing the importance of separating the PTV into two parts to improve dose homogeneity. **a** The PTV contoured as one structure (in red) with the 60-Gy isodose curve (in red) extending superiorly into the skull base and inferiorly into the mediastinum. **b** The PTV divided into two separate structures (red and green) and a subsequent reduction in the 60-Gy isodose curve superiorly and inferiorly.

Le

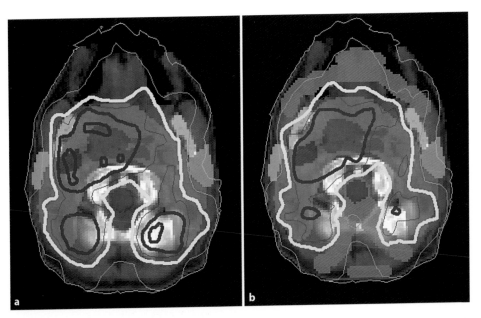

Fig. 21. Tuning structure for improving the dose distribution conformality. **a** The plan was optimized without a tuning structure. **b** The plan was optimized with a tuning structure posteriorly (in light purple). The same dose constraints were used for both cases. Dark blue: 73 Gy, purple: 66 Gy, red: 60 Gy, yellow: 54 Gy, green: 40 Gy, and light blue: 20 Gy. Note the reduction of the high-dose region posteriorly.

A useful tool for IMRT treatment planning is to create a hypothetical tissue structure, called a tuning structure, to help to conform the dose to the target. Figures 21 shows the IMRT dose distributions for a T2N2c tonsil carcinoma without or with the tuning structure placed posteriorly adjacent to the PTV. Note the improvement in the dose distribution with smaller hot spots posteriorly.

Clinical Results for IMRT of OP Cancer

IMRT results for OP carcinomas are not as mature as for NP tumors. De Arruda et al. [16] have recently published the Memorial Sloan-Kettering Cancer Center experience on IMRT for 50 patients with OP cancers. Eighty-six percent had concurrent chemotherapy. At a median follow-up of 18 months, the 2-year estimates of local progression-free, regional progression-free, distant metastasis-free and overall survival rates were 98, 88, 84 and 98%, respectively. Among the patients with greater than 9 months of follow-up, only 33% had grade 2 xerostomia (fig. 22). Esophageal stricture was noted in 3 patients.

Chao et al. [17] published on 74 patients treated with IMRT for OP carcinomas. Figure 23 summarizes their experience. At a median follow-up of 33 months, there

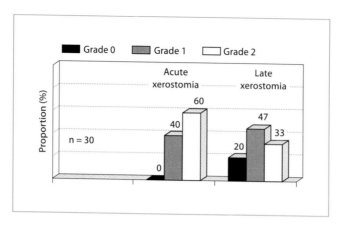

Fig. 22. Frequency of grade 0–2 xerostomia among patients with at least 9 months' follow-up after IMRT (adapted from de Arruda et al. [16]).

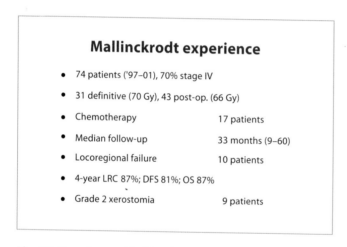

Fig. 23. Experience with IMRT for OP carcinoma at the Mallinckrodt Institute. Adapted from Chao et al. [17]. LRC = Local/regional control; DFS = disease-free survival; OS = overall survival.

were only 10 failures, giving a local/regional control rate of 87% and an overall survival rate of 87%. Only 9 out of 74 patients had grade 2 xerostomia.

At Stanford, a prospective study has compared the objective xerostomia results in patients treated with conventional radiotherapy (CRT) versus IMRT. A validated xerostomia questionnaire was administered to 29 representative IMRT patients and a matched cohort of 75 CRT patients. Tabulated responses showed a significant reduction in late salivary toxicity with the use of IMRT compared with CRT in the overall score (fig. 24), and the effect appeared to be dominated by results from treatment of OP cancers (fig. 25). When analyzed by individual questions,

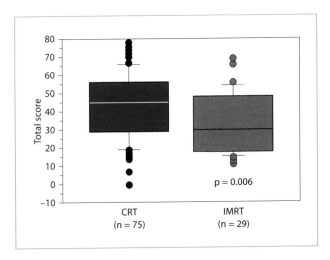

Fig. 24. Box plots showing the overall xerostomia score between IMRT- and matched CRT-treated patients.

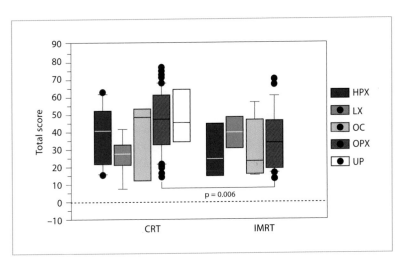

Fig. 25. Box plots showing the overall xerostomia score between IMRT- and matched CRT-treated patients by treatment site. HPX = Hypopharynx; LX = larynx; OC = oral cavity; OPX = oropharynx; UP = unknown primary.

IMRT was significantly better than CRT in terms of difficulty with talking or chewing, with mouth dryness or eating, and with the frequency of sipping liquid.

The RTOG has just completed a phase I/II feasibility study (RTOG 0022), evaluating the use of CRT and IMRT in patients with T1–2 N0–1 OP carcinomas that require bilateral neck treatment. The results of this important study will shed light on the use of IMRT in early-stage OP cancer.

Conclusions

Early results suggest that IMRT can improve local control rates and reduce xerostomia in patients with NP and OP cancers. Long-term follow-up data show that stereotactic radiotherapy used as a boost can provide excellent local control in NP cancer patients. Future considerations should focus on improving the accuracy of target delineation for these tumors, which can have quite variable presentations in their extent of disease. This will likely include the incorporation of molecular imaging studies in daily radiotherapy treatment planning. Novel systemic therapies are greatly needed to reduce the risk of distant metastases in patients with NP carcinomas.

Guidelines for Clinical Practice

- Patient setup is critical for accurate therapy delivery, and should address shoulder mobility as well as head mobility. Interfraction motion is best managed with image guidance. Tumor and normal tissue changes potentially altering dosimetry during the therapy course must be monitored, and replanning performed when they do occur.

- For therapy planning, the policy at this institution is to maintain the mean dose to the contralateral parotids less than 26 Gy.

- For nasopharynx (NP) carcinomas. Gross tumor volume (GTV): gross tumor on CT/MRI and examination. Clinical target volume (CTV): GTV plus margin including NP, retropharyngeal nodes, clivus, skull base, inferior sphenoid sinus, pterygoid fossae, parapharyngeal space, posterior nasal cavity and maxillary sinuses. Planning target volume (PTV): CTV plus 3--5 mm.

- For NP cancer: at this institution, doses are prescribed in 3 tiers. Thirty fractions are delivered, encompassing ≥95% of targets specified as PTV54, PTV60 and PTV66 followed by stereotactic boost in selected patients (54, 60, 66 Gy respectively).

- The prescription schemes for oropharynx (OP) cancers are similar to those used for NP cancer. To account for organ motion and patient setup errors, we routinely add a 3- to 5-mm margin to the GTV to generate a PTV66 (66 Gy at 2.2 Gy/fraction).

- For base of tongue and vallecular tumors, the entire base of tongue and vallecula are contoured in the PTV60, to ensure that these structures receive at least 60 Gy delivered at 2 Gy/fraction.

- For tonsil and soft palate tumors, the entire tonsillar fossa (from the pterygoid plate insertion to the pharyngoepiglottic fold) or the entire soft palate is contoured in the PTV60.

- For OP cancers, the PTV54 encompasses the clinically negative neck, which includes bilateral retropharyngeal nodes and level II through V nodes. In cases where there is level II nodal involvement, level IB nodes are also included in PTV54.

References

1 Eisbruch A, Kim HM, Terrell JE, Marsh LH, Dawson LA, Ship JA: Xerostomia and its predictors following parotid-sparing irradiation of head-and-neck cancer. Int J Radiat Oncol Biol Phys 2001;50:695–704.

2 Eisbruch A, Ship JA, Martel MK, Ten Haken RK, Marsh LH, Wolf GT, Esclamado RM, Bradford CR, Terrell JE, Gebarski SS, Lichter AS: Parotid gland sparing in patients undergoing bilateral head and neck irradiation: techniques and early results. Int J Radiat Oncol Biol Phys 1996;36: 469–480.

3 Eisbruch A, Ten Haken RK, Kim HM, Marsh LH, Ship JA: Dose, volume, and function relationships in parotid salivary glands following conformal and intensity-modulated irradiation of head and neck cancer. Int J Radiat Oncol Biol Phys 1999;45:577–587.

4 Amosson CM, Teh BS, Van TJ, Uy N, Huang E, Mai WY, Frolov A, Woo SY, Chiu JK, Carpenter LS, Lu HH, Grant WH 3rd, Butler EB: Dosimetric predictors of xerostomia for head-and-neck cancer patients treated with the smart (simultaneous modulated accelerated radiation therapy) boost technique. Int J Radiat Oncol Biol Phys 2003;56: 136–144.

5 Chao KS, Deasy JO, Markman J, Haynie J, Perez CA, Purdy JA, Low DA: A prospective study of salivary function sparing in patients with head-and-neck cancers receiving intensity-modulated or three-dimensional radiation therapy: initial results. Int J Radiat Oncol Biol Phys 2001;49:907–916.

6 Kwong DL, Pow EH, Sham JS, McMillan AS, Leung LH, Leung WK, Chua DT, Cheng AC, Wu PM, Au GK: Intensity-modulated radiotherapy for early-stage nasopharyngeal carcinoma: a prospective study on disease control and preservation of salivary function. Cancer 2004;101:1584–1593.

7 Hong TS, Tome WA, Chappell RJ, Chinnaiyan P, Mehta MP, Harari PM: The impact of daily set-up variations on head-and-neck intensity-modulated radiation therapy. Int J Radiat Oncol Biol Phys 2005;61:779–788.

8 Mohan R, Zhang X, Wang H, Kang Y, Wang X, Liu H, Ang KK, Kuban D, Dong L: Use of deformed intensity distributions for on-line modification of image-guided IMRT to account for interfractional anatomic changes. Int J Radiat Oncol Biol Phys 2005;61:1258–1266.

9 Bucci KM, Kia P, Lee N, Fischbein NJ, Kramer A, Weinberg V, Akazawa C, Cabera A, Fu KK, Quivey JM: Intensity modulated radiation therapy for carcinoma of the nasopharynx: An update of the UCSF experience. 46th Annu Meet Am Soc Ther Radiol Oncol, Atlanta, 2004.

10 Lee N, Xia P, Fischbein NJ, Akazawa P, Akazawa C, Quivey JM: Intensity-modulated radiation therapy for head-and-neck cancer: the UCSF experience focusing on target volume delineation. Int J Radiat Oncol Biol Phys 2003;57:49–60.

11 Wolden SL, Chen WC, Pfister DG, Kraus DH, Berry SL, Zelefsky MJ: Intensity-modulated radiation therapy (IMRT) for nasopharynx cancer: update of the Memorial Sloan-Kettering experience. Int J Radiat Oncol Biol Phys 2006;64:57–62.

12 Kam MK, Teo PM, Chau RM, Cheung KY, Choi PH, Kwan WH, Leung SF, Zee B, Chan AT: Treatment of nasopharyngeal carcinoma with intensity-modulated radiotherapy: the Hong Kong experience. Int J Radiat Oncol Biol Phys 2004;60: 1440–1450.

13 Zhao C, Lu TX, Han F, Lu LX, Huang SM, Deng XW, Zeng ZF, Lin CG, Cu NJ: Improved local control with intensity modulated radiation therapy in patients with nasopharyngal carcinoma. 46th Annu Meet Am Soc Ther Radiol Oncol, Atlanta, 2004.

14 Le QT, Tate D, Koong A, Gibbs IC, Chang SD, Adler JR, Pinto HA, Terris DJ, Fee WE, Goffinet DR: Improved local control with stereotactic radiosurgical boost in patients with nasopharyngeal carcinoma. Int J Radiat Oncol Biol Phys 2003;56:1046–1054.

15 Hara W, Gothnet DR, Gibbs IC, Chang SD, Puto HA, Fee WF, Le QL: The use of stereotactic radiosurgical boost to improve local control in patients with nasopharyngeal carcinoma. 87th Annu Meet Am Radium Soc, Barcelona, 2005.

16 de Arruda FF, Puri DR, Zhung J, Narayana A, Wolden S, Hunt M, Stambuk H, Pfister D, Kraus D, Shaha A, Shah J, Lee NY: Intensity-modulated radiation therapy for the treatment of oropharyngeal carcinoma: the memorial Sloan-Kettering cancer center experience. Int J Radiat Oncol Biol Phys 2006;64:363–373.

17 Chao KS, Ozyigit G, Blanco AI, Thorstad WL, Deasy JO, Haughey BH, Spector GJ, Sessions DG: Intensity-modulated radiation therapy for oropharyngeal carcinoma: impact of tumor volume. Int J Radiat Oncol Biol Phys 2004;59:43–50.

Dr. Quynh-Thu Le
Department of Radiation Oncology
Stanford University
Stanford, CA 94305-5302 (USA)
Tel. +1 650 498 5032, Fax +1 650 725 8231
E-Mail qle@reyes.stanford.edu

Meyer JL (ed): IMRT, IGRT, SBRT – Advances in the Treatment Planning and
Delivery of Radiotherapy. Front Radiat Ther Oncol. Basel, Karger, 2007, vol. 40, pp 232–238

A Discussion of the Clinical Use of Advanced Technologies in Head and Neck Radiotherapy

J.L. Meyer[a] · A. Eisbruch[b] · Q.-T. Le[c]

Departments of Radiation Oncology, [a]Saint Francis Memorial Hospital, San Francisco, Calif.,
[b]University of Michigan, Ann Arbor, Mich., [c]Stanford University, Stanford, Calif., USA

Intensity-modulated radiation therapy (IMRT) has found its greatest clinical benefit in the therapy of head and neck tumors, largely because of its effective sparing of critical normal tissues including mucosal, salivary, and neurosensory structures. At the same time, there is greater variation in the treatment programs used for tumors in this region than for other regions, as the roles of surgery, chemotherapy and radiotherapy change with the differences in anatomical presentation and disease extent for each case. Since these tumors may be radiocurable, the manner of application of these precision technologies can impact the survival of individual patients. Together, these concerns create important questions regarding the use of IMRT for curative therapy for head and neck tumors.

Intensity-Modulated Radiation Therapy for Head and Neck Tumors: Technical Concerns

What is the optimal number of gantry angles for a step-and-shoot approach to IMRT?

Dr. Eisbruch: This is an active area of investigation in physics. Of course, the greater the number of angles, the greater the conformality that can be achieved, but each field takes additional time for planning and execution, thereby reducing the efficiency of the clinic. The question is, what degree of planning provides *clin-*

ically significant benefit for the patient? At our institution, we have found that about 7 equidistant fields are sufficient for most head and neck IMRT courses. In a complex case, such as a nasopharynx tumor with involved lymph nodes, 8 or 9 equidistant fields may give a slightly better result and may be used. Beyond this, a greater number of delivery angles, and the technologies that produce them, seem unlikely to provide additional benefit and their value would need to be demonstrated in clinical evaluations.

Dr. Le: At Stanford, this has been an active research topic in our physics group. Currently, between 5 and 9 gantry angles are often used for our head and neck cases, though it will depend on the target volumes and the complexity of each case.

Immobilization is especially important for IMRT delivery in the head and neck region. What current approaches are being added to our available options?

Dr. Le: Immobilization of the shoulders is especially important when IMRT is used for comprehensive nodal irradiation. The Stanford group has evaluated three different approaches for shoulder immobilization, including a comprehensive thermoplastic mask that extends from the head to the shoulder, a separate shoulder immobilization system that is available commercially and our own shoulder immobilization system. Despite these, shoulder motion is still about 2–3 mm regardless of the kind of immobilization used. In our experience, the comprehensive thermoplastic masks that cover the shoulders can cause slightly greater skin dose in the base of neck, sometimes requiring that a portion of the mask be removed during the treatment course which reduces the degree of immobilization. Another head and neck area that is more difficult to immobilize and reproduce as a daily target is the oral cavity. Often these tumors are treated primarily with surgery; however, when they are managed with definitive radiotherapy, the tilt of the chin can vary from day to day within standard thermoplastic masks. Since the setup may be difficult to reproduce precisely even with careful immobilization, one may need to consider using an appropriately larger planning target volume in these cases.

How does one match an anterior supraclavicular field to a head and neck IMRT field? Are recurrences at the match line reported?

Dr. Le: At Stanford, most patients receive comprehensive IMRT planning of nodal irradiation, especially for postoperative patients and patients with gross disease in the lower neck. We avoid matching in the postoperative setting because we have observed at least one recurrence that spanned a match line. The Mallinckrodt group has reported similar findings. In patients receiving definitive radiotherapy with IMRT, it is important to have the IMRT fields cover all gross disease identified by imaging and physical examinations. If tumor extends into the lower neck, there should be no reason to divide the fields and introduce a match line. When treating the uninvolved neck with an anterior supraclavicular field matched to the IMRT fields, we do not use a common isocenter for both field sets. The isocenter of the IMRT fields remains at the primary site, where immobilization is more reliable. We first generate the IMRT plan using this isocenter. Then we identify the position of its 50% isodose line, in the coronal and sagittal projections, on the patient's skin and add an additional 2- to 3-mm skin gap. This becomes the isocenter for the AP (anterior-posterior) supraclavicular field, which is always half-beam blocked. As a result, the match line is dosimetrically conservative and somewhat cooler, and we are therefore cautious in using matching fields.

Dr. Eisbruch: An anterior supraclavicular field may underdose the supraclavicular nodes, as I showed before, and it is uncommon for us to use this approach. It is undertaken in a minority of cases, and only when the neck is clinically negative bilaterally. When we do, we feather the IMRT fields and the supraclavicular field. When the neck is positive, I am concerned about the higher risk for disease in the supraclavicular nodes. They are included in the IMRT target volumes in the majority of cases.

Conventional head and neck radiotherapy has used minor adaptations such as mouth guards to reduce scatter from dental fillings, and skin bolus to increase dose to scars. Are these still appropriate in the IMRT era?

Dr. Le: We routinely use mouth guards in our current immobilization system, and we perform the treatment planning CT with them in place. Admittedly, it is difficult to accurately model and correct for the increased exposure from dental artifacts, because they significantly alter the Hounsfield units on CT. Regarding bolus, the IMRT approach often uses several beams that are tangential, resulting in greater skin dose. At our institution, further skin bolus is used only if there is frank skin involvement by tumor. As before, it would be placed on the patient's skin prior to the planning CT.

Dr. Eisbruch: I would say that the indications for skin bolus with IMRT probably would be similar to those with conventional therapy. In practice, if the PTV (planning target volume) is determined to extend to the surface, then the skin becomes a target and is planned to receive full-dose therapy. Notwithstanding the dosimetric uncertainties at the surface, I have not seen recurrences in the skin and we usually do not introduce bolus before planning.

Intensity-Modulated Radiation Therapy for Head and Neck Tumors: Clinical Concerns

During the therapy course, patients may lose weight and tumors may shrink. What are practical approaches to managing these clinical changes? Should one modify the dose distributions based upon tumor shrinkage by replanning the patient sequentially during radiotherapy?

Dr. Eisbruch: If a patient's contour changes and the mask no longer fits, because of weight loss or tumor shrinkage, then it may be necessary to bring the patient back to simulation, try to reproduce the original position, and to reconstruct the mask. If the original treatment position cannot be reproduced, then occasionally the planning must be entirely repeated. Large external contour changes may also require that replanning be performed to dosimetrically maintain the original targets. However, this is not expected or intended based on tumor regression alone. Currently, my conviction is that the extent of gross tumor before irradiation continues to be the target for therapy to full dose, even as the gross disease shrinks during treatment. Investigation may guide us on this issue, which does need to be studied further, but this is our current policy.

Are the dose heterogeneities involved with IMRT more concerning for some sites in the head and neck region than other sites?

Dr. Eisbruch: Dose heterogeneity may be better tolerated in the nasopharynx than other sites, even though the treatment volumes may be larger. This is consistent with what is already known. Many groups have shown the greater tolerance of these tissues to high focal radiation doses, such as those used with brachytherapy boost techniques. These same doses would not be tolerated in other sites, especially the oral cavity or base of tongue. It appears that the clinical site may determine whether higher doses per fraction can be tolerated.

Dr. Le: The most important issue is whether one can spare the oral cavity. One must have reasonable concern about the possibility of nonhealing ulcerations when using large fraction sizes to the tongue and oral cavity tissues. This region has a very sensate mucosa, and as mentioned, dental fillings may cause focal dose changes that are not accurately modeled.

Since the NP (nasopharynx) may tolerate higher IMRT doses, is it necessary to use boost techniques involving brachytherapy or high-fraction stereotactic methods for the NP when IMRT technologies are already being used?

Dr. Le: At our institution, stereotactic radiotherapy with Cyberknife technology has been used in sequential fashion with IMRT, not concurrently. As such, it has used sequential planning that covers the residual disease following 66-Gy fractionated external beam radiotherapy. Therefore, the boost is intended for patients with larger and/or persistent tumors. Our results have been excellent in these challenging cases and we have continued this approach. It is possible that similar results might be attained with IMRT alone, and currently we are investigating a reduction of the boost dose in favor of a higher dose with the initial IMRT.

For the radiotherapy of head and neck cancers, one strategy to deliver higher dose heterogeneity within the tumor is the use of twice-per-day therapy, the second daily treatment delivering a focused 'concomitant boost'. Could IMRT technology further increase the benefit of this approach?

Dr. Le: Stanford has not attempted this, but investigators at the Memorial Sloan-Kettering Cancer Center and at the University of Florida have done so, and have reported encouraging results. One concern would be the possibility of a very high dose focus occurring, since it is more difficult to control the hot spots derived from 2 separate IMRT plans.

Dr. Eisbruch: Most institutions have not undertaken this because of the length of time involved in IMRT delivery. Twice-per-day IMRT would be even more difficult logistically. This is why the RTOG (Radiation Therapy Oncology Group) protocol preferred an approach using a larger dose per fraction and one fraction per day. It certainly might be possible to deliver IMRT to the entire target volume in a morning treatment, and in the evening treatment use IMRT to the GTV (gross tumor volume) alone. The second treatment might not need 7 or 9 beams, perhaps only 5, making it more feasible.

Surgery and Intensity-Modulated Radiation Therapy

For the patient with regionally advanced neck disease, does IMRT obviate the need for a planned neck dissection?

Dr. Eisbruch: We have an institutional policy of dissecting patients after irradiation who have nodal disease of N2 or N3 extent, regardless of their initial response. If one knows ahead of time that the patient will undergo a neck dissection according to policy, then one can consider less dose to the gross disease in the neck – perhaps 60 Gy instead of 70 Gy. However, there are other institutions that take a watch-and-wait approach following radiotherapy. This is based on evolving data that if both PET scan and clinical examination of the neck are negative 3 months after radiotherapy, then surgery may not be required.

Dr. Le: This remains an active debate everywhere, even within our own institution where different approaches are taken by different skilled surgeons. Overall, our policy is gravitating toward an approach of close observation. If there is a complete response based on physical examination and posttreatment anatomic imaging studies, which are obtained 6–8 weeks after chemoradiation, then a baseline PET-CT scan is performed at 3 months as part of the surveillance. On the other hand, if palpable or imaged adenopathy persists, then a neck dissection is usually performed.

Chemotherapy and Intensity-Modulated Radiation Therapy

Are there special concerns with the use of chemotherapy with IMRT, given the dose heterogeneity that typically occurs within these radiation fields?

Dr. Eisbruch: Whenever one uses a higher dose per fraction than is standard, patients may not tolerate the addition of concurrent chemotherapy acceptably. Concern about this has been raised over the past few years, based upon clinical reports from Baylor University and elsewhere. Certain RTOG (Radiation Therapy Oncology Group) radiation protocols are now using 2.2 Gy per fraction or more to some areas of tumor treatment. If one decides to give a higher dose per fraction than usual to the gross disease, such as 2.2 Gy or more, one should take into account that chemotherapy probably should not be given. The exception to this may be for the treatment of nasopharynx tumors, where higher doses per fraction may be better tolerated. Conversely, if one thinks that chemotherapy is indicated for a patient because of the extent of disease, then current evidence suggests that a standard dose per fraction to the gross disease is preferable.

Given the enhanced reactions that result when chemotherapy is given during a radiotherapy course, should the planning target volume or clinical target volume be reduced when concurrent therapy is the treatment program?

Dr. Eisbruch: Definitely not; the same PTV (planning target volume) and CTV (clinical target volume) are indicated as would be used without chemotherapy, and both the fields and doses should be based only on the clinical indications for that particular tumor. It is true that chemotherapy adds to the *overall* rates of local/regional control for many tumors, but one cannot reliably reduce the extent of the target volumes, or the dose to those volumes, in any individual case at this time.

If normal tissue reactions are enhanced by the use of chemotherapy, then should the radiotherapy dose constraints for the parotid gland be altered for patients receiving concurrent chemotherapy?

Dr. Eisbruch: The chemotherapy effects are not so precisely directed, and the investigations at this institution have not found a measurable effect of chemotherapy on parotid outflow. I might note that other investigators did note some effect, but our work did not and our parotid dose limitations are not changed by the use of chemotherapy.

Dr. Le: This is also true at Stanford, where there is a tradition of using chemotherapy more frequently for head and neck cancers than at other institutions. In our experience, there has been little difference in parotid radiosensitivity whether or not chemotherapy was added. For instance, this has been true in comparisons of patients treated postoperatively without chemotherapy with those treated definitively with chemotherapy. The limitation of 26 Gy mean dose to the parotid is maintained at our institution, with or without the use of chemotherapy.

Is the pharmaceutical amifostine useful for moderating radiotherapy normal tissue reaction, and is it necessary or appropriate in the context of IMRT?

Dr. Eisbruch: At our institution, amifostine is not often used, but work from other groups indicates that it can improve xerostomia. Whether amifostine will decrease mucositis and dysphagia remains unanswered and is a matter of further research.

Dr. Le: We have not used amifostine routinely in the IMRT patients. It can cause moderate nausea, which may be more difficult to manage in the IMRT patients since they are fixed in position more rigorously and longer for the treatment sessions. However, investigators at the MD Anderson Cancer Center are actively investigating the use of amifostine with IMRT.

Meyer JL (ed): IMRT, IGRT, SBRT – Advances in the Treatment Planning and
Delivery of Radiotherapy. Front Radiat Ther Oncol. Basel, Karger, 2007, vol. 40, pp 239–252

Lung Cancer: Intensity-Modulated Radiation Therapy, Four-Dimensional Imaging and Mobility Management

Frank J. Lagerwaard · Suresh Senan

Department of Radiation Oncology, VU University Medical Center, Amsterdam,
The Netherlands

Abstract

The use of image-guided radiotherapy (IGRT) for lung cancer improves target coverage and potentially reduces the risk of treatment-related toxicity. Four-dimensional radiotherapy (which refers to the explicit inclusion of temporal changes in anatomy during imaging) treatment planning and treatment delivery are important components of IGRT for lung cancer. Four-dimensional CT (4DCT) scanning is a major breakthrough that has transformed radiotherapy planning for lung cancer. Individualized internal target volumes can be directly obtained from these 4DCT scans, e.g. using maximum intensity projections. Color intensity projections of 4DCT scans provide temporal information on organ mobility within a single composite image. As only a minority of patients are likely to benefit from respiratory gating, patient-specific assessment of tumor mobility is essential.

Copyright © 2007 S. Karger AG, Basel

It has been reported that the use of two-dimensional radiotherapy for lung cancer carries a substantial risk for target miss. A review by Rosenman et al. [1] reported that major errors in irradiation of the target volume occurred in up to 31% of major lung cancer trials conducted between the 1980s and early 1990s. Two recent developments may even have increased the risk of errors in radiotherapy delivery for lung cancer since the two-dimensional era. First, the use of CT-based three-dimensional conformal radiotherapy planning results in dose distributions that closely conform to the target volume, thereby increasing the potential for a partial target miss. Second, involved fields have been recommended by the European Organization for Research and Treatment of Cancer in radiotherapy for stage III lung cancer [2], and omission of elective mediastinal fields could increase the risk of target miss.

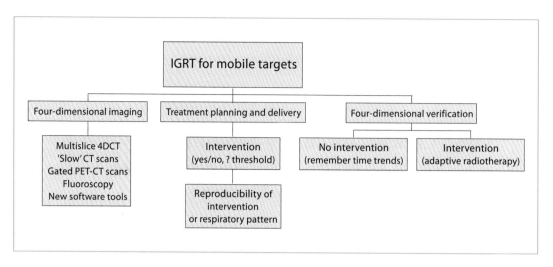

Fig. 1. Overview of the IGRT process for lung cancer.

Appropriate use of image-guided radiotherapy (IGRT) could decrease the risk of such inaccuracies in target irradiation, as well as decrease the risk of toxicity. Recent studies have reported on the feasibility of high-dose radiotherapy, in excess of 70 Gy, following induction platinum-based chemotherapy [3, 4]. However, this treatment approach was associated with grade III–IV toxicity in 8–18% of patients, including bronchial stenosis, pleural fistulae, and obstruction of the esophagus or pulmonary artery [3, 4]. Furthermore, the introduction of new molecular target agents such as VEGF inhibitors into combined treatments may lead to unexpected toxicities.

The use of IGRT for lung cancer can be complex, and several issues must be addressed ranging from the optimal imaging and treatment planning techniques for IGRT to four-dimensional delivery and treatment verification methods (fig. 1).

Four-Dimensional Imaging for Treatment Planning

Radiotherapy planning for lung cancer has traditionally been based on a single planning CT scan acquired during free breathing. Such random scans may generate artifacts of the patient's anatomy, and give an inaccurate representation of the shape, volume and position of normal organs and target volumes (fig. 2). Treatment planning on nonrepresentative scans will have an impact on all of the treatment fractions delivered and result in systematic errors. In addition, the calculated dose in a static patient model is unlikely to represent the actual dose delivery during treatment.

Lagerwaard · Senan

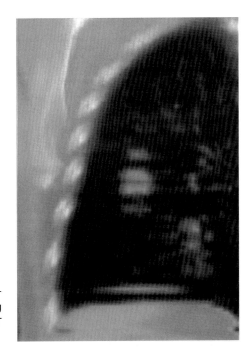

Fig. 2. Motion artifacts in the tumor and diaphragm arising from free breathing during the generation of a radiotherapy planning CT scan.

Four-Dimensional Rationale and Uses

The need for anatomic information over time to optimize radiotherapy is the underlying basis for four-dimensional radiotherapy, which refers to the explicit inclusion of such temporal changes during the imaging, treatment planning and treatment delivery phases of therapy. It has to be recognized, however, that dedicated four-dimensional treatment planning systems are not yet commercially available. Four-dimensional radiotherapy can be used for several purposes, including:

- determining the movement of target volumes for individual patients/targets,
- assessing the need for mobility intervention,
- evaluating the impact of mobility intervention,
- assessing residual mobility after mobility intervention.

Image Acquisition: Four-Dimensional Imaging Techniques

Several techniques for four-dimensional imaging are now available that allow for the generation of individualized and reproducible target volumes (table 1). A simple method for peripheral tumors is to perform a 'slow' CT scan during quiet respiration [5, 6]. The prolongation of the image acquisition time to 4 s (or longer) per CT revolution during quiet respiration allows for the incorporation of tumor mobility during 1–2 respiratory cycles in images from each table position. In order to limit the radiation exposure to patients and the scanning time, the slow CT scan

Table 1. Four-dimensional imaging techniques for lung cancer

Imaging technique	Remarks
Two-phase scans	End-inspiration and end-expiration scans may overestimate respiration-induced mobility and disregard potential hysteresis
Multiple planning scans	Labor-intensive method requiring image registration of multiple data sets; random assessment of tumor position
Breath-hold scans	Poor tolerance by patients with poor pulmonary function, as well as problems with verification during treatment
Slow CT scans	Simple, patient-friendly scanning technique but its use is limited to peripheral lung cancers
Prospective four-dimensional scans	Prior assessment of phase for gating is necessary; evaluation of different delivery strategies is not possible with a single-phase 4DCT scan
Retrospective four-dimensional scan	Performed during quiet respiration; very large amount of data is generated, which requires new software tools

can be restricted to the region of the primary tumor, and this scan can be coregistered with a standard planning scan. The main limitation of slow CT is the fact that these scans are suitable for peripheral lung lesions only, as mobile structures in the mediastinum appear blurred in these images.

The technique of respiration-correlated four-dimensional CT (4DCT) scanning on a multislice CT is in routine use at our center for treatment planning of lung cancer therapy. In a 4DCT scan, spatial and temporal information on shape and mobility are acquired synchronously in a single investigation [7–9]. At the VU University Medical Center, 4DCT scans are performed on a 16-slice GE Lightspeed scanner (General Electric Co., Waukesha, Wisc., USA). The breathing pattern is recorded using the Varian Real-Time Positioning Management System (Varian Medical Systems, Palo Alto, Calif., USA). In brief, the respiratory signals are recorded using infrared-reflecting markers on the upper abdomen of the patient during uncoached free breathing. The markers are illuminated by infrared-emitting diodes surrounding a camera, which captures the motion of these markers. Generating a single 4DCT scan during quiet respiration is relatively simple, and poses no problems to patients with poor pulmonary function. The 4DCT scanning procedure of the entire thorax takes about 90 s.

The four-dimensional data sets are retrospectively sorted into 10 phase bins within the respiratory cycle, using the Advantage 4DCT application running on an Advantage Workstation 4.1 (General Electric Co., Waukesha, Wisc., USA). Each bin represents the patient's anatomy during a single respiratory phase, and further analysis is performed using the Advantage software.

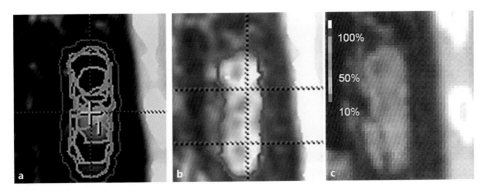

Fig. 3. ITV generation for a small mobile tumor. **a** The ITV (green contour) derived from contouring all 10 GTVs (yellow contours). **b** The result of MIP of the mobile tumor. As a result of the phase summation, the full range of tumor mobility is imaged, and a 'mobile GTV' can be directly contoured. **c** The result of CIP of the mobile tumor. The green color at the cranial side of the tumor illustrates that the tumor is at its end-expiratory position for most of the time.

Target Delineation: Four-Dimensional Internal Target Volumes for Treatment Planning

The clinical implementation of 4DCT scanning leads to a major increase in patient data that have to be reviewed for target definition. Ten respiration-correlated three-dimensional data sets (bins) are commonly derived from a single four-dimensional data set, and each represents the patient's anatomy during a single respiratory phase. Deriving a gross tumor volume (GTV) that incorporates all mobility ('mobile GTV') requires contouring the tumor in all 10 respiratory phases, which is very time consuming. This volume of data impedes routine clinical use of 4DCT scans in lung cancer and underscores the need for solutions for an efficient clinical use of four-dimensional imaging.

Instead of contouring all phases of the 4DCT, more practical solutions for deriving internal target volumes (ITVs) from 4DCT scans include contouring just the extreme phases of the 4DCT (two-phase planning), or using all phases of the 4DCT to derive a maximum intensity projection (MIP) or a color intensity projection (CIP).

Two-Phase Planning

Contouring the tumor in all separate respiratory phases (fig. 3a) is time consuming, and a simpler approach could be the contouring of only the end-expiration and end-inspiration phases of the 4DCT scan, i.e. two-phase planning. This approach presumes a linear trajectory between both extreme respiratory tumor positions, but may miss tumor hysteresis, as can occur with a different path of mobility during inspiration and expiration and has been described previously [10].

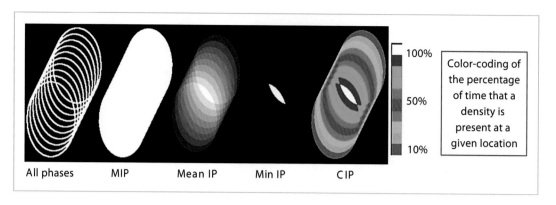

Fig. 4. Illustration of the potential use of pixel-based intensity projection protocols in 4DCT scans. From left to right: separate phases on a 4DCT scan, maximum, mean, and minimum projection of the phase bins of the 4DCT. The figure on the extreme right shows the corresponding CIP where color encodes for the period of time that the tumor (high intensity) is present at that location.

Several postprocessing tools can be used to summarize information from four-dimensional bins into a composite intensity projection data set, including a pixel-based projection of the maximum, the mean, and the minimum intensity (fig. 4). The potential clinical uses and examples of the use of these routine volume-rendering techniques applied in diagnostic radiology will be described briefly in the following sections.

Maximum Intensity Projections

A rapid and accurate method for generating reliable ITVs from 4DCT data sets for peripheral lung cancer is to use MIPs. Briefly, MIP scans reflect the highest data value encountered along the viewing ray for each pixel of volumetric data, giving rise to a full intensity display of the brightest object along each ray on the projection image. As such, MIP scans can be used to generate composite images with pixel-based phase summation of tumor positions in all phases of respiration. This, in turn, allows for the direct contouring of 'mobile GTVs', or in case of stereotactic radiotherapy where separate GTV to clinical target volume margins are not often used, the direct generation of ITVs (fig. 3b). A study in 12 patients with peripheral tumors showed MIP-based ITVs to be in agreement with ITVs derived from contouring GTVs on all phases of the 4DCT [11]. Generation of individualized ITVs on MIP images took less than 10 min per patient, and significantly reduced the clinical workload. Major limitations of MIP scans include (1) their unsuitability for accurate imaging of the mediastinum, and (2) errors in cases where tumors are adjacent to normal structures that have an equal or greater density on CT scans. Potential errors can be avoided by projecting individual GTVs

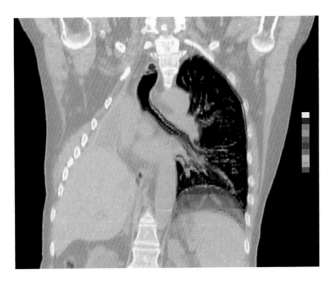

Fig. 5. Frontal CIP image of a patient with a prior right pneumonectomy. The colors illustrate the asymmetrical mobility with a virtual absence of mobility on the right side. In contrast, mobility of the left diaphragm and the left main stem bronchus is clearly visualized.

at extreme phases of respiration onto the MIP ITV for tumors that are adjacent to the mediastinum, heart, or diaphragm.

Color Intensity Projections

MIPs of 4DCT scans enable fast and patient-specific ITVs to be generated, but do not make optimal use of the temporal information contained in 4DCT data sets. At the VU University Medical Center, a CIP technique has been developed which incorporates the motion information of selected component 4DCT data sets for each slice into a single composite color image. The algorithm is based on calculation of the maximum, minimum, and mean intensity of each pixel [12]. The brightness is a measure of the intensity of each pixel; the saturation is a measure of a pixel's amount of color and the hue is the actual color, with colors covering the range of blue-green-red. Consequently, where internal mobility is present, the hue of the color in the composite image encodes the period of time a tumor or organ is present at that location (fig. 4, right). CIP images enable mobility of tumors and normal organs to be visualized and measured within a single composite image (fig. 5).

The reproducibility of 4DCT scans obtained during quiet respiration has recently been investigated in patients with stage I non-small-cell lung cancer [submitted, 2006]. Analysis of repeat 4DCT scans generated during a single CT session in 20 patients revealed that volumetric and spatial differences in planning target

Table 2. Mobility management

Method	Technique	Comments
Incorporate all movements	4DCT or slow CT	May lead to increased risk of normal tissue toxicity
Freeze movement	Breath hold	Not feasible in all lung cancer patients
Intercept movement: *gated* radiotherapy	Respiratory cycle as surrogate of tumor position	(1) Treatment time increased (2) Difficulties in target verification
Track or chase tumor	Implanted markers and specialized treatment delivery	(1) Difficult endobronchial marker insertion (2) CT-guided insertion risks pneumothorax (3) Markers migrate after insertion (4) Difficult to predict normal tissues doses

volumes (PTVs) in excess of 10% and 2 mm, respectively, were observed in a fifth of patients. Despite the use of conformal stereotactic plans using 8–12 treatment beams, the observed variations in PTVs translated into significant dosimetric differences in only 1 patient.

Mobility Management in the Lung Cancer Patient

Several strategies for mobility management are currently used in clinical practice, including fully incorporating target mobility, freezing target mobility, intercepting the moving target, and tracking the tumor (table 2). Factors that must be taken into account before deciding upon an approach include the accuracy, the workload, patient tolerance, imaging dose and resources required [13]. However, an important first question is whether motion management is necessary in the first place. The AAPM Task Group 76 [14] has suggested that tumor motion of more than 5 mm is 'significant', but the basis for this cutoff point is not clear, and it also fails to address the errors that may be introduced by interventions required by complex strategies. Tumor mobility in excess of 1 cm during quiet respiration has been reported to occur in 27–50% of patients with peripheral tumors [15–17], which suggests that intervention to modify or limit motion is clinically relevant only for a minority of patients with such lesions.

Case Study
Patient. A 72-year-old male, with medically inoperable T2N0M0 lung cancer of the right lower lobe (fig. 6).

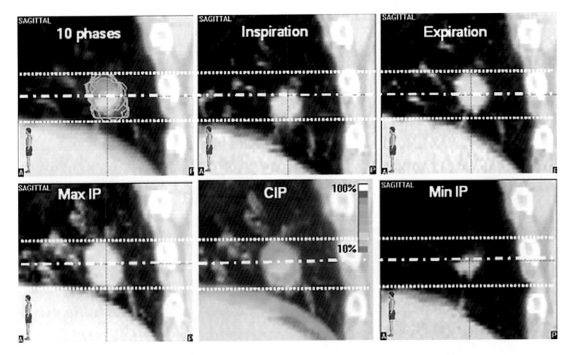

Fig. 6. Sagittal reconstruction of a mobile tumor in the left lower lobe. The figure illustrates contouring of all 4DCT phase bins on the left upper panel, the corresponding inspiration and expiration phase of the 4DCT scan (upper middle and right panel), an MIP scan (lower left panel), a CIP scan (middle lower panel) and a minimum intensity projection on the lower right.

Treatment. A 4DCT scan acquired during quiet respiration was used to generate an individualized ITV. Figure 6 shows sagittal views of the tumor in all phases, the MIP scan, and the CIP scan, respectively.

Result. The ITV for four-dimensional stereotactic radiotherapy was contoured on the MIP scan (fig. 7, left panel), and treatment was delivered in 5 fractions of 12 Gy, prescribed to the 80% isodose. The treatment was completed in 2 weeks.

The use of 4DCT to incorporate all movements into the target volume has been discussed above, and technical methods to 'track' or 'chase' the tumor (such as the Cyberknife device) are discussed in the section of this volume on stereotactic body radiation therapy. Here, two general approaches to mobility management in the lung cancer patient will be discussed further.

Breath Hold

Breath hold, usually at end-inspiration, has been used to minimize the mobility of targets in the lung [18]. Although theoretically attractive, this method has a number of practical disadvantages. Cooperative patients have to be coached in order to ensure reproducible results, and an individualized assessment is required for

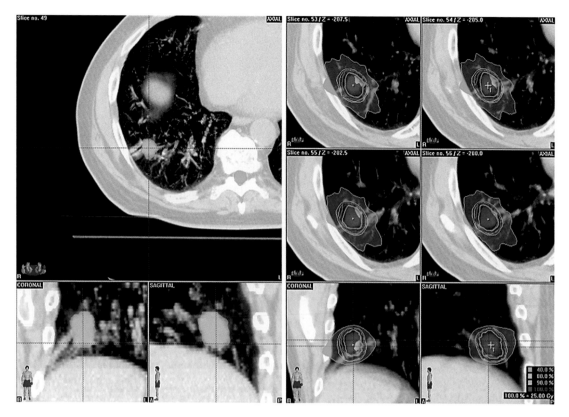

Fig. 7. Contouring the ITV on the MIP scan, stereotactic treatment planning was performed to the PTV (pink contour), which was derived from the addition of a 3-mm margin to the ITV. Stereotactic treatment planning was performed with 11 noncoplanar treatment fields with mini-multileaf shielding, resulting in a highly conformal dose distribution. The inner light-green iso-dose represents the 80% prescription isodose.

each patient. In addition, a considerable number of medically inoperable patients with compromised respiratory function cannot tolerate breath hold. When performing breath hold, some residual mobility persists due to variations in breath holding and cardiac action, and this movement must also be incorporated. In addition, tumor drifts have been reported during treatment, which is particularly relevant for stereotactic body radiation therapy in view of the long fractional treatment time [19]. Onishi et al. [20] described a self-breath-holding system, which is based on the control of the radiation beam by patients themselves. Planning CT scans during patients' self-breath-holding were repeated three times, and the tumor positions on these scans showed that the technique was reproducible within 2-mm distance. In addition to patient-controlled breath hold, several groups have restricted mobility using active breathing control [21], or even using general anesthesia and high-frequency ventilation [22].

Respiratory Gating

The use of respiratory gating permits a reduction in field sizes, as treatment can be limited to just the phases in which the mobile target is in a predetermined position. Gating at end-expiration has been reported to permit longer duty cycles and to be more reproducible [23–25]. As gating prolongs the treatment time, it is common to use a gate that allows a duty cycle of 20–40% of respiration. For patients with stage I non-small-cell lung cancer, a retrospective analysis suggested a potential benefit of respiratory gating using three consecutive phases at end-tidal expiration as it reduced the mean tumor mobility from 8.5 to 1.4 mm. The gains from gating were greatest in mobile tumors, which we arbitrarily defined as tumors with a three-dimensional mobility vector of at least 1 cm. The latter comprised about one third of the tumors in our study. The absolute volume of the PTV is also of importance, since a small benefit for a large PTV could be clinically more relevant than a large benefit for a small PTV. Although a volumetric reduction was observed for most cases, reductions in PTV of 30 and 50% were only achieved with respiratory gating in 13 patients (38%) and 5 patients (15%), respectively [17].

Similar findings were found in an analysis of gating in 15 patients with stage III lung cancer [26]. The use of respiratory gating reduced lung toxicity parameters such as the volume of normal lung receiving more than 20 Gy and the mean lung dose by 5% and 3 Gy, respectively. As could be expected, gating was most beneficial for the more mobile tumors located in the middle and lower lobes. The mean residual mobility within the selected 3–4 end-expiration phases was 4.0 ± 3.5 mm.

Fluoroscopy to Select Patients for Gating

As only a small percentage of patients are likely to benefit from respiratory gating, patient-specific assessment of tumor mobility is useful. The traditional method for estimating tumor mobility is using fluoroscopy, which is still widely used in treatment simulation and is now possible with on-board imaging devices. The main limitations of fluoroscopy are that it only gives a rough two-dimensional estimate of tumor mobility, that tumors are often not visualized in all directions, and (most importantly) that there is no linkage to planning CT scans. These limitations may persist even with advanced technology. In a study comparing virtual fluoroscopy projections derived from 4DCT with contours on actual 4DCT data for peripheral lung tumors, mobility could not be measured in one or more directions in 25% of tumors using the virtual approach [27]. Fluoroscopy also led to mobility being overestimated by clinicians ($p < 0.05$). The reliable use of fluoroscopy for monitoring the tumor position requires the endobronchial or transthoracic insertion of fiducial markers, which is associated with morbidity. With endobronchial placement, often only one marker can be placed near the tumor, while it has been reported that at least 3 markers are needed to detect rotational tumor movement [28].

CIP to Select Patients for Gating

Another approach for identifying patients suitable for respiratory gating from four-dimensional data sets includes the contouring of only the two extreme respiratory bins, where the extent of tumor overlap between these two phases is highly predictive for tumor mobility. Mobility can also be visualized using CIPs, which allow for the mobility of the tumor, diaphragm, abdominal wall, or external marker in selected phases for respiratory gating to become immediately apparent. As the CIP for a single slice can be calculated within seconds, interactive gating phase selection is simple to implement. Identifying patients who might benefit from gating using CIP is more efficient than approaches such as screening on a four-dimensional viewer or viewing multiple contoured target volumes for all patients. Although mobility screening of 4DCT data sets using dedicated software (Advantage 4D) is possible, objective screening of multiple structures simultaneously is not feasible. CIP also enables the concurrent evaluation of external markers and tumor position.

Four-Dimensional Verification

Finally, there remain unresolved issues of verifying mobility management at the treatment unit. Time trends in lung tumors during both stereotactic and conventional radiotherapy have been reported, both with respect to volumetric changes and positional changes [29, 30]. Although it is possible to perform electronic portal imaging during gated treatment delivery, it is often difficult to verify the position of the treatment portals due to a lack of anatomical detail in these images. New methods for ensuring accuracy of therapy delivery, especially through the use of four-dimensional technology, should be defined as an important and immediate goal.

Conclusions

Four-dimensional imaging, and in particular 4DCT scanning performed on a multislice CT, is a major breakthrough that has transformed radiotherapy planning for lung cancer. Improved software is required to simplify treatment planning for four-dimensional radiotherapy. Although interventions for target mobility appear appropriate in selected patients treated with high-dose radiotherapy for lung cancer, verification of IGRT at the treatment unit remains very much a work in progress. It is important to realize that locally advanced lung cancer is a systemic disease requiring early chemoradiotherapy, and the use of complex interventions for mobility should not delay the start of treatment. There remains a need to correlate the clinical use of IGRT with improved outcomes, either in terms of improved tumor control, or in terms of reduced toxicity.

Guidelines for Clinical Practice

- Image-guided radiotherapy (IGRT) for lung cancer improves target coverage and can reduce the risk of treatment-related toxicity.

- Four-dimensional radiotherapy refers to the explicit inclusion of temporal changes in anatomy during imaging, treatment planning and treatment delivery.

- Four-dimensional CT (4DCT) scanning is a major breakthrough that has transformed radiotherapy planning for lung cancer.

- Maximum intensity projections represent composite images of tumor positions in all phases of respiration, thereby allowing for direct generation of internal target volumes from 4DCT.

- Color intensity projections of 4DCT provide temporal information on organ mobility within a single composite image.

- As only a minority of patients is likely to benefit from respiratory gating, patient-specific assessment of tumor mobility is essential.

- It is important to correlate the use of IGRT with improved outcomes in terms of tumor control and/or reduced toxicity.

- Locally advanced lung cancer is often a systemic disease requiring early chemoradiotherapy, and the use of complex interventions for mobility should not delay the start of treatment.

References

1 Rosenman JG, Halle JS, Socinski MA, Deschesne K, Moore DT, Johnson H, Fraser R, Morris DE: High-dose conformal radiotherapy for treatment of stage IIIA/IIIB non-small-cell lung cancer: technical issues and results of a phase I/II trial. Int J Radiat Oncol Biol Phys 2002;54:348–356.

2 Senan S, De Ruysscher D, Giraud P, Mirimanoff R, Budach V: Literature-based recommendations for treatment planning and execution in high-dose radiotherapy for lung cancer. Radiother Oncol 2004;71:139–146.

3 Miller KL, Shafman TD, Anscher MS, Zhou SM, Clough RW, Garst JL, Crawford J, Rosenman J, Socinski MA, Blackstock W, Sibley GS, Marks LB: Bronchial stenosis: an underreported complication of high-dose external beam radiotherapy for lung cancer? Int J Radiat Oncol Biol Phys 2005;61:64–69.

4 Marks LB, Garst J, Socinski MA, Sibley G, Blackstock AW, Herndon JE, Zhou S, Shafman T, Tisch A, Clough R, Yu X, Turrisi A, Anscher M, Crawford J, Rosenman J: Carboplatin/paclitaxel or carboplatin/vinorelbine followed by acceler-

ated hyperfractionated conformal radiation therapy: report of a prospective phase I dose escalation trial from the Carolina Conformal Therapy Consortium. J Clin Oncol 2004;22: 4329–4340.

5 Lagerwaard FJ, van Sörnsen de Koste JR, Nijssen-Visser MR, Schuchhard-Schipper RH, Oei SS, Munne A, Senan S: Multiple 'slow' CT scans for incorporating lung tumor mobility in radiotherapy planning. Int J Radiat Oncol Biol Phys 2001; 51:932–937.

6 van Sörnsen de Koste JR, Lagerwaard FJ, Schuchhard-Schipper RH, Nijssen-Visser MR, Voet PW, Oei SS, Senan S: Dosimetric consequences of tumor mobility in radiotherapy of stage I non-small cell lung cancer – An analysis of data generated using 'slow' CT scans. Radiother Oncol 2001;61: 93–99.

7 Ford EC, Mageras GS, Yorke E, Ling CC: Respiration-correlated spiral CT: a method of measuring respiratory-induced anatomic motion for radiation treatment planning. Med Phys 2003;30:88–97.

8   Underberg RW, Lagerwaard FJ, Cuijpers JP, Slot-man BJ, van Sornsen de Koste JR, Senan S: Four-dimensional CT scans for treatment planning in stereotactic radiotherapy for stage I lung cancer. Int J Radiat Oncol Biol Phys 2004;60:1283–1290.

9   Pan T, Lee TY, Rietzel E, Chen GT: 4D-CT imaging of a volume influenced by respiratory motion on multi-slice CT. Med Phys 2004;31:333–340.

10 Seppenwoolde Y, Shirato H, Kitamura K, Shimizu S, van Herk M, Lebesque JV, Miyasaka K: Precise and real-time measurement of 3D tumor motion in lung due to breathing and heartbeat, measured during radiotherapy. Int J Radiat Oncol Biol Phys 2002;53:822–834.

11 Underberg RWM, Lagerwaard FJ, Slotman BJ, Cuijpers JP, Senan S: Use of maximum intensity projections (MIP) for target volume generation in 4DCT scans for lung cancer. Int J Radiat Oncol Biol Phys 2005;63:253–260.

12 Cover KS, Lagerwaard FJ, Senan S: Color intensity projections: a rapid approach for evaluating four-dimensional CT scans in treatment planning. Int J Radiat Oncol Biol Phys 2006;64:954–961.

13 Mageras GS: Introduction: management of target localization uncertainties in external-beam therapy. Semin Radiat Oncol 2005;15:133–135.

14 Report of AAPM Task Group 76: The management of respiratory motion in radiation oncology, 2005.

15 Neicu T, Shirato H, Seppenwoolde Y, Jiang SB: Synchronized moving aperture radiation therapy (SMART): average tumour trajectory for lung patients. Phys Med Biol 2003;48:587–598.

16 van Sörnsen de Koste JR, Lagerwaard FJ, Nijssen-Visser MR, Graveland WJ, Senan S: Tumor location cannot predict the mobility of lung tumors: a 3D analysis of data generated from multiple CT scans. Int J Radiat Oncol Biol Phys 2003;56:348–354.

17 Underberg RW, Lagerwaard FJ, Slotman BJ, Cuijpers JP, Senan S: Benefit of respiration-gated stereotactic radiotherapy for stage I lung cancer: an analysis of 4DCT datasets. Int J Radiat Oncol Biol Phys 2005;62:554–560.

18 Rosenzweig KE, Hanley J, Mah D, Mageras G, Hunt M, Toner S, Burman C, Ling CC, Mychalczak B, Fuks Z, Leibel SA: The deep inspiration breath-hold technique in the treatment of inoperable non-small-cell lung cancer. Int J Radiat Oncol Biol Phys 2000;48:81–87.

19 Murphy MJ, Martin D, Whyte R, Hai J, Ozhasoglu C, Le QT: The effectiveness of breath-holding to stabilize lung and pancreas tumors during radiosurgery. Int J Radiat Oncol Biol Phys 2002;53:475–482.

20 Onishi H, Kuriyama K, Komiyama T, Tanaka S, Sano N, Aikawa Y, Tateda Y, Araki T, Ikenaga S, Uematsu M: A new irradiation system for lung cancer combining linear accelerator, computed tomography, patient self-breath-holding, and patient-directed beam-control without respiratory monitoring devices. Int J Radiat Oncol Biol Phys 2003;56:14–20.

21 Wong JW, Sharpe MB, Jaffray DA, Kini VR, Robertson JM, Stromberg JS, Martinez AA: The use of active breathing control (ABC) to reduce margin for breathing motion. Int J Radiat Oncol Biol Phys 1999;44:911–919.

22 Hof H, Herfarth KK, Munter M, Hoess A, Motsch J, Wannenmacher M, Debus JJ: Stereotactic single-dose radiotherapy of stage I non-small-cell lung cancer (NSCLC). Int J Radiat Oncol Biol Phys 2003;56:335–341.

23 Balter JM, Lam KL, McGinn CJ, Lawrence TS, Ten Haken RK: Improvement of CT-based treatment-planning models of abdominal targets using static exhale imaging. Int J Radiat Oncol Biol Phys 1998;41:939–943.

24 Minohara S, Kanai T, Endo M, Noda K, Kanazawa M: Respiratory gated irradiation system for heavy-ion radiotherapy. Int J Radiat Oncol Biol Phys 2000;47:1097–1103.

25 Ford EC, Mageras GS, Yorke E, Rosenzweig KE, Wagman R, Ling CC: Evaluation of respiratory movement during gated radiotherapy using film and electronic portal imaging. Int J Radiat Oncol Biol Phys 2002;52:522–531.

26 Underberg RW, van Sornsen de Koste JR, Lagerwaard FJ, Vincent A, Slotman BJ, Senan S: A dosimetric analysis of respiration-gated radiotherapy in patients with stage III lung cancer. Radiat Oncol 2006;1:8.

27 van der Geld YG, Senan S, van Sornsen de Koste JR, van Tinteren H, Slotman BJ, Underberg RW, Lagerwaard FJ: Evaluating mobility for radiotherapy planning of lung tumors: a comparison of virtual fluoroscopy and 4DCT. Lung Cancer 2006;53:31–37.

28 Murphy MJ: Tracking moving organs in real time. Semin Radiat Oncol 2004;14:91–100.

29 Underberg RWM, Lagerwaard FJ, van Tinteren H, Cuijpers JP, Slotman BJ, Senan S: Time trends in target volumes for stage I non-small-cell lung cancer after stereotactic radiotherapy. Int J Radiat Oncol Biol Phys 2006;64:1221–1228.

30 Kupelian PA, Ramsey C, Meeks SL, Willoughby TR, Forbes A, Wagner TH, Langen KM: Serial megavoltage CT imaging during external beam radiotherapy for non-small-cell lung cancer: observations on tumor regression during treatment. Int J Radiat Oncol Biol Phys 2005;63:1024–1028.

Dr. Frank J. Lagerwaard
Department of Radiation Oncology
VU University Medical Center
De Boelelaan 1117
NL–1007 MB Amsterdam (The Netherlands)
Tel. +31 20 444 0414, Fax +31 20 444 0410
E-Mail fj.lagerwaard@vumc.nl

Meyer JL (ed): IMRT, IGRT, SBRT – Advances in the Treatment Planning and
Delivery of Radiotherapy. Front Radiat Ther Oncol. Basel, Karger, 2007, vol. 40, pp 253–271

Partial Breast Irradiation

Patient Selection, Guidelines for Treatment, and Current Results

Peter Y. Chen · Frank A. Vicini

Department of Radiation Oncology, William Beaumont Hospital, Royal Oak, Mich., USA

Abstract

Studies evaluating selected patients treated with partial breast irradiation (PBI) in accelerated fractionation schemes have demonstrated the equivalence of PBI with traditional whole-breast irradiation. The major advantage of PBI is the time compression of treatment down to less than 1 week
compared with 6.5 weeks for whole-breast external beam treatments. Four techniques are available
to deliver PBI. These include interstitial brachytherapy multicatheter systems, the Mammosite Radiation Therapy System applicator, external beam three-dimensional conformal radiation therapy and
intraoperative radiation therapy. For the two brachytherapy techniques of multicatheter implantation and the Mammosite, accurate placement is achieved with image guidance via intraoperative
ultrasonography, mammography, and/or CT scanning. Technologies such as image-guided cone
beam CT assure accurate delivery of PBI with external beam three-dimensional conformal radiation
therapy. Results of PBI show excellent control rates with mild toxicities; cosmetic outcomes are good
to excellent in the vast majority of patients.

A number of randomized trials have documented the equivalence of breast-conserving therapy and mastectomy [1, 2]. To shorten the overall treatment time, centers have been investigating the use of partial breast irradiation (PBI) in accelerated fractionation schemes, and comparing the outcomes to those of standard
whole-breast tangential beam irradiation delivered in 6–7 weeks. We present the
rationale for PBI, delineate the various techniques available for PBI, update the
data supporting such partial breast treatments, and review the highlights of the
National Surgical Adjuvant Breast Project (NSABP) B-39/Radiation Therapy
Oncology Group (RTOG) 0413 randomized phase III trial.

Definition and Rationale of Partial Breast Irradiation

PBI is the delivery of larger doses per fraction of radiation therapy to the lumpectomy cavity (plus a 1- to 2-cm margin) using brachytherapy or external beam irradiation techniques after surgery, for breast-conserving cancer therapy. The major advantage is the time compression, from the 6–7 weeks required for whole-breast radiotherapy with boost down to 4–5 days for partial breast radiotherapy.

The rationale for PBI includes the time reduction with its greater convenience, and the possible reduction in both the acute and chronic toxicities of therapy as the volume of treatment is smaller. Such reduction in morbidity should lead to improvement in the quality of life of patients. Additionally, PBI may eliminate the scheduling problems associated with integrating systemic therapies by concisely delivering the radiotherapy initially. Together, these factors may improve the utilization of breast-conserving therapy, known to be underutilized [3, 4].

What is the scientific rationale for PBI? The major effect of postlumpectomy radiotherapy is to reduce the risk of recurrence in the vicinity of the original tumor. Rates of recurrence away from the tumor bed ('elsewhere failures') are actually similar with or without radiotherapy following lumpectomy [5–7]. The expectation is that in carefully selected patients whole-breast radiotherapy may not be necessary.

Patient Selection

Eligibility criteria for the William Beaumont Hospital (WBH) PBI protocols include infiltrating ductal carcinoma measuring less than 3 cm in its greatest dimension, negative surgical margins greater than or equal to 2 mm, age greater than 40 years, and surgically staged axilla with less than or equal to three positive lymph nodes. In 1997, the last criterion was changed to negative lymph nodes, based on the documented survival benefit of larger, regional field radiotherapy for lymph node-positive postmastectomy patients, as shown in the Danish and British Columbia trials [8, 9]. Patients with an extensive intraductal component, infiltrating lobular histology, ductal carcinoma in situ, or clinically significant areas of lobular carcinoma in situ were excluded from our protocols.

As interest in PBI increased, two societies put forward their own criteria for PBI. The selection criteria endorsed by the American Brachytherapy Society include: patient age ≥45 years, invasive ductal carcinoma only, tumor size ≤3 cm, negative resection margins (defined as no tumor on ink), and no axillary metastases [10]. The eligibility criteria for PBI set forth by the American Society of Breast Surgeons include: patient age ≥50 years, invasive ductal or ductal carcinoma in situ, tumor size ≤2 cm, negative resection margins (≥2 mm in all directions), and negative axillary nodal status. In contrast, for the randomized phase III clinical trial spon-

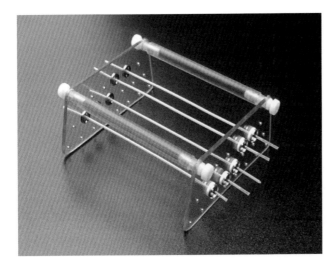

Fig. 1. Brachytherapy template.

sored by the NSABP/RTOG (B-39/0413) the criteria have been broadened to include ductal carcinoma in situ, invasive lobular carcinoma, axillary metastases in up to three nodes, and younger age (≥18 years).

Partial Breast Irradiation Techniques

Multicatheter/Multineedle Implantations
Multicatheter/multineedle-based systems for PBI have incorporated templates to guide placement of the interstitial catheters/needles for uniform geometric coverage (fig. 1). The WBH technique has included both low-dose-rate iodine-125 implants that deliver 50 Gy over 96 h at 0.52 Gy per hour, and high-dose-rate iridium-192 implants that deliver either 32 Gy in 8 fractions or 34 Gy in 10 fractions (with a minimal interfraction time interval of 6 h). Each implant has been designed to irradiate the lumpectomy cavity with at least a 1- to 2-cm margin (fig. 2). Quality control criteria have been reported previously [11, 12].

Other investigators have also used template-based systems. In the technique described by Kuske et al. [13], interstitial high-dose-rate implants are used with patients in the prone position on a stereotactic biopsy table; a table aperture allows for stereotaxis with mammographic guidance (fig. 3). Cuttino et al. [14] have included operative CT image guidance for optimal coverage of the lumpectomy cavity with a template-based system. With such CT guidance, both freehand and template-guided implants are achievable.

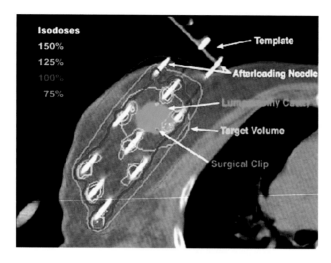

Fig. 2. Dosimetric treatment planning.

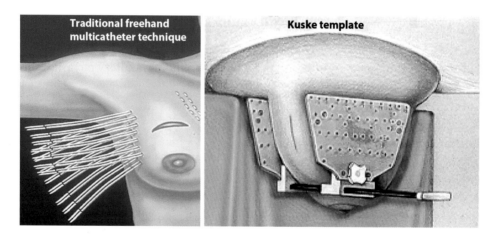

Fig. 3. Catheter-based brachytherapy.

MammoSite Radiation Therapy System

The MammoSite Radiation Therapy System (RTS) device comes in two spherical sizes: 4–5 cm or 5–6 cm diameter. The fill volumes range from 35 to 70 cm³ for the smaller balloon and from 70 to 125 cm³ for the larger one (fig. 4). As not all lumpectomy cavities are spherical, the MammoSite RTS ellipsoid balloon may be considered, which has a fill volume of 60–65 cm³.

These MammoSite balloon catheters are instilled with sterile saline to tightly fit the lumpectomy cavity. A high-activity iridium-192 source travels through the central catheter channel to a single dwell position for the spherical geometry

Chen · Vicini

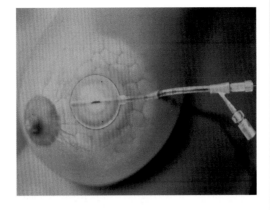

MammoSite device
(Cytyc Corporation)

Inflatable ballon placed in
lumpectomy cavity at surgery

Remote afterloading

3,400 cGy (340 cGy × 10) in 5 days

(FDA clearance)

Fig. 4. Balloon catheter: 'MammoSite'.

balloon, while multiple dwell positions are possible with the ellipsoidal device. Each of the dwell times can be varied to optimize the dosimetry for each individual. The dose is prescribed to 1 cm from the balloon surface, and the total dose is 3.4 Gy times 10 fractions for a total of 34 Gy over 5 days. Experience is being gained using the newer ellipsoid balloon catheter, as well as the original spherical ones.

The MammoSite device is placed in the lumpectomy cavity either during or after completion of breast-conserving surgery. After instillation of the sterile saline, the balloon is checked for conformance to the lumpectomy cavity to assure that the central catheter is nondisplaced, and skin spacing is adequate (the distance between the MammoSite balloon and the skin surface). The desired skin spacing is at least 7–8 mm. CT scanning after balloon placement is performed to assure geometric symmetry, adequate skin spacing, and appropriate conformance of the device to the excision cavity.

External Beam PBI
For the three-dimensional conformal radiation therapy (3DCRT) approach, treatments are individually planned for patients with the goals of meeting the dose-volume minimum constraints for the planning target volume (PTV) and maximum constraints for the normal tissues.

Target Delineation. To meet these dose-volume constraints, the contouring of targets is an important first step. The excision cavity is contoured as the gross tumor volume, and is defined by the treating physician using the surgically placed

Table 1. NSABP B-39 PBI: summary contour guidelines

Site	Anatomy	Exclusions
Excision cavity	Physician drawn	
CTV	Excision cavity + 15 mm	Exclude the first 5 mm below the skin surface Exclude chest wall and pectoralis muscles
PTV	CTV + 10 mm	
PTV for evaluation	PTV	Exclude regions outside of ipsilateral breast Exclude the first 5 mm below the skin surface Exclude chest wall and pectoralis muscles
Whole breast volume: ipsilateral	All tissues within the tangential fields, includes the chest wall	Exclude lung, heart, stomach, liver
Whole breast volume: contralateral	All tissues within the tangential fields, includes the chest wall	Exclude lung, heart, stomach, liver
Thyroid	Physician contours	All 'bright' thyroid tissues
Heart	Physician contours	Inferior surface of pulmonary artery to most inferior aspects of the heart

clips and/or the architectural distortion resulting from the operative procedure. The clinical target volume (CTV) is the gross tumor volume + 15 mm, but excludes the first 5 mm below the skin surface as well as the chest wall and pectoralis muscles deep to the breast. These target delineations have been adopted in the phase III national cooperative NSABP B-39/RTOG 0413 protocol (table 1). The CTV is uniformly expanded by 10 mm to define the PTV. Finally, the PTV for evaluation is the PTV excluding regions outside of the breast, the first 5 mm below the skin surface, chest wall and pectoralis muscles (fig. 5).

Dose Constraints. Once all of the contours are drawn, the normal tissue dose limits are set, as defined by the NSABP B-39/RTOG 0413 and shown in table 2. Note that these constraints define maximum accepted levels for the percentage of the breast receiving treatment, the dose to the opposite breast, and doses to the significant regional normal tissues including lung and heart volumes. These dose constraints, used in the NSABP B-39/RTOG 0413 protocol, are similar to those adopted by the RTOG 0319 trial, which is evaluating 3DCRT confined to the region of the lumpectomy cavity for stage I and II breast carcinoma and investigating the feasibility and reproducibility of such partial breast external beam treatments [15].

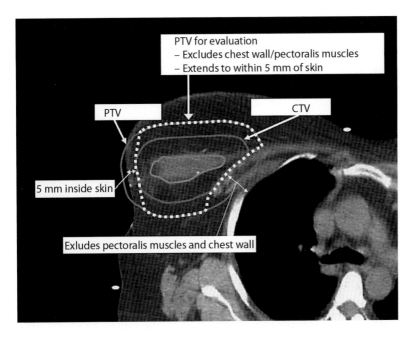

Fig. 5. NSABP B-39/RTOG 0413 contouring guidelines.

Table 2. Dose limits – normal tissues

Site	Volume	Dose
Uninvolved normal breast	<60% whole breast volume	≥50% of prescribed dose (19.25 Gy)
Uninvolved normal breast	<35% whole breast volume	100% of prescribed dose (38.50 Gy)
Contralateral breast	any point	<3% of prescribed dose (1.15 Gy)
Ipsilateral lung	<15% of the lung	30% of prescribed dose (1.15 Gy)
Contralateral lung	<15% of the lung	5% of prescribed dose (1.92 Gy)
Heart (right-sided lesions)	<5% of the heart	5% of prescribed dose (1.92 Gy)
Heart (left-sided lesions)	<40% of the heart	5% of prescribed dose (1.92 Gy)
Thyroid	maximum point dose	3% of prescribed dose (1.15 Gy)

Treatment Planning. Treatment planning is performed using a free-breathing CT scan acquired at 5-mm intervals. The isocenter is set in the center of the PTV and standardized tangent fields are established. Oblique non-coplanar 4- and 5-field beam arrangements using 6 MV photons are generated. Both arrangements use breast tangent fields with a 10–20° steeper angle for the medial beams, to maximally spare breast tissue, and couch angles of 15–70°. General guidelines, which only represent starting points in the planning process for 4-beam orientations, are shown in table 3. The collimator angle is adjusted to place the thick (heel) portion

Table 3. Gantry and couch angles (degrees) for left/right-sided 4-field beam arrangement

	Right breast				Left breast			
	left ASIO	left AISO	right PSIO	right PISO	right ASIO	right AISO	left PSIO	left PISO
Gantry	45–55	45–55	220–235	220–235	305–315	305–315	125–140	125–140
Couch	30–50	320–345	340–345	15–20	310–330	15–40	15–20	340–345

During beam arrangement, it is helpful to create a three-dimensional viewing window to visualize what the beams look like on the patient. Especially with the ASIO beam, one can check to be sure that the beam clears the patient's face/chin. Minimizing the projected surface of the PTV in the three-dimensional beam's eye view window helps to optimize the gantry and couch angles and reduce the dose to the breast. The blocks window helps to visualize the internal structures. Attention should be paid to avoid beams entering or exiting through the contralateral breast, lung, heart and thyroid gland.

of the wedge towards the central portion of the breast by the nipple. Beam weights are then manually optimized such that the CTV is encompassed by the 100% isodose line and the PTV by the 95% isodose line [16].

Prescription. The dose prescribed for the external beam PBI with 6 MV photons is 38.5 Gy, delivered in 10 fractions given twice daily and using a minimal inter-fraction time of 6 h. In other work, Dr. Formenti at New York University has planned and delivered 3DCRT for partial breast treatments [17, 18]. There, patients have been treated in the prone position, and the dose prescribed is 30 Gy in 6-Gy fractions over 10 days.

Intensity-Modulated Radiation Therapy. To date, the experience from WBH has demonstrated that the use of intensity-modulated radiation therapy (IMRT) for whole-breast tangential irradiation is feasible with excellent early results. Dose-volume histogram analysis demonstrates a significant improvement in homogeneity compared with conventional open-field tangents, with the former typically with hot spots limited to 105% of the prescribed dose. Other potential benefits include minimizing dose to the underlying lung and/or heart, more uniform dose coverage of the tumor bed, reducing both acute and late toxicities of breast irradiation and the potential application to a more complex radiation therapy [19]. In the phase III trial of the NSABP/RTOG, IMRT has been excluded because of the fact that IMRT methodologies are presently not entirely standardized and providing oversight for the technical aspects of delivery is inordinately time consuming with currently available tools. Moreover, to date, no long-term published data exist on the use of IMRT for PBI.

Image-Guided Radiation Therapy. At WBH, each of the 10 fractions given twice daily is verified by imaging the tumor cavity clips, initially using an electronic portal imaging device and now using cone beam CT [20]. Placement of clips is a requirement for all potential candidates for PBI and in particular those treated on the 3DCRT protocols at WBH. Prior to each fraction, the position of the clips is imaged using an electronic portal imaging device for an orthogonal pair (anterior-posterior and lateral) and for each of the beams employed in the 3DCRT plan. These images are then correlated with the original simulation films for accuracy. In addition, implementation of cone beam image-guided radiation therapy has been ongoing at WBH, and the present policy is to acquire a cone beam image before each of the planned 10 fractions given twice daily with necessary adjustments made based upon the cone beam image of each particular fraction [21]. Treatment proceeds if the clip positions are within 2 mm of the simulated clip positions, as compared with the original helical planning CT scan data set. Otherwise, necessary translations of the couch are made and the accurate position of the clipped target volume is assured with a repeat cone beam CT.

Intraoperative PBI

In Europe, two groups have extensive experience using intraoperative radiotherapy to deliver PBI (fig. 6, 7). In the approach developed by Veronesi et al. [22], an electron cone is used intraoperatively. This allows irradiation to be directed to the tumor bed at a set depth. Breast tissue can be mobilized from all sides and directly placed within the cone to ensure coverage during treatment. The dose given is 21 Gy in 1 fraction.

In another approach, Vaidya et al. [23] use a spherical applicator that treats the entire lumpectomy cavity in three dimensions. It is a spherical applicator with a geometry similar to that achieved by the MammoSite RTS (fig. 8). However, treatment is given intraoperatively. The spherical applicator delivers a single-fraction dose of 5 Gy prescribed at 1 cm, and a dose of 20 Gy at 0.2 cm from the tumor bed.

Treatment Results of the Various Partial Breast Irradiation Techniques

Multicatheter System PBI Results
Local Control. Published PBI results of catheter-based brachytherapy approaches are listed in table 4. As noted, the local recurrence rates range from 0 as reported by the Massachusetts General Hospital to 6% as reported by Tufts-Brown University. Representative results are shown for the WBH series of 199 patients with a median follow-up period of 6.5 years. The local control rate is 98.8%. Compared with a cohort of matched controls receiving whole-breast irradiation, all outcome endpoints including local control, cause-specific survival, and overall survival are not significantly different with PBI [24].

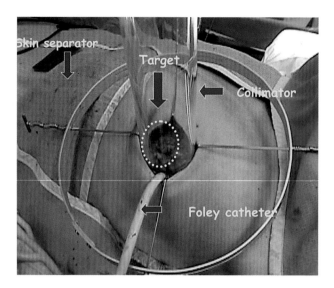

Fig. 6. Intraoperative electron cone.

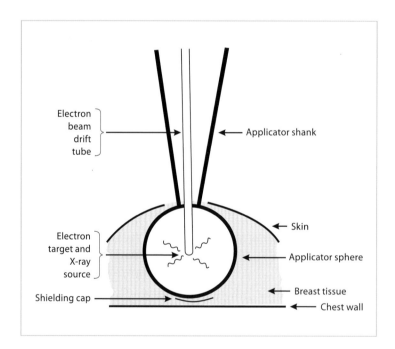

Fig. 7. Intraoperative spherical applicator (approach developed by Vaidya et al. [23] at the University College London).

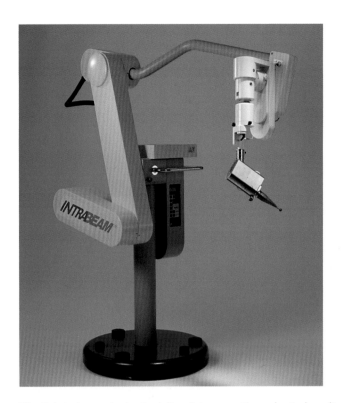

Fig. 8. Intrabeam device to deliver intraoperative spherical applicator treatments.

Table 4. Published PBI results: catheter-based brachytherapy

Institution	Patients	Follow-up months	Local recurrence, %
WBH: low-dose-rate patients [24]	120	82	0.9
Oschner Clinic [30]	51	75	2.0
WBH: all patients [24, 25]	199	65	1.2
National Institute of Oncology Hungary [31]	45	60	4.4
Tufts-Brown University [32]	33	58	6
WBH: high-dose-rate patients [24, 25]	79	52	2.1
Virginia Commonwealth University [33]	44	42	0
RTOG 95-17	99	44	3.0
University Kansas [34]	25	47	0
National Institute of Oncology Hungary phase III [35]	181	30	1.1
Florence, Italy	90	27	4.4
Massachusetts General Hospital [36]	48	23	0
Total	815		0–6

Table 5. Toxicities (%) with resolution or stabilization over time with interstitial catheter needle-based brachytherapy

	<6 months (n = 165)			2 years (n = 128)			Follow-up >5 years (n = 79)		
	I	II	III	I	II	III	I	II	III
Breast pain	27	0	0	13	1	0	8	1	0
Breast edema	50	1	0	12	0	0	6	1	0
Erythema	35	1	0	11	0	0	11	0	0
Hyperpigmentation	67	2	0	39	2	0	37	0	0
Fibrosis	22	1	0	48	2	1	46	5	1
Hypopigmentation	18	0	0	34	0	0	38	0	0

Toxicity grades: I = mild; II = moderate; III = severe.

Table 6. Cosmetic outcome at three time points with accelerated PBI

≤6 months (n = 165)			2 years (n = 128)			≥5 years (n = 79)		
excellent	good	fair	excellent	good	fair	excellent	good	fair
10%	85%	1%	29%	68%	2%	33%	66%	1%
Total 95%			Total 97%			Total 99%		

Total percentage equals excellent and good outcomes combined. Note: 4 and 1% of unreported cosmesis for ≤6 months and 2 years, respectively.

Toxicity. The toxicity profiles over time generally have been mild and typically have diminished with longer follow-up (table 5) [25]. These include breast pain, edema, erythema, and hyperpigmentation. Mild breast fibrosis and hypopigmentation increase until the 2-year mark and then stabilize (table 5). Fat necrosis and telangiectasia increase with the passage of time, with fat necrosis increasing from 1% at ≤6 months to 9% at 2 years and 11% at 5 years. Nearly all the telangiectasias are small (<2 mm) and increase in incidence from 5% at ≤6 months to 21% at 2 years and 34% at 5 years [25]. Assessment of cosmetic results at three time points after treatment (greater than 6 months, and at 2 and 5 years) reveals that more than 95% of patients have good to excellent results at all time points (table 6). There is stabilization of the percentage with combined good-to-excellent results at 2 years, but an increase in those with excellent results out to 5 years [25].

Table 7. Published clinical data: Mammosite

Institution	Cases	Follow-up months	Local recurrence %	Cosmetic results (good/ excellent), %	Infection %
Multi-institutional trial	43	21	0	88	3.7
Mammosite Registry Trial	106	NR	0	90	6
Tufts-New England Medical Center	28	19	0	93	NR
St. Vincent's Comprehensive Cancer Center	32	11	0	86	16
Breast Care Center of the Southwest	21	NR	NR	NR	NR
Rush University Medical Center	112	NR	0	80	6

NR = Not reported.

MammoSite PBI Results

As reported by Dr. Keisch at the ASTRO meeting in 2004, the Food and Drug Administration trial of the use of the MammoSite RTS device treated 43 patients to 34.0 Gy in 10 fractions, twice per day over 5 days [26]. With a median follow-up period approaching 3 years, no recurrences had been observed at the time of the report. With skin spacing of 5 mm or greater, 88% of the patients had good to excellent cosmesis. Based on this trial sponsored by the manufacturer, the MammoSite RTS was approved for clinical use by the US Food and Drug Administration in May 2002.

Additional patients have been treated with the MammoSite RTS using these recommended doses, and their outcomes have been entered into a registry managed by the American Society of Breast Surgeons. This registry trial completed patient accrual and closed in November 2004. Fifteen hundred patients were enrolled from 87 institutions encompassing 233 investigators. To date, the reported rates of cosmesis for all patient visits showed an overall 95% good to excellent score. Over time, at 24 months, the good to excellent cosmesis rate was maintained at 94.7%. Variables analyzed that showed an adverse effect on early cosmesis were skin spacing less than 7 mm, a smaller breast volume/size (cup size A and B), and the occurrence of infection at the treatment site.

Table 7 lists the published clinical data for the MammoSite RTS applicator. Most remarkably, across all institutions and with a median follow-up varying from 11 to 21 months, there are no local recurrences reported. The range for good to excellent cosmesis is 80–93% with the multi-institutional registry trial reporting 88% [27].

3DCRT PBI Results

The WBH [16, 28] and New York University [17, 18] have reported their results with this approach. Both institutions have reported on a limited number of patients, and with a minimum follow-up of 8–10 months at WBH and 18 months at New York University. Both groups report no local recurrences, and 100% good to excellent cosmetic results. However, the follow-up interval for both studies is quite short, and long-term results in terms of both morbidity and cosmesis are awaited.

In both studies, patients were treated with complex field arrangements, and this raises concern about the reproducibility and feasibility of such treatment techniques at multiple institutions. However, the validity of using such approaches more widely has been investigated by the RTOG 0319 trial. The field arrangements, which are rather complex, have been scored for reproducibility and feasibility at 24 institutions. Only 4 out of the first 42 evaluable treatments were scored as unacceptable [15, 28]. Thus, the technique has been shown to be reproducible in >90% of these treatment courses. Based on the results of this RTOG 0319 trial, the technique has been adopted for the randomized phase III trial of the NSABP B-39/RTOG 0413 study, which is investigating accelerated PBI in early-stage breast cancer patients compared with standard whole-breast irradiation.

Intraoperative PBI Results

Approaches using intraoperative radiotherapy are yet being tested in randomized settings by Veronesi et al. [22] with the European Institute of Oncology and by Vaidya et al. [23] at the University College of London. Neither has reported results of the intraoperative single-fraction PBI experience.

Ongoing Studies and Future Directions

Current Studies

As of March 2005, the randomized trial cosponsored by the NSABP and RTOG was open for patient accrual. Compared with the entry criteria of the earlier prospective, single-institution studies, this randomized phase III trial includes patients with ductal carcinoma in situ and invasive lobular carcinoma. Margin status is defined as no tumor on ink. Patients may have up to three axillary lymph nodes involved. Patients with an extensive intraductal component can be included, but this must be fully excised with negative margins. Patients must be more than 18 years old. Randomization is to either whole-breast irradiation or accelerated PBI. If the patient is randomized to PBI, each institution may perform one of three forms of partial breast treatment: interstitial multicatheter brachytherapy, MammoSite RTS

Table 8. Prospective randomized trials: PBI

Institution, trial	Trial design	Patients	Control arm	Experimental arm	Status
NSABP B-39/ RTOG 0413	equivalence, detect 50% difference, assume 6% LR at 10 years	3,000	50–50.4 Gy whole breast, ±10–16 Gy boost	(1) interstitial brachytherapy, or (2) Mammosite, or (3) three-dimensional conformal EBRT	activated March 21, 2005
National Institute of Oncology, Budapest, Hungary [31]	noninferiority	570	50 Gy whole breast, no boost	(1) interstitial brachytherapy (5.2 Gy × 7) or (2) electrons (50 Gy)	260 enrolled
European Brachytherapy Breast Cancer GEC-ESTRO Working Group	noninferiority, nonirrelevant, detect a 3% difference	1,170	50–50.4 Gy whole breast +10 Gy boost	(1) brachytherapy only: 32.0 Gy 8 fractions HDR 30.3 Gy 7 fractions HDR 50 Gy PDR	activated May 2004
European Institute of Oncology [37]	equivalence, assume 3% LR, detect <7.5%	824	50 Gy whole breast (+) boost	intraoperative single-fraction EBRT 21 Gy × 1	587 patients enrolled
University College of London [38]	equivalence, assume 9% LR, detect 13.5%	1,600	whole-breast radiotherapy per institution	intraoperative single-fraction EBRT 5 Gy × 1	120 enrolled

EBRT = External beam radiation therapy; HDR = high dose rate; PDR = pulsed dose rate; LR = local recurrence.

applicator, or 3DCRT. The primary endpoint measures will be breast tumor recurrence, with secondary endpoint measures including distant disease-free survival, overall survival, quality of life, cosmetic outcome, fatigue, local breast symptoms, burden of care, and direct nonmedical costs, i.e. lost income.

The sample size was determined to be 3,000 patients based on an estimated 10-year cumulative instance of in-breast tumor recurrence for whole-breast therapy of 6.1%. Accrual is expected to take 2.5 years. Analysis will occur after the first 175 in-breast tumor recurrences, estimated to occur at 11 years after the trial opens. Standards of pathology review will be required. Quality of life and cosmesis assessments will be made as well. Each institution will be credentialed, certifying technical quality for performing both interstitial therapy and 3DCRT. There will be reviews of performance for the first case (rapid review), the subsequent 4 cases (timely review), following completion of 5 cases (approval for accrual), as well as randomly following this (random case review). This ongoing randomized trial of the NSABP/RTOG will offer additional class I data/evidence with respect to the efficacy of PBI. Table 8 delineates the prospective randomized trials that are investigating PBI.

Genetic Imprinting

Ongoing clinical research involves ascertaining the type of local recurrence, whether it is a true, clonally identical tumor as the original index lesion, or a clonally different tumor and thus a new primary carcinoma. Such identification is done via deletion mutations using primers directed to DNA within specific target genes. If one has no gene (allele) deletions that are noted, 2 signals (heterozygosity present) of the target gene(s) exist. This would represent a normal cell with no deletions of any genes. However, if a deletion mutation of one allele of a target gene is present, 1 signal is lost leading to loss of heterozygosity (LOH); this would therefore signify a carcinoma cell with a deletion mutation that has lost one signal peak.

Each carcinoma has a unique pattern of LOH gene mutations. A composite pattern of LOH gene mutations is the DNA fingerprint of any particular neoplasm. Comparison of the LOH pattern between the index lesion and the ipsilateral breast tumor recurrence establishes whether or not it is a recurrence or new primary lesion. Thus, the LOH gene mutation profile allows for carcinoma comparisons. Specifically, in defining the type of breast recurrence, those which are clonally related (derived from the same primary clone of neoplastic cells) would represent persistence/recurrence of the index carcinoma. In contrast, clonally distinct LOH profiles would confirm distinct and separate primary carcinomas, that is, a new, unique primary lesion derived from a different clone of neoplastic cells.

The implications of such genetic fingerprinting for patients treated with PBI are striking. The in-breast failure patterns can be designated not only in terms of the clinical failure pattern, but also the molecular pattern of failure – via LOH being the more accurate method (compared with clinical and/or light microscopic assessment) to establish the type of failure. Indeed, with such LOH analysis 43% of the PBI in-breast recurrences have been reclassified at WBH. We found that 2 patients with clinical 'elsewhere failures' in the breast were in reality true recurrences/marginal misses [29].

Conclusions

Many single-institutional series employing various PBI techniques and one published randomized trial from Hungary have demonstrated the efficacy and safety of PBI. These selected patients, treated with PBI in accelerated fractionation schemes, have shown control rates equal to or exceeding those of conventional external beam tangential irradiation delivered over 6.5 weeks. The latest technologies in both brachytherapy and external beam (3DCRT, image-guided radiation therapy) offer the tools to achieve PBI. Several phase III trials including the NSABP

B-39/RTOG 0413 protocol are in progress to provide class I evidence for the efficacy of PBI compared with whole-breast therapy. Beyond clinical efficacy, genetic clonality studies will enable more definitive molecular fingerprinting of failure patterns of PBI.

Acknowledgement

The authors would like to thank Ms. Margaret Calhoun for her assistance in the preparation of this paper.

Guidelines for Clinical Practice

- Studies evaluating selected patients treated with partial breast irradiation (PBI) in accelerated fractionation schemes delivered over 4–5 days have shown control rates comparable with those of standard whole-breast external beam treatment given over 6–7 weeks.

- Single institutional experiences have had selection criteria similar to those used at the William Beaumont Hospital including pure infiltrating ductal carcinoma of ≤3 cm, negative surgical margins of ≥2 mm, age >40 years and pathological staging of the axilla with ≤3 positive nodes, which in 1997 was changed to all sampled nodes negative for any metastasis. However, the criteria for entry into the NSABP B-39/RTOG 0413 phase III randomized trial have been broadened to include ductal carcinoma in situ, infiltrating lobular carcinoma, axillary metastases in up to 3 nodes and younger age (≥18 years).

- Four techniques are available to deliver PBI: interstitial brachytherapy multicatheter systems, the Mammosite Radiation Therapy System (RTS) applicator, external beam three-dimensional conformal radiation therapy (3DCRT), and intraoperative radiation therapy. In general, for interstitial multicatheter techniques, the target volume is defined as 1–2 cm beyond the excision cavity, while for the Mammosite RTS the planning target volume is 1 cm beyond the balloon surface. For 3DCRT, the clinical target volume is a 1.5-cm expansion beyond the excision cavity with an additional 1-cm expansion for the planning target volume. For intraoperative radiation therapy, the dose prescription varies between the user groups. The time-dose fractionation scheme is 3.40 Gy given twice daily in 10 fractions over 5 treatment days with both the multicatheter system or Mammosite RTS; the external beam 3DCRT is delivered at 3.85 Gy twice daily in 10 fractions over the same time period.

- Cosmetic and toxicity results, whether with external beam or interstitial brachytherapy, demonstrate that the vast majority of patients have good to excellent cosmetic outcomes with stabilization of cosmesis at 2 years from completion of treatment. The majority of morbidities with PBI are mild and stabilize or resolve over time.

- The ongoing United States phase III clinical trial (NSABP B-39/RTOG 0413) along with other randomized trials being conducted overseas should provide class I evidence with respect to the efficacy of PBI.

References

1 Fisher B, Anderson S, Bryant J, Margolese RG, Deutsch M, Fisher ER, et al: Twenty-year follow-up of a randomized trial comparing total mastectomy, lumpectomy, and lumpectomy plus irradiation for the treatment of invasive breast cancer. N Engl J Med 2002;347:1233–1241.

2 Veronesi U, Cascinelli N, Mariani L, Greco M, Saccozzi R, Luini A, et al: Twenty-year follow-up of a randomized study comparing breast-conserving surgery with radical mastectomy for early breast cancer. N Engl J Med 2002;347:1227–1232.

3 Morrow M, White J, Moughan J, Owen J, Pajack T, Sylvester J, et al: Factors predicting the use of breast-conserving therapy in stage I and II breast carcinoma. J Clin Oncol 2001;19:2254–2262.

4 Nattinger AB, Hoffmann RG, Kneusel RT, Schapira MM: Relation between appropriateness of primary therapy for early-stage breast carcinoma and increased use of breast-conserving surgery. Lancet 2000;356:1148–1153.

5 Sector resection with or without postoperative radiotherapy for stage I breast cancer: a randomized trial. Uppsala-Orebro Breast Cancer Study Group. J Natl Cancer Inst 1990;82:277–282.

6 Clark RM, McCulloch PB, Levine MN, Lipa M, Wilkinson RH, Mahoney LJ, et al: Randomized clinical trial to assess the effectiveness of breast irradiation following lumpectomy and axillary dissection for node-negative breast cancer. J Natl Cancer Inst 1992;84:683–689.

7 Veronesi U, Marubini E, Mariani L, Galimberti V, Luini A, Veronesi P, et al: Radiotherapy after breast-conserving surgery in small breast carcinoma: long-term results of a randomized trial. Ann Oncol 2001;12:997–1003.

8 Overgaard M, Hansen PS, Overgaard J, Rose C, Andersson M, Bach F, et al: Postoperative radiotherapy in high-risk premenopausal women with breast cancer who receive adjuvant chemotherapy. Danish Breast Cancer Cooperative Group 82b Trial. N Engl J Med 1997;337:949–955.

9 Ragaz J, Jackson SM, Le N, Plenderleith IH, Spinelli JJ, Basco VE, et al: Adjuvant radiotherapy and chemotherapy in node-positive premenopausal women with breast cancer. N Engl J Med 1997;337:956–962.

10 Arthur DW, Vicini FA, Kuske RR, Wazer DE, Nag S: Accelerated partial breast irradiation: an updated report from the American Brachytherapy Society. Brachytherapy 2002;1:184–190.

11 Kestin LL, Jaffray DA, Edmundson GK, Martinez AA, Wong JW, Kini VR, et al: Improving the dosimetric coverage of interstitial high-dose-rate breast implants. Int J Radiat Oncol Biol Phys 2000;46:35–43.

12 Vicini FA, Kestin LL, Edmundson GK, Jaffray DA, Wong JW, Kini VR, et al: Dose-volume analysis for quality assurance of interstitial brachytherapy for breast cancer. Int J Radiat Oncol Biol Phys 1999;45:803–810.

13 Kuske RR: Brachytherapy techniques. The university of Wisconsin/Arizona approach; in Wazer DE, Arthur DW, Vicini FA (eds): Accelerated Partial Breast Irradiation. Techniques and Clinical Implementation. Heidelberg, Springer, 2006, pp 105–128.

14 Cuttino LW, Todor D, Arthur DW: CT-guided multi-catheter insertion technique for partial breast brachytherapy: reliable target coverage and dose homogeneity. Brachytherapy 2005;4:10–17.

15 Vicini F, Winter K, Straube W, Wong J, Pass H, Rabinovitch R, et al: A phase I/II trial to evaluate three-dimensional conformal radiation therapy confined to the region of the lumpectomy cavity for stage I/II breast carcinoma: initial report of feasibility and reproducibility of Radiation Therapy Oncology Group (RTOG) Study 0319. Int J Radiat Oncol Biol Phys 2005;63:1531–1537.

16 Baglan KL, Sharpe MB, Jaffray D, Frazier RC, Fayad J, Kestin LL, et al: Accelerated partial breast irradiation using 3D conformal radiation therapy (3D-CRT). Int J Radiat Oncol Biol Phys 2003;55:302–311.

17 Formenti SC, Rosenstein B, Skinner KA, Jozsef G: T1 stage breast cancer: adjuvant hypofractionated conformal radiation therapy to tumor bed in selected postmenopausal breast cancer patients – Pilot feasibility study. Radiology 2002;222:171–178.

18 Formenti SC, Truong MT, Goldberg JD, Mukhi V, Rosenstein B, Roses D, et al: Prone accelerated partial breast irradiation after breast-conserving surgery: preliminary clinical results and dose-volume histogram analysis. Int J Radiat Oncol Biol Phys 2004;60:493–504.

19 Vicini FA, Sharpe M, Kestin L, Martinez A, Mitchell CK, Wallace MF, et al: Optimizing breast cancer treatment efficacy with intensity-modulated radiotherapy. Int J Radiat Oncol Biol Phys 2002;54:1336–1344.

20 Jaffray DA, Siewerdsen JH, Wong JW, Martinez AA: Flat-panel cone-beam computed tomography for image-guided radiation therapy. Int J Radiat Oncol Biol Phys 2002;53:1337–1349.

21 Letourneau D, Wong JW, Oldham M, Gulam M, Watt L, Jaffray DA, et al: Cone-beam-CT-guided radiation therapy: technical implementation. Radiother Oncol 2005;75:279–286.

22 Veronesi U, Gatti G, Luini A, Intra M, Orecchia R, Borgen P, et al: Intraoperative radiation therapy for breast cancer: technical notes. Breast J 2003;9:106–112.

23 Vaidya JS, Tobias JS, Baum M, Wenz F, Kraus-Tiefenbacher U, D'Souza D, et al: TARGeted Intraoperative radiotherapy (TARGIT): an innovative approach to partial-breast irradiation. Semin Radiat Oncol 2005;15:84–91.

24 Vicini FA, Kestin L, Chen P, Benitez P, Goldstein NS, Martinez A: Limited-field radiation therapy in the management of early-stage breast cancer. J Natl Cancer Inst 2003;95:1205–1210.

25 Chen PY, Vicini FA, Benitez P, Kestin LL, Wallace M, Mitchell C, et al: Long-term cosmetic results and toxicity after accelerated partial-breast irradiation: a method of radiation delivery by interstitial brachytherapy for the treatment of early-stage breast carcinoma. Cancer 2006;106:991–999.

26 Keisch M, Vicini F, Kuske RR, Hebert M, White J, Quiet C, et al: Initial clinical experience with the MammoSite breast brachytherapy applicator in women with early-stage breast cancer treated with breast-conserving therapy. Int J Radiat Oncol Biol Phys 2003;55:289–293.

27 Vicini FA, Beitsch PD, Quiet CA, Keleher A, Garcia D, Snider HC, et al: First analysis of patient demographics, technical reproducibility, cosmesis, and early toxicity: results of the American Society of Breast Surgeons MammoSite breast brachytherapy trial. Cancer 2005;104:1138–1148.

28 Vicini FA, Remouchamps V, Wallace M, Sharpe M, Fayad J, Tyburski L, et al: Ongoing clinical experience utilizing 3D conformal external beam radiotherapy to deliver partial-breast irradiation in patients with early-stage breast cancer treated with breast-conserving therapy. Int J Radiat Oncol Biol Phys 2003;57:1247–1253.

29 Goldstein NS, Vicini FA, Hunter S, Odish E, Forbes S, Kraus D, et al: Molecular clonality determination of ipsilateral recurrence of invasive breast carcinomas after breast-conserving therapy: comparison with clinical and biologic factors. Am J Clin Pathol 2005;123:679–689.

30 King TA, Bolton JS, Kuske RR, Fuhrman GM, Scroggins TG, Jiang XZ: Long-term results of wide-field brachytherapy as the sole method of radiation therapy after segmental mastectomy for T(is,1,2) breast cancer. Am J Surg 2000;180:299–304.

31 Polgar C, Sulyok Z, Fodor J, Orosz Z, Major T, Takacsi-Nagy Z, et al: Sole brachytherapy of the tumor bed after conservative surgery for T1 breast cancer: five-year results of a phase I-II study and initial findings of a randomized phase III trial. J Surg Oncol 2002;80:121–128.

32 Wazer DE, Berle L, Graham R, Chung M, Rothschild J, Graves T, et al: Preliminary results of a phase I/II study of HDR brachytherapy alone for T1/T2 breast cancer. Int J Radiat Oncol Biol Phys 2002;53:889–897.

33 Arthur DW, Koo D, Zwicker RD, Tong S, Bear HD, Kaplan BJ, et al: Partial breast brachytherapy after lumpectomy: low-dose-rate and high-dose-rate experience. Int J Radiat Oncol Biol Phys 2003;56:681–689.

34 Krishnan L, Jewell WR, Tawfik OW, Krishnan EC: Breast conservation therapy with tumor bed irradiation alone in a selected group of patients with stage I breast cancer. Breast J 2001;7:91–96.

35 Polgar C, Major T, Fodor J, Nemeth G, Orosz Z, Sulyok Z, et al: High-dose-rate brachytherapy alone versus whole breast radiotherapy with or without tumor bed boost after breast-conserving surgery: seven-year results of a comparative study. Int J Radiat Oncol Biol Phys 2004;60:1173–1181.

36 Lawenda BD, Taghian AG, Kachnic LA, Hamdi H, Smith BL, Gadd MA, et al: Dose-volume analysis of radiotherapy for T1N0 invasive breast cancer treated by local excision and partial breast irradiation by low-dose-rate interstitial implant. Int J Radiat Oncol Biol Phys 2003;56:671–680.

37 Veronesi U, Gatti G, Luini A, Intra M, Ciocca M, Sanchez D, et al: Full-dose intraoperative radiotherapy with electrons during breast-conserving surgery. Arch Surg 2003;138:1253–1256.

38 Vaidya JS, Tobias JS, Baum M, Keshtgar M, Joseph D, Wenz F, et al: Intraoperative radiotherapy for breast cancer. Lancet Oncol 2004;5:165–173.

Dr. Peter Y. Chen
William Beaumont Hospital
3601 W. 13 Mile Road
Royal Oak, MI 48073 (USA)
Tel. +1 248 551 7038, Fax +1 248 551 0089
E-Mail pchen@beaumont.edu

Meyer JL (ed): IMRT, IGRT, SBRT – Advances in the Treatment Planning and
Delivery of Radiotherapy. Front Radiat Ther Oncol. Basel, Karger, 2007, vol. 40, pp 272–288

Upper Abdominal Malignancies: Intensity-Modulated Radiation Therapy

Mojgan Taremi · Jolie Ringash · Laura A. Dawson

Department of Radiation Oncology, Princess Margaret Hospital, University of Toronto, Toronto, Canada

Abstract

Local control and survival of most upper abdominal malignancies are poor. Challenges associated with the safe delivery of tumoricidal doses of radiation therapy to these malignancies include organ motion due to breathing, gastrointestinal filling and peristalsis, and the presence of many normal tissues with a low tolerance to radiation. Intensity-modulated radiation therapy (IMRT) can facilitate normal tissue sparing and dose escalation to these tumors, which has the potential to reduce toxicity and improve local control. Planning studies have demonstrated the potential for dose escalation with IMRT. However, degradation of upper abdominal IMRT plans in the presence of organ motion has also been demonstrated. Thus, organ motion reduction and image guidance strategies should be implemented in conjunction with IMRT. Clinical experience with dose-escalated IMRT is limited, and IMRT should continue to be studied in clinical trials before it is routinely used for upper abdominal malignancies.

Background

Upper abdominal malignancies represent some of the most challenging cancers to treat. Overall survival may be poor due to the development of distant metastases early in the natural history and to delayed detection. Although radiation therapy has an important role in the treatment of upper abdominal malignancies, treatment delivery has been challenging due to organ motion and the proximity of sensitive normal tissues. Improvements in radiation therapy planning and delivery have the potential to improve tumor control and reduce toxicity for all upper abdominal malignancies. Intensity-modulated radiation therapy (IMRT) facilitates high-precision dose escalation and possibly dose reduction to adjacent normal tissues. In this paper, the clinical rationale for IMRT in the upper abdomen, the potential pitfalls and the existing literature are discussed. The primary tumor sites discussed include hepatocellular carcinoma, liver metastases, gastric cancer, pancreatic cancer, cholangiocarcinoma, and upper abdominal sarcoma. Although some radiotherapy planning and delivery issues are similar for upper abdominal lymphomas, the challenges are reduced by the lower doses required for the lymphomas and they are not discussed here.

As outcomes in metastatic disease from colorectal cancer are improving with chemotherapy, local control of oligometastases in the liver has become more important. Ablative therapies such as radio frequency ablation, percutaneous ethanol injection or interstitial laser photocoagulation may be used to treat liver metastases [1]. However, many of these techniques are not suitable for tumors larger than 5 cm or tumors located adjacent to large vessels [2].

Similarly, for hepatocellular carcinoma, only a subset of patients are eligible for surgery, transplant or ablative approaches. With a better understanding of the partial organ tolerance of the liver to radiation, and with technical advances, high-dose conformal radiation therapy is an alterative option for some patients [3].

Adjuvant chemoradiation therapy is included in the standard of care for gastric cancer [4]. However, conventional techniques are associated with substantial normal tissue irradiation. The optimal technique to irradiate the stomach with minimal morbidity has yet to be established.

Pancreatic cancer is the fourth most common cause of death from cancer, and local failure is a frequent problem. A recent ESPAC randomized trial of adjuvant radiation therapy showed no benefit from adjuvant chemoradiation; local recurrences occurred in 61% of patients, and late toxicities may have contributed to late death [5]. These results may have been due to the large fields and/or low doses of radiation therapy used. High-precision radiation therapy may improve the therapeutic ratio. Additionally, primary chemoradiotherapy is an option for patients with unresectable disease; the role of radiotherapy dose escalation in this setting has been incompletely explored.

Most patients with cholangiocarcinoma also develop locoregional recurrences. Radiation dose escalation may improve local control; however, liver, small bowel and renal toxicity remain major obstacles in conventional radiation planning.

Other tumors may also present in the upper abdomen, such as retroperitoneal and paraspinal sarcomas. A dose response exists for sarcoma, and local recurrence is related to survival [6]. Close proximity of these tumors to the spinal cord and other critical normal tissues makes conventional planning challenging. High-precision techniques can facilitate delivery of high-dose radiation to these tumors

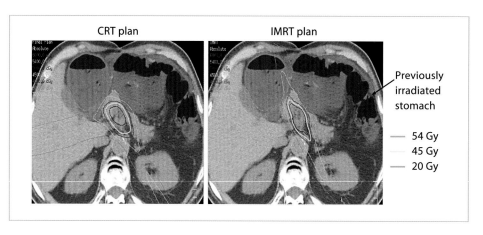

Fig. 1. Example of potential benefits of IMRT versus conformal radiation for a patient with an isolated nodal recurrence from esophageal cancer. The patient was previously irradiated, and thus the doses to the previously irradiated stomach had to be kept to below 20 Gy in 2 Gy per fraction, adding complexity to the planning process.

while sparing the adjacent normal tissues. Finally, isolated nodal recurrences in the upper abdomen may benefit from radical radiotherapy if disease is controlled elsewhere. Re-irradiation of upper abdominal malignancies is another situation where IMRT may be advantageous, as shown in figure 1.

Historically, the role of external beam radiation therapy in upper abdomen malignancies has been limited due to the above issues. The patients most likely to benefit from high-precision radiation, including IMRT, are those with diseases for which conventional radiation provides poor local control, evidence of a dose response exists, local recurrence is related to morbidity or survival, and/or toxicities from radiation therapy are dose limiting factors. The majority of these criteria apply to upper abdominal malignancies. Despite the rationale for high-precision radiotherapy and IMRT for upper abdominal malignancies, there is less experience with IMRT in the upper abdomen compared with other tumor sites. Possible reasons for the (appropriate) slow introduction of IMRT to the upper abdomen include organ motion due to breathing, challenges with target delineation and lack of soft tissue image guidance strategies until recently.

New Technologies for the Radiotherapy of Abdominal Tumors

Intensity-Modulated Radiation Therapy
IMRT facilitates delivery of highly conformal radiation to targets. IMRT refers to the use of variable radiation fluence patterns from multiple beam angles. Most often, IMRT is used in conjunction with automated computer-assisted optimiza-

Taremi · Ringash · Dawson

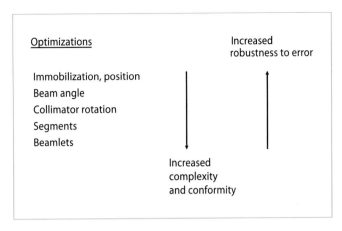

Fig. 2. Types of optimization relative to plan complexity and sensitivity to uncertainties. As the complexity increases, the sensitivity to uncertainties increases.

tion. Commercial IMRT planning systems optimize the fluence pattern of beamlets(1 × 1 cm segments within a beam angle). Computer-aided optimization is an iterative process that mimics what a dosimetrist does when planning, but at a high efficiency, with more degrees of freedom (e.g. 1 × 1 cm beamlet weights can be varied, allowing an extremely large number of possible fluence patterns). IMRT may be delivered without computer-aided optimization [7]. Other aspects of radiation therapy planning may not always be optimized. For example, positioning a tumor at a distance from a dose-limiting normal tissue may provide greater gains than those possible from beamlet fluence pattern optimization alone. Automated optimization may also be used to improve beam angle, number of beams, non-intensity-modulated field beam weight, or collimator rotation. As the complexity of optimization increases, the robustness decreases, while the sensitivity to error increases (fig. 2). Methods to develop robust IMRT plans are being investigated [8].

Although IMRT and automated optimization provide the opportunity for dose to be distributed more precisely than previously possible, IMRT does not eliminate dose to normal tissues (fig. 1, 3, 4). Hence, the partial volume tolerance of normal tissues needs to be better understood. Currently, technological advances have surpassed our clinical knowledge. Despite some progress in the understanding of partial volume effects for normal tissues, the decision of how much dose is to be delivered to one organ versus another is often subjective. Is dose to one organ more acceptable than to another organ? Is a higher dose to a smaller volume more tolerable than a lower dose to a larger volume? Maximizing the clinical gains from IMRT requires such knowledge.

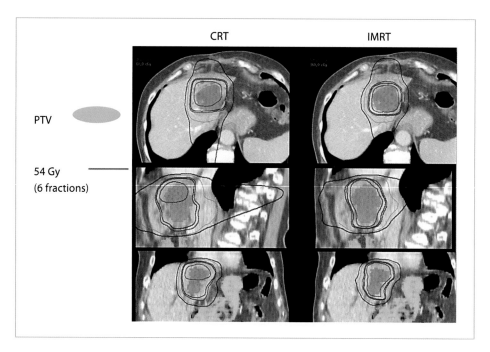

Fig. 3. Example of potential benefits of IMRT versus conformal radiation therapy for a patient with unresectable cholangiocarcinoma. Tumor coverage is improved with IMRT.

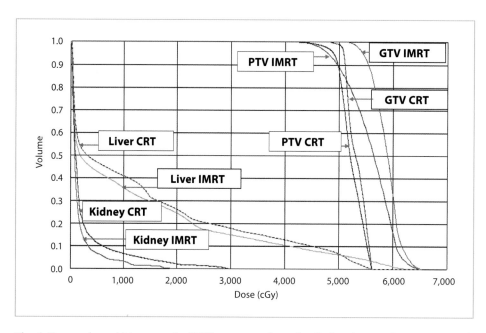

Fig. 4. Dose-volume histograms for IMRT versus conformal radiation therapy for a patient with unresectable cholangiocarcinoma. Tumor coverage is improved, while doses to critical normal tissues are reduced.

Once IMRT can be used to reduce the risk of normal tissue injury from radiation therapy, the dose to tumor may be escalated, leading to possible improved tumor control. Ultimately, the goal of IMRT is to improve local control, while reducing toxicity, thus leading to improved quality of life and survival.

The IMRT Process

IMRT cannot be introduced to the clinic without consideration of all other aspects of high-precision radiation planning and delivery, including patient positioning, immobilization, target delineation, organ motion, setup error and image guidance. As dose gradients are steeper and doses may be higher with IMRT, the consequences of errors in tumor delineation, dosimetry or geometric uncertainties may be more deleterious.

Computerized Tomography Simulation

At the time of simulation, patient positioning, the imaging modality (CT, MR), resolution (e.g. CT thickness), and phase of contrast (e.g. arterial IV contrast for hepatocellular carcinoma) must be chosen carefully. Motion must be considered at this time, as breathing introduces artifacts in the definition of tumor and normal tissue that affect tumor control probability and normal tissue complication probability. Furthermore, if motion is not considered, there is potential for a systematic error due to differences between simulation and treatment.

One method to manage motion is to eliminate it, for example with a breath-hold scan. An effort to conduct all imaging to be used for planning with the patient in the same position, and in the same phase of breath hold is required. If breath hold is not possible, reduction of breathing motion may help to reduce the negative impact of breathing motion.

An alternative to breath-hold imaging is to obtain a four-dimensional imaging data set, in which patients breathe normally and the images are automatically sorted into multiple phases of the respiratory cycle. From this, any position could be used for planning and image guidance (e.g. mean tumor position) [9]. Planning on the exhale data set with asymmetric planning target volume (PTV) margins is an option [10]. The phase of the breathing cycle in which the patient is planned should correspond to the phase of breathing cycle used for image guidance and treatment.

Target Volumes

Delineation of the gross tumor volume (GTV) and clinical target volume (CTV) should be done using diagnostic quality imaging. For example, the use of triphasic intravenous contrast is important in defining primary and metastatic liver cancers, which often are not visible on non-contrast CT scans. For each case, a decision has to be made regarding what volumes are at risk for microscopic disease. These regions require inclusion in the CTV.

The PTV margins must incorporate setup uncertainty and internal organ motion. Individual institution setup uncertainty data should be used if available. Individual patient internal organ motion (e.g. breathing motion) should be used if this information is known.

Organ Motion

The organs in the upper abdomen move due to physiologic change such as breathing. Motion of the liver is predominantly in the superior-inferior direction with an average displacement of 12 ± 7 mm, and displacements of the liver and kidneys may be as great as 5 cm in some patients [11, 12]. Nonbreathing motion due to variable filling of hollow organs and peristalsis is poorly characterized. Motion must be reduced and considered in IMRT planning. Uncertainties in target definition and position are more important in IMRT, because dose gradients are often much steeper around the PTVs than would be the case with conventional plans. As motion can result in alterations in target and normal organ volume definitions, PTV margins and the entire dose distribution, interventions to reduce the impact of intrafraction organ motion are required.

Strategies to compensate for breathing motion include the use of abdominal pressure, voluntary shallow breathing, voluntary deep inspiration, voluntary breath hold at variable phases of the respiratory cycle, active breathing control (ABC), gated radiotherapy and real-time tumor tracking. Although voluntary breath holds may be beneficial for some patients, there is potential for leaking air and patient error. ABC refers to organ immobilization with breath holds that are controlled, triggered and monitored by a caregiver. In approximately 60% of patients with liver cancer, ABC was successful, with intrafraction reproducibility ($\sigma = 1.5–2.5$ mm) [13, 14]. However, with ABC, from day to day the position of the immobilized liver varies relative to the bones (interfraction reproducibility, $\sigma = 3.4–4.4$ mm), indicating the importance of daily image guidance when ABC is used.

Gated radiotherapy, with the beam on only during a predetermined phase of the respiratory cycle, usually utilizes an external surrogate for tumor position (as opposed to direct tumor imaging) to gate the radiation beam. This can reduce the volume of normal tissue irradiated, but changes in baseline organ position can occur from day to day [15]. Again, image guidance is important to avoid geographic misses, especially in the setting of hypofractionated therapy with few treatment sessions.

Tumor tracking is another approach to reduce the effects of organ motion. An elegant real-time tumor tracking system was first described by Shirato et al. [16]. This system consisted of fluoroscopic X-ray tubes in the treatment room, allowing visualization of radiopaque markers in tumors. The linear accelerator was triggered to irradiate only when the marker was located within the planned treatment region.

For gating, breath hold and tracking the exhalation phase of the respiratory cycle has advantages over the inhalation phase for tumors of the upper abdomen. The exhalation phase tends to be more reproducible and more time is spent in exhalation than inhalation.

Image-Guided Radiation Therapy

Image guidance at the time of treatment can improve setup accuracy and precision, increasing the chance that the radiotherapy dose is delivered as planned. This may result in a reduced PTV margin, reduced volume of normal tissue irradiated, and may ultimately facilitate safe dose escalation. On-line correction strategies reduce both systematic and random setup errors, with a greater reduction in error compared with the off-line approach, at the expense of more time and cost. These correction strategies are most appropriate for IMRT plans that are likely to degrade in the presence of realistic setup uncertainties.

Most upper abdominal malignancies cannot be accurately localized with the use of skin marks or bone anatomy. Options for locating internal anatomy include the use of implanted radiopaque fiducial markers as surrogates for the target, visualization of tissues adjacent to the tumor (e.g. the diaphragm) or imaging the tumor itself. Fiducial markers may also be used to measure organ motion and or track/gate the beam, as with the real-time tumor tracking system used by Shirato et al. [16]. Another system (Novel's BrainLAB, Heimstetten, Germany) acquires kilovoltage (kV) orthogonal images and matches to digitally reconstructed radiographs obtained from the planning CT.

Volumetric image guidance immediately prior to treatment using the tumor or an adjacent soft tissue organ is now possible. One advantage of volumetric imaging systems is the visualization of adjacent normal tissues for more accurate avoidance. Ultrasound has been used for image guidance of liver and pancreas IMRT, with resultant reductions in residual setup error (residual error vector of 4.6 ± 3.4 mm) [17]. The placement of a diagnostic CT scanner in the treatment room is another approach for volumetric imaging [18, 19]. The CT scanner is in close proximity to the linear accelerator, allowing the couch to be moved from the imaging position to the treatment position. Specialized linear accelerators that allow soft tissue image guidance are now available. For example, kV cone beam CT units combine kV X-ray imaging and megavoltage radiation delivery into one integrated gantry-mounted system (Synergy, Elekta Oncology, Stockholm, Sweden; Trilogy, Varian Medical Systems, Palo Alto, Calif.; Artiste, Siemens, Concord, Calif.; Tomotherapy, Madison, Wisc., USA). Planar kV image projections are obtained as the gantry rotates about the patient on the linear accelerator table, over 30 s to 4 min. Cone beam CT three-dimensional volume reconstruction images may then be obtained for position verification or guidance. Doses delivered to obtain cone beam CT scans typically range from 0.5 to 2 Gy, which is substantially less than the dose from megavoltage orthogonal images. We have recently demonstrated the feasibility of using kV cone beam CT image guidance in liver cancer [20].

Intensity-Modulated Radiation Therapy for Abdominal Tumors: Planning Studies

Liver Cancer

Dvorak et al. [21] compared IMRT to forward-planned conformal radiation for 7 patients with lung lesions and 3 with liver lesions. All patients were treated with the same beam arrangements (5–7 noncoplanar and individually weighted multi-leaf collimator shaped beams), using 3×12 Gy fractions, prescribed to the 65% isodose level. Not surprisingly, no improvement was observed with the IMRT approach, since the tumors were relatively small and spherical. In contrast, irregularly shaped tumors such as the unresectable cholangiocarcinoma shown in figure 3 may benefit more from IMRT.

In a study from Taiwan, conformal radiotherapy plans (43–58 Gy, using up to 8 noncoplanar fields) were compared with 5-field axial IMRT plans in 12 of 68 patients with hepatocellular carcinoma who had developed radiation-induced liver disease after receiving conformal radiation therapy [22]. The authors concluded that IMRT was capable of preserving acceptable target coverage while improving or maintaining the nonhepatic organ sparing. However, the mean liver dose was higher in 10 of 12 IMRT plans.

University of Michigan investigators demonstrated the potential benefit of using equivalent uniform dose and normal tissue complication probability in IMRT optimization for hepatic malignancies [23]. IMRT optimization improved plans in 15 challenging cases for which the delivered dose using conformal radiation therapy had been limited due to either adjacent normal tissue tolerance (7 cases, 'overlap cases') or liver tolerance (8 cases, 'nonoverlap cases'). For the same risk of liver toxicity, the mean PTV equivalent uniform dose increase with IMRT was 11 Gy (for high-grade tumors) and 18 Gy (for low-grade tumors) for overlap cases and 10 Gy for nonoverlap cases (in 1.5-Gy fractions). For the overlap cases, a 6-field noncoplanar beam arrangement was better than the original conformal beam arrangement in the majority of cases. For the nonoverlap cases, the original conformal beam arrangement was most suitable. In 2/15 cases, beamlet sizes >1 cm had to be used due to the large tumor size, and IMRT plans failed to protect the normal liver better than conformal radiation therapy.

Gastric Carcinoma

A comparison of 45-Gy (median dose to target volume) step-and-shoot IMRT versus conventional 8-beam and noncoplanar plans showed best kidney sparing with noncoplanar anterior-posterior (AP) and posterior-anterior (PA) fields and best liver sparing with IMRT [24]. The same group [25] then compared techniques in 15 patients with gastric cancer: 8-field step-and-shoot IMRT, conformal radiation planning, an AP opposed beam arrangement (AP-PA), and intensity-modulated arc therapy/tomotherapy plans using 1- or 2-cm collimation. Step-and-shoot IMRT and tomotherapy were found to improve the target coverage while at the same time reducing the dose to sensitive normal structures. However, the smallest volume of liver was irradiated with the AP-PA technique. IMRT plans were less dependent on individual anatomy. The main problems with IMRT were long treatment time (about 20 min) and increased inhomogeneity of dose within the target volume.

Ringash et al. [26] evaluated observer preference for IMRT versus conformal radiation plans. Twenty patients who had undergone treatment planning with 5-field conformal plans were replanned with 7- to 9-axial-field IMRT. Two independent radiation oncologists specializing in gastrointestinal malignancies reviewed the cumulative dose-volume histograms and organ-dose summaries for each plan. The IMRT plan was preferred in 17 of 19 cases (89%). In 86% of IMRT plans, the target coverage was improved, while spinal cord, liver, kidney and heart dose was reduced in 74, 71, 69 and 69%, respectively. In 4 of the 20 IMRT plans, at least one radiation oncologist had safety concerns due to a higher spinal cord dose and/or the volume of small bowel irradiated.

One difficulty in interpreting comparative studies in gastric cancer is that the partial volume tolerance of the kidney is not well understood. Few studies exist in which patients have been followed for many years after radiotherapy to allow manifestation of kidney injury.

Esophageal Cancer

In a recent study involving 10 patients with cancer of the distal esophagus and gastroesophageal junction [27], 4 treatment plans were generated including conformal radiation therapy, 4-beam IMRT (with the same beam arrangement as conformal radiation therapy), 7-beam IMRT, and 9-beam IMRT. The target dose was 50.4 Gy in 28 fractions. IMRT reduced the mean lung dose and target heterogeneity was improved in 8/10 patients. The conformity index improved with IMRT plans, more so as beam number increased. The conformality advantage with more beams has to be weighed against longer treatment time and a larger volume of normal tissue exposed to low doses.

Photons versus Protons

Advances in radiation therapy technology, particularly IMRT, proton beam or other charged-particle radiation therapy have led to improved treatment for patients with bone and soft tissue sarcomas. In one study [28], plans for 5 patients with paraspinal sarcoma were computed comparing intensity-modulated photon therapy (7 coplanar fields) and intensity-modulated proton therapy (3 coplanar beams). Prescribed dose was 77.4 Gy (1.8 Gy/fraction) to the GTV. For all intensity-modulated proton plans, dose escalation [to 92.9 CGE (cobalt gray equivalent: proton Gy × 1.1)] was possible without exceeding the normal tissue dose limits.

Another study showed the potential benefit of proton therapy [29] in 4 patients (2 inoperable pancreatic tumors, 1 inoperable and 1 postoperative biliary duct tumor). Comparison plans included conformal photon plans, IMRT photon plans and proton plans ('spot-scanning technique'). The aim was to irradiate a large PTV to 50 Gy, and to boost a smaller PTV to 70–75 Gy. None of the conformal plans could deliver 50 Gy to large PTVs while respecting the dose-volume constraints on critical organs. IMRT photon plans nearly achieved dose constraints to critical structures for 2/3 inoperable patients and for the postoperative patient. For all patients, 4-field proton plans achieved reduced doses to normal tissues for the same PTV coverage as the photon IMRT plans.

Intensity-Modulated Radiation Therapy for Abdominal Tumors: Clinical Experience

There are few published reports of clinical outcomes following IMRT treatment of upper abdominal malignancies. Fuss et al. [30] reported on the accuracy of setup in 62 patients treated with daily ultrasound image-guided IMRT [cholangiocarcinoma and gall bladder cancer (n = 10), hepatocellular carcinoma (n = 10), liver metastases (n = 11), pancreatic cancer (n = 20), other (n = 18)]. The tumor itself or adjacent vascular structures were used for image guidance. The daily image guidance improved the accuracy of setup (mean magnitude of residual setup error 4.6 ± 3.4 mm).

Liver Cancer

Fuss and Thomas [31] demonstrated several cases of liver cancer in which IMRT reduced the mean liver dose compared to conformal techniques. No radiation-induced liver toxicity was observed in 10 patients treated with conventionally fractionated (54–76 Gy) IMRT or in 2 patients treated with hypofractionated (36 Gy in 3 fractions) IMRT.

Pancreatic Cancer

Ben-Josef et al. [32] reported on 15 patients with pancreatic cancer who were treated adjuvantly (n = 7) or for primary treatment (n = 8), with IMRT delivered over 5 weeks. The dose to the highest-risk volume was 45–54 Gy for adjuvant therapy and 54–55 Gy for unresectable disease, while 45 Gy was delivered to regional nodes. Systemic therapy was used concurrently in all patients (capecitabine in all and gemcitabine in 73%). One patient (7%) developed a grade 3 gastric ulcer.

Milano et al. [33] reported clinical outcomes in 25 patients with pancreatic or cholangiocarcinoma treated with IMRT to a dose of 45–59.4 Gy. Median follow-up was 10.2 months and median survival was 9.3 months. Only 1 patient with unresectable cancer had a local recurrence. In comparison to patients treated with conformal radiation therapy, IMRT reduced the mean dose to the liver, kidneys, stomach and small bowel. However, grade 4 toxicities occurred in 2 patients (ileus, fistula), and grade 3 in 3 patients (acute cholecystitis, hypovolemia). The author concluded that IMRT could increase the toxicity to the small bowel by increasing the volume exposed to low-dose radiotherapy.

In another study, 10 patients with pancreatic cancer were planned with conformal radiation therapy and inverse-planned IMRT [34]. The aim of the treatment plan was to deliver 61.2 Gy to the GTV and 45 Gy to the CTV. The median volume of small bowel exceeding 50 and 60 Gy was 19.2 ± 11.2 and 12.5 ± 4.8% for IMRT, respectively, compared with 31.4 ± 21.3 and 19.8 ± 18.6% for conformal radiation therapy.

In a phase 2 prospective study, 19 patients were treated with 45 Gy in 1.8 Gy per fraction to the pancreas tumor and regional lymph nodes using IMRT, concurrent with either 5-fluorouracil (200 mg/m^2/day, protracted venous infusion) or capecitabine (1,000 mg/m^2 per os, Monday to Friday) [35]. Within 1 month, 25-Gy stereotactic radiosurgery using Cyberknife was administered to the primary tumor. Of 16 patients who completed the treatment, 2 patients had grade 3 gastrointestinal toxicity (gastroparesis). The median survival was 33 weeks; the site of first progression was distant (liver) in all patients. Only 1 patient had local failure 34 weeks after treatment and the remaining 15 patients who completed treatment were free of local progression until death. It was suggested that local control in pancreatic cancer would not likely translate to improved survival.

In another phase 1 study, patients with pancreatic cancer were treated with IMRT (33 Gy/11 fractions) and concurrent gemcitabine (350 mg/m^2) [36]. Due to dose-limiting toxicity (myelosuppression and upper gastrointestinal toxicity requiring a hospital admission), the dose of gemcitabine was reduced to 250 mg/m^2, radiation dose escalation was not feasible and the trial was closed early.

Sarcoma

Outside the abdomen, sarcoma is treated with doses of up to 66 Gy combined with surgery. However, the prescribed dose for retroperitoneal sarcoma is limited due to the large volume and proximity of normal radiosensitive structures.

Musat et al. [37] investigated 5 IMRT plans in patients with retroperitoneal sarcoma. With IMRT, dose escalation was possible to 54 Gy and dose homogeneity to PTV improved compared to conformal plans. Moreover, the protection factor for normal tissues and the conformity index improved by 20 and 25%, respectively.

Yamada et al. [38] investigated noninvasive immobilizing devices for 35 patients with paraspinal tumors being treated with IMRT. The patient population included 11 cases of recurrent primary sarcoma, 3 cases of primary chondroma and 21 cases of metastatic malignancies mainly from renal cell carcinoma. In 24 patients with prior radiotherapy, the median dose had been 3,000 cGy in 10 fractions and the median dose prescribed was 2,000 cGy/5 fractions (2,000–3,000 cGy). In 11 previously unirradiated patients, the median prescribed dose was 7,000 cGy. More than 90% of patients experienced improvement in pain, weakness, or paresthesia; 75 and 81% of secondary and primary lesions, respectively, exhibited local control after a median follow-up of 11 months. There was no radiation-induced myelopathy or radiculopathy observed. The authors concluded that high-precision stereotactic and image-guided paraspinal IMRT allowed the delivery of high doses of radiation in multiple fractions to tumors within close proximity to the spinal cord while respecting cord tolerance.

Cautions for IMRT Use in the Upper Abdomen

IMRT plans are more sensitive to uncertainty than conventional radiation therapy plans. Thus, errors in target definition are more likely to lead to marginal recurrences. Geometric uncertainties including motion, setup error and dosimetric uncertainty are also more likely to introduce heterogeneity, including cooler doses in the tumor and/or hotter doses in normal tissues as compared with the planned dose distribution. Another disadvantage of IMRT is the necessity for greater expertise, validation and quality assurance measures.

Experience in clinical situations indicates that there is value to careful selection of beam orientation in IMRT treatment planning. Conformality improves with additional beams, however, the associated increase in treatment time could decrease tumor control probability and increase error due to intrafraction movement.

IMRT in isolation, i.e. without management of organ motion and setup error, could in fact be more likely to cause tumor recurrence or normal tissue injury than a conventional plan. Gierga et al. [39] investigated the effect of individual patient motion due to breathing on IMRT plans. Patients with pancreatic cancer (n = 6) or cholangiocarcinoma (n = 1) who had surgically implanted clips underwent fluoroscopic simulation to verify the location of the treatment isocenter before beginning radiotherapy. Motion degraded the plans, and in one case, there was a 28% reduction in PTV minimum dose.

Another caution for IMRT is that the partial volume tolerances of the normal tissues in the upper abdomen are not all well understood, especially for hypofractionated radiation therapy schedules. Thus, the technological advances in IMRT that allow dose to be deposited very carefully have bypassed our understanding of what the most biologically effective dose distributions may be.

With IMRT, there is a substantial increase in monitor units per target dose. Depending on treatment energy, IMRT may require 3.5–4.9 times more monitor units compared with conventional radiotherapy. This increase in monitor units along with the increased volume of tissue receiving low doses leads to an increased risk of second malignancies with IMRT, especially for younger patients.

Furthermore, as treatment time increases, there is a theoretical risk of increased tumor cell survival. This is highlighted in a study from China, in which the clonogenic survival of two hepatoma cell lines was studied [40]. The alpha/beta ratio and repair half-time of the HepG2 and Hep3b cell lines were 3.1 and 7.4 Gy, and 22 and 19 min, respectively. The prolonged fraction delivery time decreased the cell killing in HepG2 but not in Hep3b, suggesting that in tumors with a low alpha/beta ratio, increased radiation delivery time may be associated with increased clonogenic survival.

Conclusions

High-precision radiation therapy has the potential to improve outcomes in upper abdominal malignancies. IMRT is one method of high-precision radiation therapy. Planning studies have demonstrated the potential benefits of IMRT, with reduced doses to normal tissues facilitating dose escalation.

Upper abdominal IMRT plans are more sensitive to uncertainties than conventional plans, and thus patient position, motion, tumor delineation, and image guidance need particular attention. Gains in tumor coverage and normal tissue sparing may be possible with simple interventions such as appropriate immobilization and optimization of beam angle. Beamlet fluence automated optimization is not likely to be required in all clinical scenarios. There is a need to develop robust IMRT planning solutions that are less sensitive to uncertainties. Finally, the full potential of IMRT will not be realized until there is a better understanding of partial volume radiation effects on normal tissues.

Preliminary clinical experience demonstrates that dose-escalated IMRT can be used safely in upper abdominal malignancies. However, clinical outcomes are mixed, and the potential gains and toxicities should be studied further in clinical trials before IMRT is routinely used to treat upper abdominal malignancies.

Guidelines for Clinical Practice

- Upper abdominal malignancies are some of the most challenging cancers to treat due to organ motion and the presence of many dose-limiting normal tissues.

- Intensity-modulated radiation therapy (IMRT) is one component of the radiation therapy process that has the potential to facilitate dose escalation and dose reduction to normal tissues.

- Upper abdominal IMRT plans are more sensitive to uncertainties than conventional plans, and thus patient position, motion and tumor delineation need to be carefully considered. Image-guided radiation therapy should also be used if IMRT is implemented.

- There is a need to develop robust IMRT planning solutions less sensitive to uncertainties.

- Planning studies have shown the potential benefits of IMRT in the upper abdomen, with reduced doses to normal tissues facilitating dose escalation, in some, but not all, patients with upper abdominal malignancies.

- Patients with small spherical target volumes appear to have less dosimetric benefit from IMRT versus conformal radiation therapy.

- Dose-escalated IMRT has been used in clinical trials of upper abdominal malignancies; however, severe toxicities have been reported following IMRT, and clinical experience is limited.

- The clinical gains and toxicities following IMRT need to be studied further in clinical trials before IMRT is routinely used for upper abdominal malignancies.

References

1 Hargreaves GM, Adam R, Bismuth H: Results after nonsurgical local treatment of primary liver malignancies. Langenbecks Arch Surg 2000;385: 185–193.
2 Curley SA: Radiofrequency ablation of malignant liver tumors. Oncologist 2001;6:14–23.
3 Dawson LA, McGinn CJ, Lawrence TS: Conformal chemoradiation for primary and metastatic liver malignancies. Semin Surg Oncol 2003;21: 249–255.
4 Macdonald JS, Smalley SR, Benedetti J, et al: Chemoradiotherapy after surgery compared with surgery alone for adenocarcinoma of the stomach or gastroesophageal junction. N Engl J Med 2001; 345:725–730.
5 Neoptolemos JP, Stocken DD, Friess H, et al: A randomized trial of chemoradiotherapy and chemotherapy after resection of pancreatic cancer. N Engl J Med 2004;350:1200–1210.

6 Fein DA, Corn BW, Lanciano RM, Herbert SH, Hoffman JP, Coia LR: Management of retroperitoneal sarcomas: does dose escalation impact on locoregional control? Int J Radiat Oncol Biol Phys 1995;31:129–134.
7 Eisbruch A, Dawson LA, Kim HM, et al: Conformal and intensity-modulated irradiation of head and neck cancer: the potential for improved target irradiation, salivary gland function, and quality of life. Acta Otorhinolaryngol Belg 1999; 53:271–275.
8 Chu M, Zinchenko Y, Henderson SG, Sharpe MB: Robust optimization for intensity-modulated radiation therapy treatment planning under uncertainty. Phys Med Biol 2005;50:5463–5477.
9 Sonke JJ, Zijp L, Remeijer P, van Herk M: Respiratory-correlated cone beam CT. Med Phys 2005; 32:1176–1186.

10 Balter JM, Lam KL, McGinn CJ, Lawrence TS, Ten Haken RK: Improvement of CT-based treatment-planning models of abdominal targets using static exhale imaging. Int J Radiat Oncol Biol Phys 1998;41:939–943.

11 Booth JT, Zavgorodni SF: Set-up error and organ motion uncertainty: a review. Australas Phys Eng Sci Med 1999;22:29–47.

12 Davies SC, Hill AL, Holmes RB, Halliwell M, Jackson PC: Ultrasound quantitation of respiratory organ motion in the upper abdomen. Br J Radiol 1994;67:1096–1102.

13 Dawson LA, Brock KK, Kazanjian S, et al: The reproducibility of organ position using active breathing control (ABC) during liver radiotherapy. Int J Radiat Oncol Biol Phys 2001;51:1410–1421.

14 Eccles C, Brock KK, Hawkins MA, Bissonnette J, Dawson LA: Reproducibility of liver using active breathing control. Int Jo Radiat Oncol Biol Phys 2005;64:751–759.

15 Smitsmans MH, de Bois J, Sonke JJ, et al: Automatic prostate localization on cone-beam CT scans for high precision image-guided radiotherapy. Int J Radiat Oncol Biol Phys 2005;63:975–984.

16 Shirato H, Shimizu S, Kitamura K, et al: Four-dimensional treatment planning and fluoroscopic real-time tumor tracking radiotherapy for moving tumor. Int J Radiat Oncol Biol Phys 2000;48:435–442.

17 Fuss M, Salter BJ, Cavanaugh SX, et al: Daily ultrasound-based image-guided targeting for radiotherapy of upper abdominal malignancies. Int J Radiat Oncol Biol Phys 2004;59:1245–1256.

18 Court L, Rosen I, Mohan R, Dong L: Evaluation of mechanical precision and alignment uncertainties for an integrated CT/LINAC system. Med Phys 2003;30:1198–210.

19 Onishi H, Kuriyama K, Komiyama T, et al: A new irradiation system for lung cancer combining linear accelerator, computed tomography, patient self-breath-holding, and patient-directed beam-control without respiratory monitoring devices. Int J Radiat Oncol Biol Phys 2003;56:14–20.

20 Hawkins MA, Bissonnette JP, Eccles C, Lockwood G, Cummings B, Ringash J, Sherman M, Knox J, Gallinger S, Dawson LA: Preliminary results of a phase I study of stereotactic radiotherapy for unresectable primary and metastatic liver cancer. 41st Annu Meet Am Soc Clin Oncol, Orlando, 2005.

21 Dvorak P, Georg D, Bogner J, Kroupa B, Dieckmann K, Potter R: Impact of IMRT and leaf width on stereotactic body radiotherapy of liver and lung lesions. Int J Radiat Oncol Biol Phys 2005;61:1572–1581.

22 Cheng JC, Wu JK, Huang CM, et al: Dosimetric analysis and comparison of three-dimensional conformal radiotherapy and intensity-modulated radiation therapy for patients with hepatocellular carcinoma and radiation-induced liver disease. Int J Radiat Oncol Biol Phys 2003;56:229–234.

23 Thomas E, Chapet O, Kessler ML, Lawrence TS, Ten Haken RK: Benefit of using biologic parameters (EUD and NTCP) in IMRT optimization for treatment of intrahepatic tumors. Int J Radiat Oncol Biol Phys 2005;62:571–578.

24 Lohr F, Dobler B, Mai S, et al: Optimization of dose distributions for adjuvant locoregional radiotherapy of gastric cancer by IMRT. Strahlenther Onkol 2003;179:557–563.

25 Wieland P, Dobler B, Mai S, et al: IMRT for postoperative treatment of gastric cancer: covering large target volumes in the upper abdomen: a comparison of a step-and-shoot and an arc therapy approach. Int J Radiat Oncol Biol Phys 2004;59:1236–1244.

26 Ringash J, Perkins G, Brierley J, et al: IMRT for adjuvant radiation in gastric cancer: a preferred plan? Int J Radiat Oncol Biol Phys 2005;63:732–738.

27 Chandra A, Guerrero TM, Liu HH, et al: Feasibility of using intensity-modulated radiotherapy to improve lung sparing in treatment planning for distal esophageal cancer. Radiother Oncol 2005;77:247–253.

28 Weber DC, Trofimov AV, Delaney TF, Bortfeld T: A treatment planning comparison of intensity-modulated photon and proton therapy for paraspinal sarcomas. Int J Radiat Oncol Biol Phys 2004;58:1596–1606.

29 Zurlo A, Lomax A, Hoess A, et al: The role of proton therapy in the treatment of large irradiation volumes: a comparative planning study of pancreatic and biliary tumors. Int J Radiat Oncol Biol Phys 2000;48:277–288.

30 Fuss M, Salter BJ, Herman TS, Thomas CR Jr: External beam radiation therapy for hepatocellular carcinoma: potential of intensity-modulated and image-guided radiation therapy. Gastroenterology 2004;127(5 suppl 1):S206–S217.

31 Fuss M, Thomas CR Jr: Stereotactic body radiation therapy: an ablative treatment option for primary and secondary liver tumors. Ann Surg Oncol 2004;11:130–138.

32 Ben-Josef E, Shields AF, Vaishampayan U, et al: Intensity-modulated radiotherapy (IMRT) and concurrent capecitabine for pancreatic cancer. Int J Radiat Oncol Biol Phys 2004;59:454–459.

33 Milano MT, Chmura SJ, Garofalo MC, et al: Intensity-modulated radiotherapy in treatment of pancreatic and bile duct malignancies: toxicity and clinical outcome. Int J Radiat Oncol Biol Phys 2004;59:445–453.

34 Landry JC, Yang GY, Ting JY, et al: Treatment of pancreatic cancer tumors with intensity-modulated radiation therapy (IMRT) using the volume at risk approach (VARA): employing dose-volume histogram (DVH) and normal tissue complication probability (NTCP) to evaluate small bowel toxicity. Med Dosim 2002;27:121–129.

35 Koong AC, Christofferson E, Le QT, et al: Phase II study to assess the efficacy of conventionally fractionated radiotherapy followed by a stereotactic radiosurgery boost in patients with locally advanced pancreatic cancer. Int J Radiat Oncol Biol Phys 2005;63:320–323.

36 Crane CH, Antolak JA, Rosen II, et al: Phase I study of concomitant gemcitabine and IMRT for patients with unresectable adenocarcinoma of the pancreatic head. Int J Gastrointest Cancer 2001;30:123–132.

37 Musat E, Kantor G, Caron J, et al: Comparison of intensity-modulated postoperative radiotherapy with conventional postoperative conformal radiotherapy for retroperitoneal sarcoma. Cancer Radiother 2004;8:255–261.

38 Yamada Y, Lovelock DM, Yenice KM, Bilsky MH, Hunt MA, Zatcky J, Leibel SA: Multifractionated image-guided and stereotactic intensity-modulated radiotherapy of paraspinal tumors: a preliminary report. Int J Radiat Oncol Biol Phys 2005;62:53–61.

39 Gierga DP, Chen GT, Kung JH, Betke M, Lombardi J, Willett CG: Quantification of respiration-induced abdominal tumor motion and its impact on IMRT dose distributions. Int J Radiat Oncol Biol Phys 2004;58:1584–1595.

40 Zheng XK, Chen LH, Yan X, Wang HM: Impact of prolonged fraction dose-delivery time modeling intensity-modulated radiation therapy on hepatocellular carcinoma cell killing. World J Gastroenterol 2005;11:1452–1456.

Dr. Laura Dawson
Princess Margaret Hospital
University of Toronto
610 University Ave.
Toronto, Ont. M5G 2M9 (Canada)
Tel. +1 416 946 2124, Fax +1 416 946 6566
E-Mail laura.dawson@rmp.uhn.on.ca

Prostate Cancer

Meyer JL (ed): IMRT, IGRT, SBRT – Advances in the Treatment Planning and
Delivery of Radiotherapy. Front Radiat Ther Oncol. Basel, Karger, 2007, vol. 40, pp 289–314

Prostate Cancer: Image Guidance and Adaptive Therapy

Patrick Kupelian[a] · John L. Meyer[b]

[a]Department of Radiation Oncology, MD Anderson Cancer Center Orlando,
Orlando, Fla., [b]Department of Radiation Oncology, Saint Francis Memorial Hospital,
San Francisco, Calif., USA

Abstract

Image-guided radiation therapy implies the use of a variety of imaging techniques in the treatment room to determine the location of target areas with the patient in the treatment position. This is particularly relevant for prostate cancer radiation therapy since the prostate gland can differ in its position within the pelvis from one treatment to another. The different imaging techniques include transabdominal ultrasound, in-room X-rays with and without the use of intraprostatic implanted fiducials, kilovoltage and megavoltage CT techniques, and even in-room MRI. The workflow and capabilities of each imaging system need to be evaluated and investigated individually.

There are several image guidance methods now available or being developed for use in radiotherapy, and often these guidance systems have been used first in the management of prostate cancer. Each method needs to be studied and validated separately for its unique characteristics. Early insights into the use of image guidance for prostate cancer are important for improving therapy of this major tumor site, and for understanding the applicability of these new technologies for other tumor sites.

This discussion will review the different technologies used for target localization in the pelvis, discuss the dosimetric impact of prostate movement during radiation therapy, and consider future applications of image guidance and adaptive radiotherapy in the treatment of prostate and other cancers.

Immobilization

The first step in image guidance is simply to place the target in the proper position relative to the treatment machine. Effective image guidance depends on careful immobilization. Even with the use of a variety of careful external immobilization devices, external methods do not achieve immobilization of the prostate itself because it continues to move within the internal anatomy. Efforts have been made to reduce prostate motion with the placement of an *endorectal balloon*, and many institutions continue to use this technique. The use of an endorectal balloon for most fractions in a treatment course, or at least some fractions, is an idea that is appealing because the balloon can pin and hold the prostate against the pelvic bone during treatment. Also, there are reports showing that the rectal distention from the balloon can reduce the rectal exposure seen on dose-volume histograms (DVHs) and the possible late rectal complications. The University of Wisconsin group documented that patients who had an endorectal balloon at the time of treatment had a lower frequency of late rectal bleeding [1]. Following a prescribed dose of 76 Gy using three-dimensional conformal radiation therapy (3DCRT), the frequency of grade 2 rectal bleeding was reduced from nearly 30 to 15%, and grade 3 bleeding was slightly reduced as well, though it was uncommon in both groups.

There are questions about the daily reproducibility of the balloon placement and the stability of the balloon volume and shape. A paper from the Netherlands reported on 52 patients, all with intraprostatic markers placed before treatment [2]. Twenty-two were treated with a balloon in place and 30 without. Daily imaging on an electronic portal imaging device (EPID) was performed for localization, and movie loops analyzed prostate motion and rectal filling. These images documented prostate motion as shown by movement of the markers despite the use of the balloon. Their imaging shows the variation in the rectal filling from day to day, as well as the movement of the markers. It also shows that the position of the balloon in the pelvis is not exactly the same every day. Finally, one can occasionally see gas moving behind the balloon and causing a shift of the prostate.

Translating this imaging information into graphic data, figure 1 shows a scatter plot of the prostate displacement, with and without the balloon in place. The movement of the prostate can be seen in both cases, and in fact the plots are quite similar. It does not appear that the prostate was better immobilized by the balloon. Even with more sophisticated systems, others have seen variation in the day-to-day anatomy of the prostate and rectum despite the use of endorectal balloons. More of these types of studies are needed to confirm that the use of a rectal balloon can reduce prostate motion.

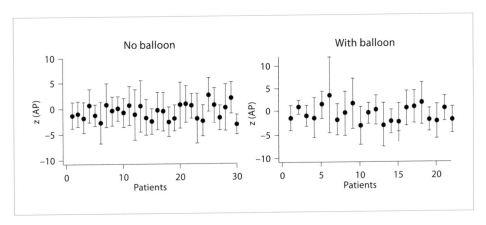

Fig. 1. Prostate immobilization using an intrarectal balloon [2]. Prostate offset motion is shown in the anterior/posterior (AP) dimension, and shows no significant improvement with the use of the balloon. Very similar results are obtained in the other 2 dimensions. Dose recalculation based on CT can be of significant benefit in defining quality assurance of treatment courses. We have evaluated treatment courses based on replanning of dosimetry taking into account the actual gland anatomy during therapy. Our results document uniformly high rates of accurate prostate targeting, assessed by the D95 (dose to 95% of the target volume) to the gland. Similarly, our recalculation presents the actual doses to the rectum and bladder, which will be of significant help in the following evaluation of the actual outcomes.

Tools for Image Guidance of Prostate Irradiation

There are many image guidance methods using ultrasound, X-rays at megavoltage (MV) or kilovoltage (kV) levels including in-room CT, and now even MRI technologies. These guidance devices may be monitoring implantable markers, either radiodense or active transponders, or soft tissue prostate anatomy.

Ultrasound
Transabdominal ultrasound was the first widely used technique for daily prostate localization in the treatment room. In some respects, it initiated the image guidance era, though experience led to questioning its efficacy. In reports evaluating the acceptability of these images for daily treatment alignment, the rates of usable images varied from 97 down to 68% [3].

How well does it work? Table 1 shows the results of a study presented recently comparing the BAT™ ultrasound device (North American Scientific) with in-room CT in a large number of comparison pairs [4]. The two approaches gave different results, with large differences in all anatomic directions and with large standard deviations. Dong et al. [4] concluded that the overall performance of the ultrasound seemed less satisfactory compared with in-room CT guidance.

Table 1. Transabdominal ultrasound: comparison with CT [4] and implanted markers [5, 6]

Transabdominal ultrasound: comparison with CT

BAT vs. in-room CT-on-rails [4]

Evaluation	15 patients, each imaged with 3 CTs per week and BAT; 342 CT/ultrasound pairs (average 23 scans/patient); physician contours were placed on each CT
Results	BAT vs. CT differences (mean ± SD)
	Lateral 0.5±3.6 mm
	Vertical 0.7±4.5 mm
	Longitudinal 0.4±3.9 mm

Transabdominal ultrasound: comparison with implanted markers

(1) BAT vs. markers (EPID) [5]

Evaluation	11 patients, 10 alignments per patient
Results	Differences (average ± SD)
	Vertical −0.7±5.2 mm
	Longitudinal 2.7±4.5 mm
	Lateral 1.8±3.9 mm

(2) SonArray vs. markers (ExacTrac) [6]

Evaluation	40 patients, 1,019 alignments, average 25 alignments per patient
Results	Frequency of misalignments
	0–5 mm 26%
	5–10 mm 48%
	10–15 mm 17%
	15–20 mm 5%
	>20 mm 4%

There are also comparisons between ultrasound and implanted markers. Table 1 also presents the results of a study from the University of California San Francisco reported in 2002 [5]. One can see that the standard deviations between ultrasound and implanted markers are also significant. Finally, additional data were presented in 2005 that evaluated differences between another ultrasound system (SonArray™, Varian Medical Systems) and markers detected by kV X-rays in the room, in a very large number of clinical observations. The differences between ultrasound and markers were again quite large. These results suggest that radiographic methods of detecting the daily position of the prostate may prove superior to those using ultrasound.

Implanted Markers

The use of markers and other methods have shown that bone anatomy is not a dependable surrogate for prostate anatomy, and that markers give more reliable in-

Table 2. Prostate marker stability

	Patients	Markers	Intermarker distances	Intermarker distance, mm
Dehnad et al. [7]	9	19	453	0.5 (SD)
Poggi et al. [8]	9	45		1.2±0.2 (mean ± SD)
Aubin et al. [9]	7	21	103	−0.01±0.87 (mean ± SD)
Litzenberg et al. [10]	10	30		0.7–1.7 (range SD)
Pouliot et al. [11]	11	33	110	1.3 (mean SD) 0.44–3.04 (range SD)
Kupelian et al. [12]	56	168	6,111	1.01±1.03 (mean ± SD) 0.3–4.2 (range SD)

formation. Their placement is relatively simple, typically using a transrectal ultrasound-guided procedure very similar to prostate biopsy. Brachytherapy needles (18 gauge) are typically used, and the preparation of the patients is relatively simple: the patients take an antibiotic on the day before and the day of the insertion. Three markers are often placed, typically one at each base and one at the apex. The procedure takes only a few minutes, and can be done on the day of the simulation.

The markers can be detected using kV X-rays or an EPID in the treatment room; somewhat larger markers may be necessary for clear MV imaging on an EPID. Markers are easy to see on kV X-rays, and several systems use them for accurate X-ray localization (ExacTrac™ by BrainLab, and others). There are software systems based on EPID – less than full-scale image-guided radiation therapy (IGRT) systems – which can determine the offsets of couch movement to apply (Acculoc™ by Northwest Medical Physics, and others).

Implanted markers can only be considered as the gold standard for position verification if they are stable within the prostate. There are many publications suggesting that they are, by using evaluation of the intermarker distance over time. Calculations of the intermarker distance variation provided by several published studies are presented in table 2. These studies show that the mean and standard deviations of these variations are very small (fig. 2). Since the variation noted is for just one marker and typically there are three, the actual center of mass of the three markers will be much less than the reported single variation. Also, the movement that does occur is not usually from migration, but rather from organ deformation, seen on CT imaging. Careful studies of individual cases show that the positions of the markers are generally stable from day to day, though on occasional days one can see prostate deformation, such as from gas in the rectum.

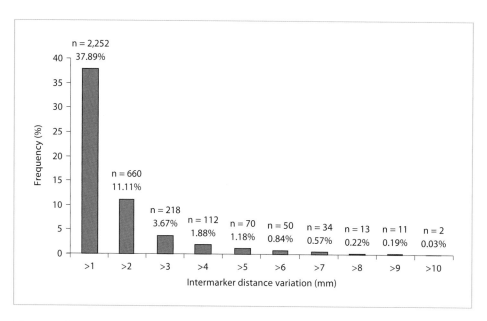

Fig. 2. Marker stability: frequency distribution of intermarker distance variation [12].

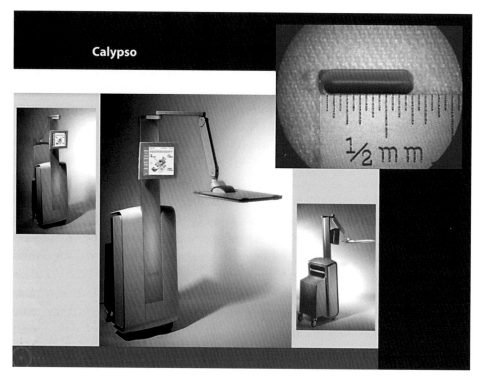

Fig. 3. Calypso System. The system utilizes an electromagnetic signal to detect the position of implanted transponders.

Kupelian · Meyer

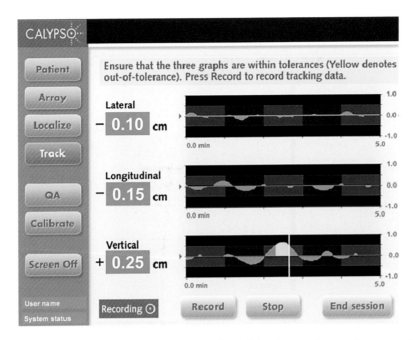

Fig. 4. A sample track from the user interface of the Calypso System demonstrating the lateral, longitudinal and vertical variations in position of the implanted transponders as a function of time. See active display online at *WEB*.

Technologies have been developed recently that are more sophisticated than simple radiodense markers. An implantable electromagnetic marker, known as the *Calypso™ System*, is now being investigated (Calypso Medical) (fig. 3). It is a wireless 15-gauge permanent implant, its position being detected by a radio-frequency signal, which refreshes at a rate of 10 Hz. The attraction of this design is that it is not associated with any radiation dose, and the tracking can continue indefinitely. However, it does not provide an image, but rather the three-dimensional coordinates of each marker. Their positions are reported relative to their original reference positions over time (fig. 4).

How accurate is this system? In in vivo measurements, these transponders are shown to be easily detected. One large study reported 979 comparisons between the positions of the transponders as reported by the system and as determined on X-rays. The length of the three-dimensional vector between the two, the Calypso System and X-ray localization, was only 1.9 ± 1.1 mm (p < 0.001). These results show very good accuracy.

Many patients have been treated with this system in place, giving real-time tracking of the prostate during the beam-on period. Examples of such tracking are shown in figures 5–7. In the first case, the prostate showed very little movement. In the second case, it drifted quite significantly; the lateral position showed

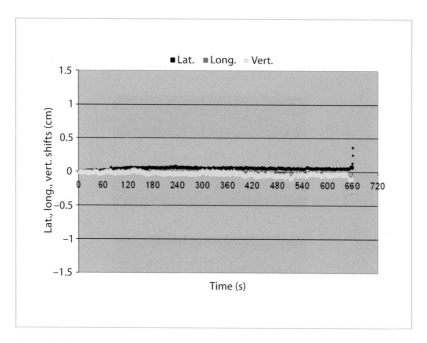

Fig. 5. Tracking using the Calypso System, case 1. Prostate position is stable during treatment in this case. Lat. = Lateral; long. = longitudinal; vert. = vertical.

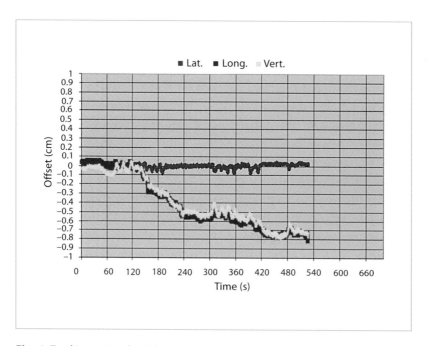

Fig. 6. Tracking using the Calypso System, case 2. Prostate position drifts during treatment in this case. Lat. = Lateral; long. = longitudinal; vert. = vertical.

Kupelian · Meyer

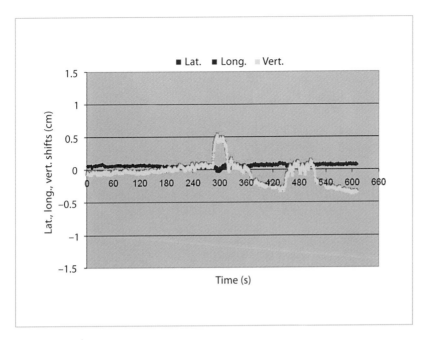

Fig. 7. Tracking using the Calypso System, case 3. Prostate position shows transient excursions in this case.

little displacement, as expected, but the longitudinal and vertical positions moved considerably. Over 9 min, the prostate actually drifted about 8 mm. Consider that if an X-ray or CT was taken to assess this same drift, the result would entirely depend on exactly when the snapshot of information had been obtained. Besides the drift of the prostate, this system has documented brief excursions of the gland during treatment, sometimes more than 1 cm. These may last only 30 s or less, but may have highly significant effects if they occur during the radiation exposure time.

A summary of approximately 1,150 sessions with this device used in different patients has been reported [13], evaluating the percentage of fractions in which the three-dimensional offset is outside of a limit of either 3 or 5 mm, for periods greater than either 10 or 30 s. For the overall weighted average of 179 fractions with tracking data, the results indicate that for a 3-mm limit, the tracking was outside of this limit in 56% of cases for >10 s (range, 41–82%), and in 47% of cases for >30 s (range 36–77%). Even for a 5-mm limit, tracking was outside of this limit for 27% of cases for >10 s, and 17% of cases for >30 s. These results show that prostate motion during therapy is a matter of concern with regard to commonly used planning target volume (PTV) expansion margins.

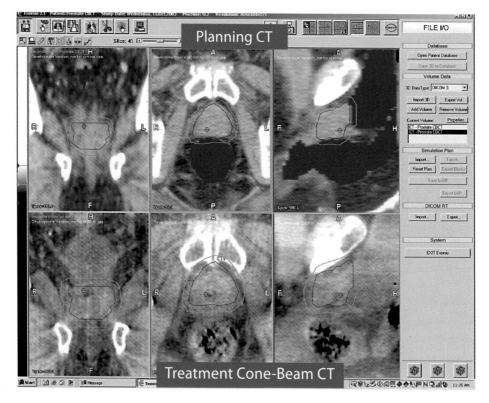

Fig. 8. Cone beam kV CT display. Note projection of planning GTV and CTV on treatment CT. Courtesy of Larry Kestin.

The above results represent aggregate data from different patients. If the results for individual patients are evaluated, looking at the percentage of fractions with more than 5 mm of displacement, they vary a great deal between patients. One patient had only 2% of fractions with displacements of over 3 mm. On the other hand, another patient had 56% of his fractions with displacements of more than 5 mm. These results indicate that the displacements are patient specific, and vary from day to day.

A paper from the William Beaumont Hospital summarizes the data on intrafraction prostate motion using real-time measurements [14]. In different reports, the results on prostate motion will vary according to the techniques used to measure it: fluoroscopy, ultrasound before or after treatment, CT real-time motion, cine MRI or implanted transponders. Of these, the Calypso System can provide nearly continuous data and has contributed the largest number of observations made.

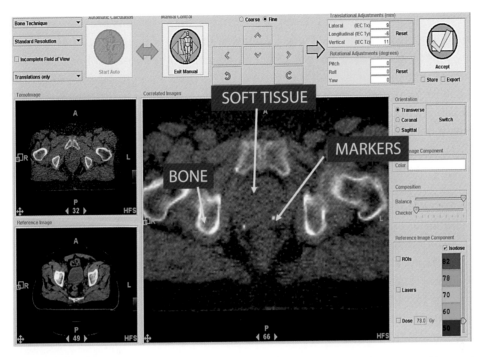

Fig. 9. Prostate IGRT. Prostate soft tissue, implanted markers and bone anatomy can all be used for localization.

In-Room MRI

In-room MRI is a concept that is being developed at the University of Florida, and there is an effort to build an operational unit that can obtain MRI sequences during radiation treatment. Movement of the anatomy can be imaged during therapy, and this will be the only device able to obtain volumetric soft tissue images while the beam is on. At this time, it is unclear whether the data can also include real-time information about the radiotherapy field or target position within the MR image. However, image analysis will still be needed. It is an interesting and promising device.

In-Room CT

In-room CT is now available. Much work has been done in this approach, and there have been different solutions including kV or MV CT in axial or cone beam configurations. Figure 9 shows the interface for a prostate case using the Elekta system at the William Beaumont Hospital, and demonstrates the approximate quality of the images that can be obtained. The alignment here is done with the contours from the initial simulation CT, and the target is aligned based on soft tissue three-dimensional images.

With the availability of CT soft tissue images, many options become available for alignment of the prostate target volume at the time of treatment. After acquiring a set of in-room CT images, target alignment can be chosen to bone, soft tissues or implanted markers if they are used. This presents a great deal of information to be evaluated by radiation therapy technologists, often in different ways and possibly with different results. Alignment may be straightforward if therapists have automatic tools for target localization to bone anatomy or markers. However, if relying on soft tissue information, they will need much more time to do the alignment and probably more dependence on physician level staff. Looking at the image quality, one can see enough anatomy on the axial images in figure 9 to make appropriate adjustments. But in the other views, it might be difficult to determine the inferior and superior borders of the prostate, and three-dimensional image registration may become challenging.

There are also MV CT solutions using helical tomotherapy or cone beam technologies. Image quality with MV CT is discussed in the article by J. Pouliot [this vol., pp 132–142]. Looking at the quality of the images obtained using helical tomotherapy at the MD Anderson Cancer Center Orlando, Fla., USA (fig. 9), one can see that the images with MV CT are generally grainier than with kV CT, but a good deal of anatomy can be visualized.

In order to use CT imaging information for practical implementation of IGRT, an important question is whether there will be enough anatomical information to perform accurate alignment. It is very similar to the situation faced in utilizing ultrasound information for daily alignment. At the MD Anderson Cancer Center Orlando, implanted prostate markers continue to be used because they make the alignment process faster and add additional information to the CT soft tissue imaging.

Managing Prostate Motion and Deformation

The cause of intrafraction prostate displacement is associated with bowel activity, peristalsis. Using MRI or cone beam CT information, with scans obtained in the same patient with only a few minutes' separation, the prostate motion can be observed, and often gas is seen passing through the rectum and causing this displacement.

Dosimetric Analysis and Active Intervention
How should information on prostate mobility be used? For instance, an implanted Calypso System transducer may provide information that a prostate has moved 5 mm during treatment for 3 s before it returns to its original location. Is this a dosimetric problem? One must be able to efficiently evaluate the potential dosimetric significance of such motion, and it is important to develop a methodology to do so.

Table 3. Intrafraction movement and treatment margins for prostate cancer

	Treatment margins, mm		
	lateral	vertical	longitudinal
Skin marks			
Ignore intrafraction motion	8.0	7.3	10.0
With intrafraction motion	8.2	10.2	12.5
Markers	1.8	5.8	7.1
Interbeam adjustments	0.4	2.3	1.8
Intrafraction tracking, correction (3-mm threshold)	0.3	1.5	1.5

Transponder tracks: 11 patients, 1 tracking session per patient, 8-min session per patient.

When transient prostate motion during therapy has been detected, how should it be managed? In current approaches, some form of expansion of the target volume would be undertaken as part of the PTV to include this motion. Table 3 shows data that have recently been presented [15]. Eleven patients were studied, and each had one 8-min tracking session using the Calypso System. The authors then enacted different scenarios using these data, to try to compensate for the prostate motion that was recorded. Their work looked at the expansion of each treatment margin in the three dimensions. First, if they simply increased field sizes based on localization to skin marks without image guidance, fields would need to be dramatically increased by 7.3–10.0 mm (ignoring intrafraction motion) or even by 8.2–12.5 mm (with intrafraction motion considered). Second, if they aligned to intraprostatic markers before treatment, margins still would need to be increased by 1.8–7.1 mm. Third, if they readjusted to intraprostatic markers during treatment, margins would need to be increased much less. Finally, if they readjusted during treatment after a 3-mm threshold was transgressed, margins would need to be increased very much less – only by 0.3–1.5 mm (fig. 8).

This analysis provides strong support for real-time tracking of the prostate during therapy. With real-time information about the prostate position, one may be able to use very small margins. Making initial PTV margins very large, risking greater normal tissue exposure because of worry about intrafraction motion, is the one option that should not be chosen.

Prostate Deformation
After volumetric soft tissue images of the prostate during treatment began to be obtained, it was realized that a great deal of prostate deformation occurs in addition to overall prostate motion. In our own work, we have seen that the pros-

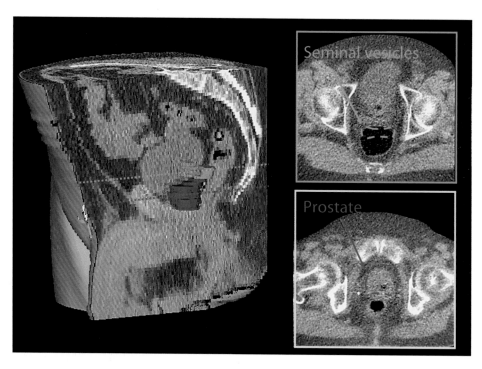

Fig. 10. Motion and deformation. See active display online at *WEB*.

tate can be lined up acceptably using daily in-room CT images. But even when the prostate itself has been lined up quite well, the seminal vesicles may not be aligned (fig. 10, and active display online at *WEB*). Because of the daily changes in the anatomy in the pelvis, not all regions of the target volume may be treated equally. More documentation of organ deformation throughout the body should be anticipated once in-room CT soft tissue imaging becomes widely available, and clinicians must develop solutions to adapt the radiotherapy process to these active changes in anatomy.

Adaptive Therapy: On-Line versus Off-Line Solutions
Off-Line Solutions
An off-line solution to motion might include planning with somewhat larger margins initially, obtaining daily scans with the initiation of treatment for some number of treatment days, then generating a final margin that is specific to that patient and continues to be used from that point forward without much additional imaging. This strategy avoids systematic errors, primarily in patient positioning. Such off-line solutions will require much less clinical effort than on-line solutions (fig. 11).

Kupelian · Meyer

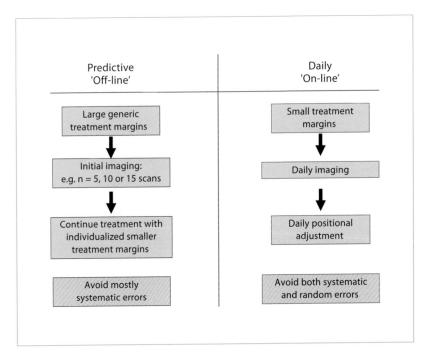

Fig. 11. Clinical strategies using adaptive IGRT. Daily on-line approach permits smaller treatment margins but requires daily imaging *and* adjustment compared with off-line approach.

On-Line Solutions

An on-line solution might be to initiate therapy with small initial margins, image the patient daily, and make daily positional adjustments of the patient. This is the best possibility of avoiding both systematic and random errors, but the clinical workload will be dramatically greater. These are practical issues for the clinic to be considered.

Practical Integration of Prostate Image-Guided Radiation Therapy into the Clinic

IGRT has a clinical impact on the work flow, as well as on patient outcomes. For both, the degree of the effect always depends on the clinical strategy used. What procedural plans will be undertaken? How often will images be obtained? How will these images be used, and who will do this work?

Clinical Impact: Work Flow

In the clinic, with systems becoming more and more efficient, it may be practical to obtain full CT guidance scans every day in at least some patients, and perhaps

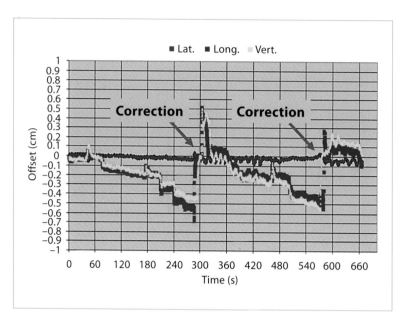

Fig. 12. Adjustment during therapy using the Calipso System. Treatment is interrupted and adjusted if position change exceeds predefined limits. Lat. = Lateral; long. = longitudinal; vert. = vertical.

in many patients. At MD Anderson Cancer Center, Orlando, the work flow process for prostate cases treated using helical tomotherapy has been analyzed. Daily imaging using this device takes 2 min, and image registration and setup takes an additional 5 min. Beam-on time is 4 min, and the entire treatment time is kept within a 15- to 20-min time slot. With increasing staff efficiency, the number of patients treated has gradually increased. Analysis of time patterns shows that with this technology, it is possible to do more and more imaging on more and more patients. In 2005, this department delivered 4,554 treatment fractions with MV CT guidance, with every patient imaged every day for every fraction.

Clinical Impact: Outcomes

Outcomes will entirely depend upon what procedures are actually performed; there will not be one result for all image-guided approaches. One study has simulated the impact of different approaches. Prostate patients had markers placed and then different treatment scenarios were modeled [16]. Their conclusion was that 'off-line setup correction procedures, especially those directed at prostate localization using markers, will result in limited benefit to a minority of patients. The relative benefit of on-line localization is still potentially significant if the intrafraction motion is relatively small'.

There are few examples of clinical outcome data to date. However, we can begin to understand the possible outcome benefits of IGRT indirectly. Consider, for instance, a series of 127 patients treated at the MD Anderson Cancer Center from 1993 to 1998 with no daily image guidance [17]. These authors analyzed long-term outcomes of patients based simply on whether the initial planning CT showed a distended rectum or not. Five or more years later, these two groups showed a huge difference in biochemical control: more than 20% worse for patients with an initially distended rectum.

This evaluation demonstrates that if there is rectal distension during simulation, then a systematic error is introduced during treatment. The most obvious conclusion would be that it is necessary to have the rectum empty at the time of simulation. But how would one know that it is empty at the time of treatment? IGRT is the obvious choice. The above evaluation suggests that the overall benefits for prostate cancer disease control substantially increase with the use of effective image guidance systems.

In addition to improvement in biochemical control, we hope to achieve improvement in normal tissue late effects. At MD Anderson Cancer Center, Orlando, rectal toxicity scored as grade 0, 1, 2 or 3 has been evaluated following treatment with 3DCRT or intensity-modulated radiation therapy (IMRT) using three different technologies that have evolved over time. The most current IMRT technologies using linear accelerator-based or helical tomotherapy approaches have shown a reduction in grade 1 rectal toxicity from 58% with 3DCRT to 27% with IMRT, and grade 2 toxicity has decreased from 18 to 7%. This work in progress has already shown that better clinical outcomes will be achieved through improvements in technology.

Future Directions in Image-Guided Radiation Therapy for Prostate Cancer

It is expected that future advances will derive from our ability to evaluate and even modify actual dose delivery during the course of treatment. There are several challenges to overcome in order to achieve these goals. First, a program to organize the daily or periodic in-room CT data and the DVHs of all regions of interest needs to be developed. It should be coupled with an efficient evaluation technique for daily dose recalculations and reconstruction of the exit dosimetry. Second, this CT and DVH data processing will require methods of registering and fusing the moving and deforming anatomy, and the daily doses corresponding to the changing anatomy. Finally, a logical strategy of dose adaptation during the therapy course needs to be developed, so that the entire distribution of finally delivered doses very closely approximates the originally planned dosimetry. Each of these three concepts will be briefly presented below.

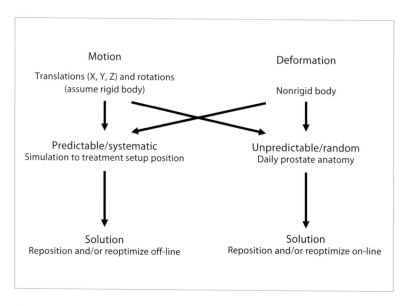

Fig. 13. Factors affecting dose delivery during a course of treatment. Adaptive approaches must address both organ motion and deformation in off-line and on-line solutions.

Evaluation of Dose Delivered during a Course of Radiotherapy

Many factors affect dose delivery during a course of treatment (fig. 13). Using a rigid model of anatomy, there are XYZ coordinate changes as well as rotational changes that can occur between simulation and treatment. Image registration tools are now available for assessing these coordinate changes and calculating the required table shifts appropriately on a daily treatment basis. The treatment plans may be revised for any systematic errors detected. However, the body is highly mobile, and additional treatment variations will occur in more random fashion based upon the daily deformation of the prostate anatomy and its position. Solutions to these changes are more challenging, and require on-line approaches, or at least methods to cumulate the actually delivered doses and periodically adapt the delivered therapy distributions.

Daily On-Line DVHs

How can the deforming anatomy and the doses given on each fraction be evaluated? Since the soft tissues can be imaged every day, and if the dose distributions are recalculated quickly, one can obtain a 'DVH of the day' (fig. 14–15). In the simplest form of dose guidance, this could be used for daily repositioning of the patient. For instance, if the rectal doses were judged unacceptable, a patient move could be modeled virtually to improve the rectal dose and a second DVH generated. If the new DVH is judged acceptable, the appropriate couch offsets could be

Kupelian · Meyer

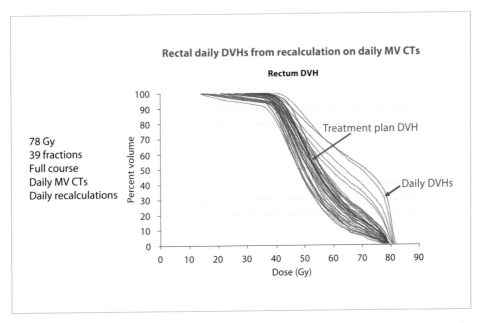

Fig. 14. Daily dose recalculation: prostate radiation therapy, rectal DVHs [18]. Actual daily DVH can be acquired, and used for daily position adjustment or cumulative dose modification.

generated and applied. In this approach, a full reoptimization plan would not be performed, but rather the dose-volume information would be used only to adjust the patient position.

Cumulative DVHs
While such daily DVH information is undoubtedly useful, and might be used for daily couch adjustments, its importance for a series of treatments cannot become clinically meaningful until there are better three-dimensional tools for cumulating this dose information. It is appealing to look at DVHs like those shown in figure 16, but it is still difficult to comprehend what dose a given point in the rectum or a specific point in the prostate has received in a series of fractions. The only way to process all of this DVH information is to develop reliable and useable deformable registration methods [18].

Deformable Registration
Anatomic changes recorded on daily CT imply that structures are being deformed, and these changes result in dosimetric changes. The process of translating these anatomic changes into a cumulative view coupled with a dosimetric pattern is called deformable dose registration (see review of these concepts by Dr. K. Brock

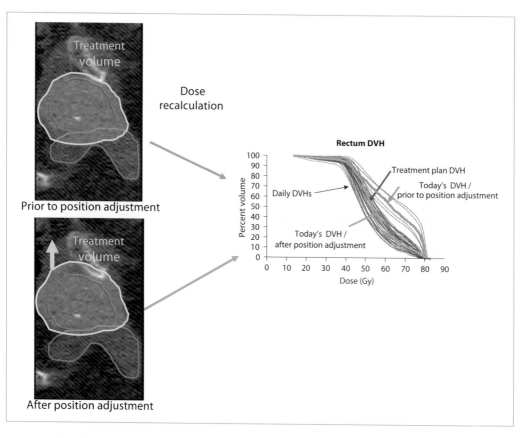

Fig. 15. Dose-guided radiotherapy. Daily DVH can be used for position adjustments.

[this vol., pp. 94–115]). The general idea is as follows. Let us suppose that the prostate looks a little different on 2 CT scans – the original CT and the daily treatment CT. With a deformation algorithm, the CT voxels of one can then be individually adjusted until they correspond to the other. This is called generating a deformation map. Once that map is generated, the doses delivered to those voxels can follow, creating an overall dose pattern (fig. 17). These methods are currently under practical development at several centers [19–21].

Adaptive Radiotherapy

With adaptive radiotherapy, we look forward to the possibility of radiation delivery modification during the course of treatment (fig. 18). While the implementation of these approaches needs to be developed fully, their background concepts can be mentioned here.

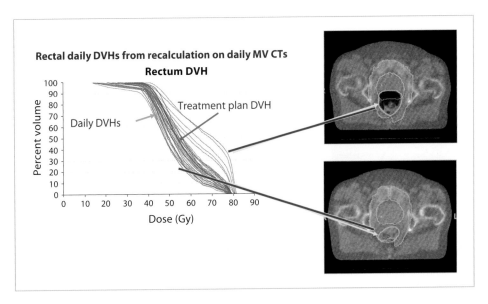

Fig. 16. Cumulative dosimetry. Adaptive strategy needs to cumulate DVH information in an anatomically meaningful way, since organs are deforming on a daily basis.

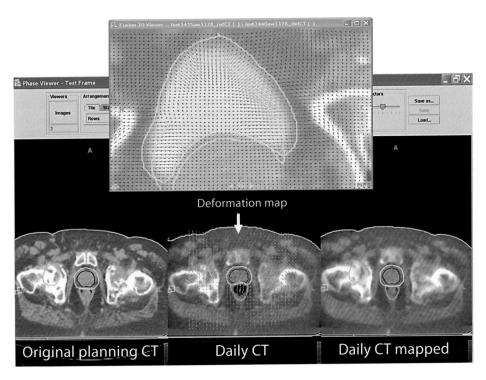

Fig. 17. Deformable registration. The process of registering images of deformable structures generates a deformation map that is used to adjust deforming anatomy, contours and enables dose accumulation.

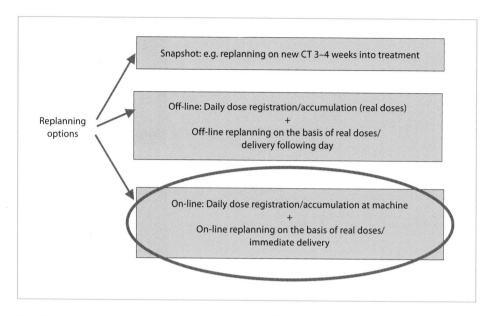

Fig. 18. Adaptive radiotherapy. Radiation delivery modification during the course of radiotherapy.

The snapshot CT method is simply a treatment replanning based on a new CT scan obtained partway through the therapy course. This procedure is now widely used for some tumors such as lung cancers.

The off-line approach requires cumulating all of the actually delivered doses, and adjusting the plan accordingly for a modified delivery the next day. This might be organized as follows. The initial CT is used for the original treatment planning and for comparison with a daily CT, acquired with image registration. The DVH of the original CT and the daily CT can then be compared. Repeating this process every day, a DVH profile of the overall therapy course can be generated that describes the actual treatment delivered. It might be performed approximately half-way through treatment, as in the example given in figure 19. After 26 fractions, the rectal DVH showed that this organ was receiving a higher dose than planned. On the basis of all the actual doses from those prior 26 fractions, a second plan could be generated adjusting these doses which resulted in a final dose profile that closely matched the originally planned distribution (fig. 20).

Fig. 19. DVH of the initial plan (planned: solid line) and cumulative DVH using daily CT scans after 26 fractions (actual: dotted line).
Fig. 20. DVH of the initial plan (planned: solid line) and cumulative DVH using daily CT scans after all fractions including one reoptimization after 26 fractions (actual: dotted line).

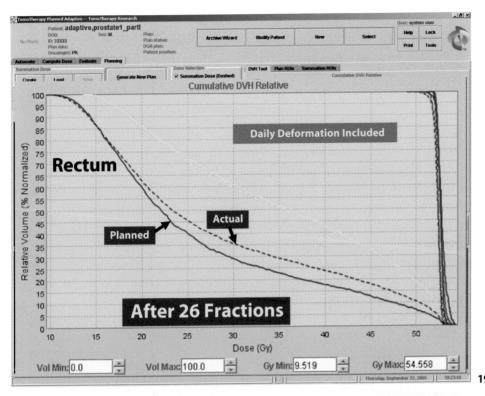

19

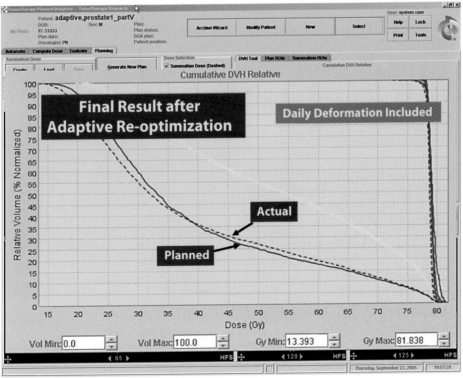

20

Ultimately, there is no reason why this entire process could not be performed while the patient is still on the treatment table, which would be the on-line approach. For prostate radiotherapy, this may well be the preferred approach.

Conclusion

Although probably infrequent and limited in duration, real-time motion of the prostate gland can have a significant effect on the distribution of radiotherapy dose. Because of prostate movement, the bone anatomy cannot be used as a proxy for the prostate gland position. For accurate daily localization, X-ray-based techniques should be coupled with the use of intraprostatic markers, which have been found to be stable within the gland in the majority of cases. However, such markers cannot show deformation of the gland that might result in altered geometry of the markers. Such real-time motion and its impact are beginning to be characterized. Quantitative, data-based solutions provide the most anatomic information, and will allow the development of true adaptive radiotherapy.

Acknowledgment

The author would like to thank Katja Langen, PhD, Sanford Meeks, PhD and Twyla Willoughby, MS.

Guidelines for Clinical Practice

- Image-guided radiation therapy (IGRT) for prostate cancer may include several different types of imaging modalities used in a wide variety of approaches. Each method must be studied individually, and the outcomes of IGRT will entirely depend on the particular approach employed.

- Image guidance methods do not replace the need for careful immobilization techniques. Similarly, the use of immobilization techniques such as endorectal balloons does not replace the need for image guidance. Whether or not balloon devices reduce prostatic motion partially, they are unlikely to eliminate it.

- Of the currently available image guidance technologies, transabdominal ultrasound may be the most prone to interuser variability.

- Bone anatomy cannot be used as a proxy for prostate gland position.

- X-ray-based image guidance techniques should be coupled with the use of intraprostatic markers, which are stable within the gland in the majority of cases. However, deformation of the gland can result in altered geometry of the markers.

- Although infrequent and limited in duration in most cases, real-time motion of the prostate gland can be significant in some cases. Such motion and its impact are beginning to be characterized.

- Continuous monitoring of the position of the prostate during treatment using implanted transducers may prove useful. Regardless, the daily treatment time from the initial imaging for IGRT to the end of treatment delivery should be minimized.

- Quantitative data-based solutions to image guidance that provide the most anatomic information will allow the development of true adaptive radiotherapy.

References

1 Patel RR, Orton N, Tome WA, Chappell R, Ritter MA: Rectal dose sparing with a balloon catheter and ultrasound localization I conformal radiation therapy for prostate cancer. Radiotherapy Oncol 2003;67:285–294.

2 Van Lin ENJT, van der Vight LP, Witjes JA, Huisman HJ, Leer J W, Visser AG: The effect of an endorectal balloon and off-line correction on the interfraction systematic and random prostate position variations: a comparative study. Int J Radiat Oncol Biol Phys 2005;61:278–288.

3 Serago CF, Chungbin SJ, Buskirk SJ, Vora SA, McLaughlin MP, Ezzell GA: Initial experience with ultrasound localization for positioning prostate cancer patients for external beam radiotherapy. Int J Radiat Oncol Biol Phys 2001;51: S94.

4 Dong l, de Crevoisier R, Bonnen M, Lee A, Cheung R, Wang H, O'Daniel J, Mohan R, Cox J, Kuban D: Evaluation of an ultrasound-based prostate target localization technique with an in-room CT-on-rails. Int J Radiat Oncol Biol Phys 2004;60:S332.

5 Langen KM, Pouliot J, Anezinos C, Aubin M, Gottschalk AR, Hsu IC, Lowther D, Liu YM, Shinohara K, Verhey LJ, Weinberg V, Roach M 3rd: Evaluation of ultrasound-based prostate localization for image-guided radiotherapy. Int J Radiat Oncol Biol Phys 2003;57:635–644.

6 Scarborough T, Golden NM, Fuller CD, Kupelian PA, Ting JY, Wong A, Thomas CR: Ultrasound versus seed marker prostate localization. Int J Radiat Oncol Biol Phys 2005;63:S196.

7 Dehnad H, Nederveen AJ, van der Heide UA, van Moorselaar JA, Hofman P, Lagendijk JJW: Clinical feasibility study for the use of implanted gold seeds in the prostate as reliable positioning markers during megavoltage irradiation. Radiother Oncol 2003;67:295–302.

8 Poggi MM, Grant DA, Sewchand W, Warlick WB: Marker seed migration in prostate localization. Int J Radiat Oncol Biol Phys 2003;56:1248–1251.

9 Aubin M, Pouliot J, Millender L, Shinohara K, Pickett B, Anezinos C, Lerhey L, Roach M: Daily prostate targeting with implanted gold markers and an a-SI panel EPID at UCSF: a five-year clinical experience. Int J Radiat Oncol Biol Phys 2004;60:S266–S267.

10 Litzenberg D, Dawson LA, Sandler H, Sanda MG, McShan DL, Balter JM: Daily prostate targeting using implanted radiopaque markers. Int J Radiat Oncol Biol Phys 2002;52:699–703.

11 Pouliot J, Aubin M, Langen KM, Liu Y-M, Pickett B, Shinohara K, Roach M: (Non)-migration of radiopaque markers used for on-line localization of the prostate with an electronic portal imaging device. Int J Radiat Oncol Biol Phys 2003;56:862–866.

12 Kupelian PA, Willoughby TR, Meeks SL, Forbes A, Wagner T, Maach M, Langen KM: Intraprostatic fiducials for localization of the prostate gland: monitoring intermarker distances during radiation therapy to test for marker stability. Int J Radiat Oncol Biol Phys 2005;62:1291–1296.

13 Kupelian P, Willoughby T, Litzenberg D, Sandler H, Roach M, Levine L, van Waardenburg M: Clinical experience with the Calypso™ 4D localization system in prostate cancer patients: implantation, tolerance, migration, localization and real-time tracking. Int J Radiat Oncol Biol Phys 2005;63:S197.

14 Willoughby TR, Kupelian PA, Pouliot J, Shinohara K, Aubin M, Roach M, Skrumeda LL, Balter JM, Litzenberg DW, Hadley SW, Wei JT, Sandler HM: Target localization and real-time tracking using the Calypso 4D localization system in patients with localized prostate cancer. Int J Radiat Oncol Biol Phys 2006;65:528–534.

15 Litzenberg D, Balter J, Hadley S, Sandler H, Willoughby T, Kupelian P, Levine L: The influence of intra-fraction motion on prostate margins. Int J Radiat Oncol Biol Phys 2005;63:S4.

16 Litzenberg DW, Balter JM, Lam KL, Sandler HM, Ten Haken RK: Retrospective analysis of prostate cancer patients with implanted gold markers using off-line and adaptive therapy protocols. Int J Radiat Oncol Biol Phys 2005;63:123–133.

17 de Crevoisier R, Tucker SL, Dong L, Mohan R, Cheung R, Cox JD, Kuban DA: Increased risk of biochemical and local failure in patients with distended rectum on the planning CT for prostate cancer radiotherapy. Int J Radiat Oncol Biol Phys 2005;62:965–973.

18 Langen KM, Meeks SL, Poole DO, Wagner TH, Willoughby TR, Kupelian PA, Ruchala KJ, Haimerl J, Olivera GH: The use of megavoltage CT (MVCT) images for dose recomputations. Phys Med Biol 2005;50:4259–4276.

19 Wang H, Dong L, Lii MF, Lee AL, de Crevoisier R, Mohan R, Cox JD, Kuban DA, Cheung R: Implementation and validation of a three-dimensional deformable registration algorithm for targeted prostate cancer radiotherapy. Int J Radiat Oncol Biol Phys 2005;61:725–735.

20 Foskey M, Davis B, Goyal L, Chang S, Chaney E, Strehl N, Tomei S, Rosenman J, Joshi: Large deformation three-dimensional image registration in image-guided radiation therapy. Phys Med Biol 2005;50:5869–5892.

21 Lu W, Chen ML, Olivera GH, Ruchala KJ, Mackie TR: Fast free-form deformable registration via calculus of variations. Phys Med Biol 2004;3067–3087.

Dr. Patrick Kupelian
Department of Radiation Oncology
MD Anderson Cancer Center Orlando
1400 S Orange Avenue
Orlando, FL 32806 (USA)
Tel. +1 321 841 8666, Fax +1 407 649 6895
E-Mail patrick.kupelian@orhs.org

Meyer JL (ed): IMRT, IGRT, SBRT – Advances in the Treatment Planning and
Delivery of Radiotherapy. Front Radiat Ther Oncol. Basel, Karger, 2007, vol. 40, pp 315–337

New Technologies for the Radiotherapy of Prostate Cancer

A Discussion of Clinical Treatment Programs

J.L. Meyer[a] · S. Leibel[b] · M. Roach[c] · S. Vijayakumar[d]

Departments of Radiation Oncology, [a]Saint Francis Memorial Hospital,
San Francisco, Calif., [b]Stanford University, Stanford, Calif., [c]University of California,
San Francisco, Calif., [d]University of California, Davis, Calif., USA

New radiation therapy planning and delivery technologies have often been applied first to the treatment of localized prostate cancer. The development and optimization of these new applications for prostate cancer therapy can make this site a model for their use at other tumor sites. For prostate cancer or other tumors, the process of defining new roles for technology can lead to a reassessment of the basic goals of the treatments themselves. What clinical advances need to be made? What changes in the target volumes, their delineation and treatment doses are these technologies to be used for? These questions are central themes in the current investigations with intensity-modulated radiation therapy (IMRT) and image-guided radiation therapy (IGRT) for prostate cancer treatment. In the following two sections, two of the authors give their insights into the use of advanced technologies for prostate cancer therapy. In the final section, provocative questions about the current directions of radiotherapy for prostate cancer are addressed in a roundtable discussion.

Target Definitions and Lessons in Clinical Treatment Planning (M. Roach)

The goals of this section are to discuss evidence for selecting targets and defining normal tissue constraints in the radiotherapy of prostate cancer. It must be recognized that there is a lack of evidence-based consensus on many of the issues involved. There are several problems that are faced in evaluating the literature on

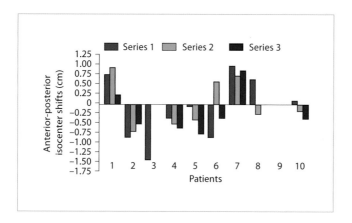

Fig. 1. Defining target volumes and the role of 3DCRT-IMRT for prostate cancer. Anterior-posterior isocenter shifts in patients receiving radiotherapy and rescanned every 2 weeks [1].

prostate radiotherapy. In assessing issues surrounding quality of life, there are large discrepancies between what physicians report and what patients report, and one must be careful in accepting complication rates that are reported without using validated quality of life instruments. Also, the ability to draw conclusions from studies is often limited by the duration and completeness of patient follow-up, since long follow-up periods are required but difficult to obtain. Finally, the radiation techniques are critical to the outcome results achieved, and yet the treatment methods for prostate radiotherapy have not been standardized. Despite these concerns, available data do support certain general recommendations, and clinical trials are continuing to develop additional conclusions.

Patient Setup and Target Localization
More than 10 years ago, the University of California, San Francisco (UCSF) group first performed studies evaluating prostate position during radiotherapy treatment courses [1]. Serial CT scans were obtained every 2 weeks during the radiotherapy, bony anatomy was used to register the scans, and the prostate position was compared between the scans. The results for individual patients are shown in figure 1. As an example, the results for the first patient show that his prostate was 0.75 cm more anterior on the second scan than the first, 2 weeks after treatment had started. Similar results were observed in other patients. Since this initial work, many other groups have obtained comparable findings. It is clear that the prostate does move during the therapy course, and its position is more variable than previously appreciated.

To address this issue and attempt to adjust for it, our group has used gold seed fiducial markers implanted into the prostate for the past 5 years. These are 1.1 ×

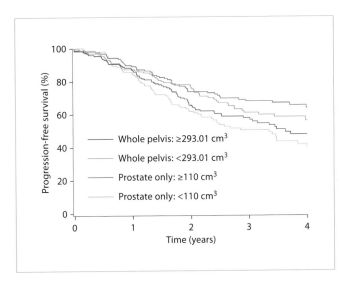

Fig. 2. RTOG 9413: progression-free survival in the 4-arm study [3].

3 mm in size; two are placed in the prostate base and one at the apex. Prior to each daily treatment, they are imaged, and adjustments are made to correct for setup error and organ movement, which can be significant problems. This is especially true in some patients. Our group has recently published a report on 3 patients with morbid obesity, indicating that if a patient is severely obese and internal markers are not used, therapy beams can miss the prostate when setup is based on skin marks alone [2]. Internal markers are especially recommended for these patients.

Planning Target Volume

The results of the Radiation Therapy Oncology Group (RTOG) protocol 9413 have been published and are relevant for patients at risk for lymph node involvement [3]. This double randomization study evaluated the effect of hormonal therapy timing (prior to or after radiotherapy), and the effect of radiotherapy field size (pelvis plus prostate or prostate alone). Pertinent outcome results are shown in figure 2. Superior progression-free survivals were achieved in patients receiving whole pelvic radiotherapy and neoadjuvant hormonal therapy. One must conclude that it is important to irradiate the regional pelvic lymph nodes when they are at risk for involvement.

Since this protocol permitted some differences in the actual size of the fields used, the RTOG 9413 results have been further analyzed by evaluating the results according to the actual fields [4]. These have been divided into groups: prostate-only, prostate-plus-mini-pelvis, and prostate-plus-whole-pelvis fields. Reanalysis shows two findings. First, the complication rates with the prostate-plus-mini-

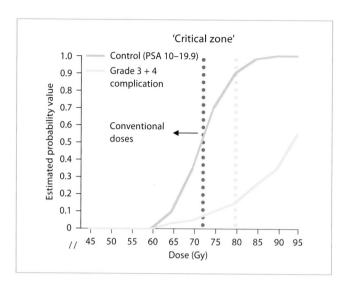

Fig. 3. 3DCRT dose-response functions: actuarial biochemical 5-year disease control and grade 3 and 4 complication rates with increasing radiation dose. Modified from Hanks et al. [5].

pelvis fields were nearly the same as with the larger prostate-plus-whole-pelvis fields. Second, the control rates did correlate with the size of the fields: 4-year progression-free survival rates were 60% for the prostate-plus-whole-pelvis, 48% for the prostate-plus-mini-pelvis and 40% for the prostate-only groups. Thus, the larger the field (and logically the more nodes treated), the greater the control rate.

Normal Tissue Effects of Treatment and Radiation Planning
In figure 3, Dr. Hanks et al. [5] show useful information about the risk of grade 3 and 4 complications after increasing radiation doses, as well as the relationship between dose and tumor control in patients with intermediate-risk disease. For high rates of tumor control, it is apparent that radiation doses need to exceed 70 Gy and perhaps approach 80 Gy or possibly higher. It is also known that the shape of the complication curve is such that the rates of complication climb steeply when these dose levels are approached. In order to spare normal tissues, it is critical to evaluate and understand the technique of treatment used to deliver the doses that are required.

In this volume, Dr. Vijayakumar et al. [pp. 180–192] report on the use of benchmarking with dose-volume histogram (DVH) analysis for assessing and guiding the use of new technologies in the clinic. This type of approach has been used at UCSF for introducing treatment programs for prostate cancer therapy, first with conformal therapy dose escalation. Prior to dose escalating any patient, a treat-

Meyer · Leibel · Roach · Vijayakumar

Table 1. Dose to the bulb of the penis and risk of impotence: change in potency based on a survey of men treated with 3DCRT at UCSF for localized prostate cancer [6]

Impact of 3DCRT on potency	Dose to 5% of bulb Gy		Dose to 70% of bulb Gy		Dose to 95% of bulb Gy	
	median	range	median	range	median	range
No change	48.5	40–70	29.0	22–69	14.0	7–47
Decline = 1	69.8	56–75	56.1	45–75	33.2	0–74
Decline >1	67.3	62–90	66.8	42–88	51.1	16–84
Kruskal-Wallis test	p = 0.08		p = 0.17		p = 0.05	

ment plan using a standard therapy technique was constructed. A three-dimensional conformal radiation therapy (3DCRT) plan was also generated, and the normal tissue DVHs compared. Dose escalation was allowed to proceed when the dose to normal tissues did not significantly increase. This approach has proved reliable, and over the past 15 years the complication rates for prostate radiotherapy at UCSF have remained low with ever more advancing external beam radiation techniques and treatment doses. One is using what one already knows to prevent higher complication rates.

Impotence

Urologists often refer to sexual function after radical prostatectomy as an improving outcome; patients are initially impotent, but this gradually resolves. The opposite is true with radiation therapy. Rates of impotence increase after treatment, and are even worse when combined with hormone therapy. Ultimately, there may be little outcome difference in sexual function between these approaches. However, one must evaluate this literature carefully, because the baseline characteristics of the patients may be different. The age of the patient and his degree of infirmity can be major considerations in the initial treatment selection.

Recent data show that it is probably important to avoid irradiating the base of the penis. Dr. Fisch et al. [6] published our data that indicated that the risk of impotence increased as the dose to the penis increased, whether measured as dose to 5% of the bulb, or 70%, or 95% (table 1). If the dose was over about 50–52 Gy, there was a higher risk of impotence. To substantiate these results, data from the RTOG 9406 dose escalation study were analyzed [7]. Without knowing the outcomes of patients in terms of sexual functioning, the planning scans of approximately 150 cases were evaluated and the bulb of the penis was delineated. A statistician then used a threshold dose to that area of 52.5 Gy, based on other studies at our institution, and found that the risk of becoming impotent after radio-

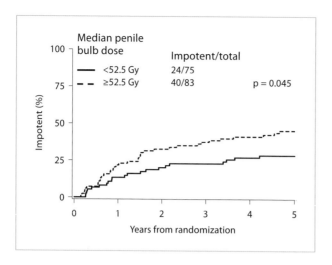

Fig. 4. RTOG 9406 dose levels: time to impotence.

therapy was significantly higher above that dose (fig. 4). Avoiding high radiotherapy doses to the penile bulb is an easy yet important aspect of defining the target volumes. IMRT can achieve this sparing somewhat more efficiently, although acceptable results can be obtained with 3DCRT.

Rectal Toxicity

The RTOG and other groups have reported their toxicity results in treating patients to 78–80 Gy for prostate cancer [8]. In general, a modest risk of greater than grade 2 rectal complications has been reported, about 2% or less at a median of 3.0 years after therapy. Often these were physician-reported rates, and measures using validated quality of life instruments could report more accurate results. As reviewed below, investigators at the Memorial Sloan-Kettering Cancer Center (MSKCC) have done perhaps the most work with IMRT for prostate cancer, and have made important observations about the value of IMRT compared with conventional 3DCRT in terms of reducing the risk of complications, especially of rectal toxicity. It is important to have longer-term follow-up in assessing these late risks of complication. Nevertheless, there is little question that improvements derived from IMRT are valid, based upon our own experience at UCSF and elsewhere.

Several groups have investigated the risks of rectal toxicity based on dose/volume assessments. For example, work published by Kuban et al. [9] is shown in figure 5, and demonstrates that 70 Gy to ≥26% of the rectal volume correlated with a higher risk of grade 2 or higher complications to the rectum. An interesting observation made by the William Beaumont group is that patients who had more

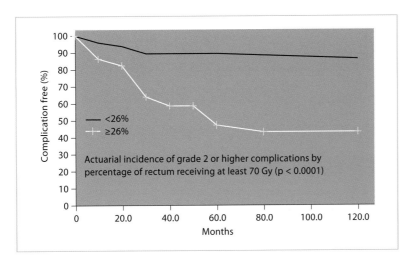

Fig. 5. Hazards of dose escalation in prostate cancer radiotherapy [9].

acute toxicity also tended to have more late toxicity. This has not been well described before, and not all series observe this phenomenon. However, if a patient is having significant acute toxicity, a reevaluation of the treatment approach may be worth considering.

If one cumulates several late rectal toxicity studies together, one can derive a threshold curve as shown in figure 6. At UCSF, the dose constraints for IMRT have been based on this curve, and the goal is set to be about 30% below what the literature suggests will be the threshold for complication. It is possible to achieve this goal with IMRT. Based upon the data of several groups [9–12], reasonable goals include keeping the radiation dose to 25% of the rectum at <70 Gy and the mean dose at <50 Gy.

Bladder Toxicity

Bladder toxicity is not as common as rectal toxicity, but can be a very late phenomenon, several years after therapy. The determination of bladder dose constraints is complicated by the changing volume of the bladder during treatment. A patient's bladder may be full during planning but will rarely be full to the same degree during therapy, and the bladder DVH that was initially planned will often not reflect the actual treatment experience. This is especially true toward the end of therapy; because of developing inflammation, patients may think that their bladder is full when it is not, resulting in an even larger dose to the bladder than planned. While these are identified problems, treatment planning investigations do show that IMRT can achieve significantly better sparing of bladder tissues than 3DCRT.

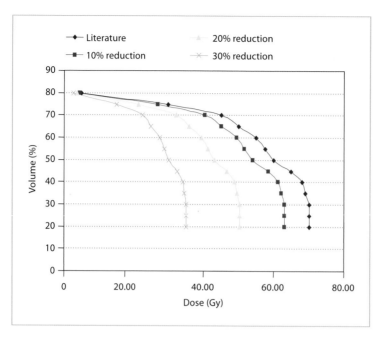

Fig. 6. Rectum dose constraints. Evidence-based constraints for rectal complications at UCSF.

Comments

In summary, accuracy is important in prostate radiotherapy to achieve the doses required for cure without increasing normal tissue damage. Validated instruments that address quality of life issues are needed. To reduce the risk of impotence, it is important to limit the radiation doses to the penile bulb. It is equally important to limit the rectal doses, and studies suggest that no more than 25% of the rectum should receive 70 Gy or more, and the mean rectal dose should be less than 50 Gy. Bladder toxicity can also occur, though not as frequently and often later than rectal effects. Finally, the future of our new technology depends on improving the quality assurance of the treatment procedures, to guarantee that everyone is treated appropriately.

The Development of Dose Objectives for Prostate Radiotherapy (S. Leibel)

What is necessary to improve local tumor control with radiotherapy in prostate cancer? First, dose levels must be sufficiently high to eliminate the most resistant tumor clonogens. Conformal treatment techniques are required if high doses are to be administered without increasing normal tissue toxicity. Another approach to improving local tumor control is to use agents that enhance the sensitivity of

Meyer · Leibel · Roach · Vijayakumar

Table 2. MSKCC dose escalation study in prostate cancer: patient characteristics (n = 1,684)

	Number	Percent
Stage		
T1c	573	34
T2a	309	18
T2b	271	16
T2c	217	13
T3	314	19
Dose		
64.8 Gy	96	
70.2 Gy	274	
75.6 Gy	476	
81 Gy	764	
86.4 Gy	74	

Age: median = 68 years, range = 46–86 years; follow-up: median = 68 months; range = 36–168 months; neoadjuvant androgen deprivation = 746 patients (44%).

tumor clonogens to the biological effects of irradiation. Some of these agents may cause a general increase in the level of radiosensitivity of tissues. Thus, the ability to deliver combined-modality therapy without overlapping toxicities represents another rationale for conformal therapy. Based on these two ideas, the hypothesis of dose escalation with conformal radiotherapy was formed: that conforming the high-dose region to the shape of the tumor will enable an increase in the tumor dose without an increase in toxicity, and an increase in the tumor dose will improve local tumor control and ultimately patient survival.

Dose Escalation for the Radiotherapy of Prostate Cancer

To test this hypothesis in the treatment of prostate cancer, a dose escalation study, designed to assess the morbidity of 3DCRT and to establish the maximum feasible dose, was initiated at MSKCC in 1988 [13, 14]. Patients with stage T2c–T3 disease were eligible for the study and evaluated for late complications at incremental dose levels of 75.6, 81 and 86.4 Gy (table 2). Forty patients were treated at each dose level and escalation to the next level was permitted if the rate of grade 3 toxicity remained less than 10%. Between 1988 and 1992, patients were treated at conventional dose levels of 64.8–70.2 Gy to establish baselines for acute tolerance and late toxicity. The 75.6-Gy arm was opened in April 1991. The dose for all other patients treated during this period was 70.2 Gy. Once it was determined that there was no excess in toxicity, the investigational dose in October 1992 was escalated to 81 Gy, and all other patients received 75.6 Gy. In October 1995, the first patient was

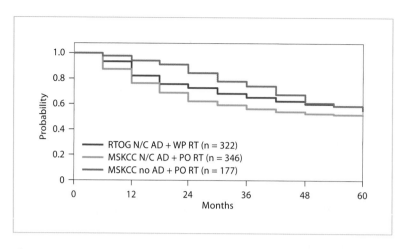

Fig. 7. Progression-free survival in prostate cancer patients with >15% risk of pelvic lymph node metastases. RTOG 9413 patients [3] treated with whole-pelvis (WP) radiotherapy (RT). MSKCC patients treated with prostate-only (PO) radiotherapy, with or without neoadjuvant (N/C) androgen deprivation (AD) (reported by Zelefsky et al. at the ASTRO-ASCO Prostate Conference, 2005).

treated with IMRT, first as a boost approach. Six months later, all patients with prostate cancer were treated to 81 Gy with IMRT. Finally, the 86.4-Gy arm was opened in May 1996. A total of 1,684 patients were treated in this fashion through July 2001.

Field Size and Dose Constraints
The planning target volume (PTV) encompassed the prostate and seminal vesicles but did not include the regional pelvic lymph nodes. Pelvic nodal irradiation was omitted because of the absence at that time of any proven benefit to prophylactic pelvic lymph node irradiation. Also, data already existed indicating that outcome was not affected by local control in patients with biopsy-proven pelvic lymph node metastases [15]. Further, there was concern that the larger volume of irradiated tissue might restrict the ability to safely escalate the dose to the prostate. The results of our study continue to support this approach, as reported by Zelefsky et al. at the ASTRO-ASCO Prostate Conference in 2005 and shown in figure 7. This compares data from the RTOG 9413 study (shown in red) with patients at MSKCC who had greater than a 50% risk of pelvic lymph node metastases and were treated to 81 Gy without neoadjuvant androgen deprivation (shown in green). There does not appear to be a significant decrement in outcome by omitting the pelvic lymph nodes from treatment.

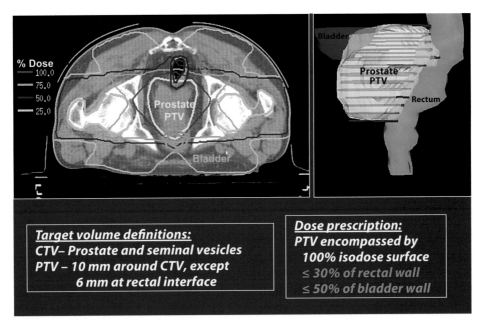

Fig. 8. Six-field 3DCRT plan for prostate cancer at MSKCC.

IMRT for Additional Dose Escalation

Early in our dose escalation study, it was recognized that the volume of rectal wall irradiated to high dose impacted the risk of treatment-related complications. After careful analysis of the dose profiles, a constraint was introduced that no more than 30% of the rectum and no more than 50% of the bladder could receive the prescription dose (fig. 8). If the DVHs indicated that this would occur, patients received a 3-month course of neoadjuvant androgen deprivation therapy before beginning radiotherapy.

Evaluating patients at 30 months following radiotherapy using 3DCRT in the MSKCC and other series, the rectal toxicity rates increased steeply after 75.6 Gy (fig. 9) [16]. Thus, dose escalation using conventional conformal techniques appears to be limited by rectal toxicity indicating that if the dose was to be escalated to a higher level, an improvement in the conformality of the dose distribution would be necessary. The new IMRT methodologies provided a solution. The physics group at MSKCC developed algorithms to calculate the dose distribution from dynamic multileaf collimation, allowing intensity-modulated fields to be implemented. After evaluating a series of different IMRT treatment plans, a 5-field plan was selected and implemented as a standard radiotherapeutic approach for prostate cancer (fig. 10).

For patients treated with the 3DCRT approach, it was shown that the mean rectal wall DVH was significantly different in those who did or did not develop rectal

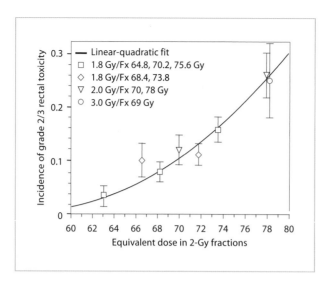

Fig. 9. Dose-response for grade 2–3 rectal toxicity after 3DCRT [16].

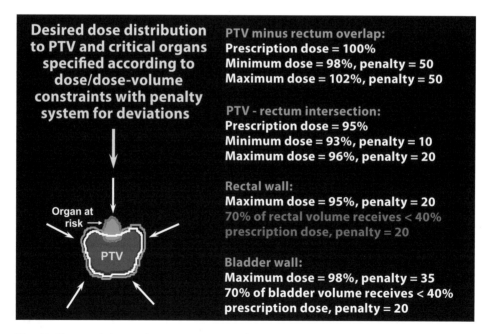

Fig. 10. Dose and dose-volume constraints and penalties for the 81-Gy IMRT prostate plan at MSKCC.

Meyer · Leibel · Roach · Vijayakumar

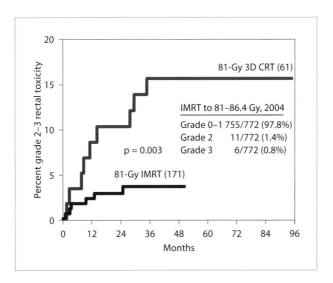

Fig. 11. Incidence of grade 2–3 rectal toxicity in prostate cancer patients treated with 3DCRT and IMRT to 81 Gy (1 case of grade 3 rectal bleeding in each treatment group) [17].

bleeding. This information helped to define the rectal dose-volume constraint in our inverse planning algorithm for the 81-Gy level prostate treatment plans. Figure 11 shows a study comparing patients treated to 81 Gy using 3DCRT (with two plans during the course) versus 81 Gy with IMRT. There is a significant decrease in the incidence of grade 2–3 rectal toxicity with the IMRT approach. At 7 years of follow-up, these values remain the same. In 772 patients treated to 81–86.4 Gy with IMRT, the incidence of grade 2 rectal toxicity was only 1.4%, and grade 3 toxicity was 0.8% [18].

Results of Dose Escalation

To examine the relationship of prostate-specific antigen (PSA) profiles after radiotherapy with local control, sextant prostate biopsies were obtained at 2.5 years or longer after treatment. The biopsies were fortuitously obtained during the time that dose escalation was in progress, permitting dose-response curves to be calculated based on biopsy findings. Figure 12 shows the percent of patients with negative biopsies for patients treated to 64.8, 70.2, 75.6 and 81 Gy [19]. A dose-response curve has been fitted for each risk group, and these differ in slope. The TCD_{50} is approximately 68 Gy for low-risk, 73 Gy for intermediate-risk and 77 Gy for high-risk groups. This is important information. It shows that radioresistance increases as the tumor phenotype becomes more malignant. Further, the evidence shows that the TCD_{90} values are 76 Gy for low-risk, 81 Gy for intermediate-risk and 86 Gy for high-risk groups, indicating that the dose levels needed to control prostate

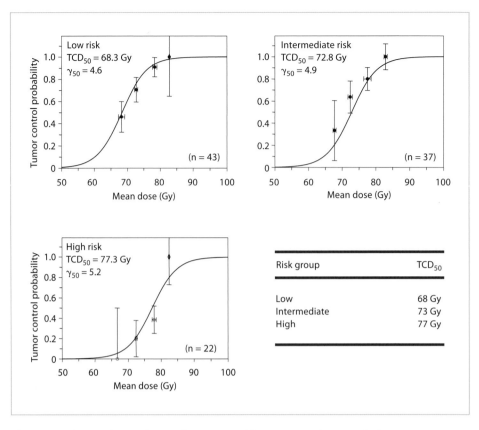

Fig. 12. Local control according to dose assessed from prostate biopsies [19].

cancer are considerably higher than the traditional 65–70 Gy and supporting the efforts to improve the precision of prostate cancer radiotherapy using sophisticated image-guided techniques.

What is the relationship of the PSA outcome profiles of patients following therapy to these biopsy data? Investigations here have shown that if a patient's PSA at nadir is 1 or less, and the PSA profile is not rising over time, then a negative biopsy is likely. Long-term PSA results in the different treatment groups are shown in figure 13. These results can be compared with those obtained using other approaches. Figure 13 also shows PSA outcomes for patients who underwent radical prostatectomy at Baylor University as reported by Dr. Scardino [20]. The other three charts show PSA outcomes by risk group for 64.8- to 70-Gy, 75.6-Gy and 81-Gy radiotherapy. The indication is that if one wishes to achieve outcomes with radiotherapy that are similar to those with surgery, then 64.8–70 Gy is not enough, nor is 75.6 Gy; one needs at least 81 Gy. Simply stated, if you treat for cure, the dose must be high enough to cure those you treat.

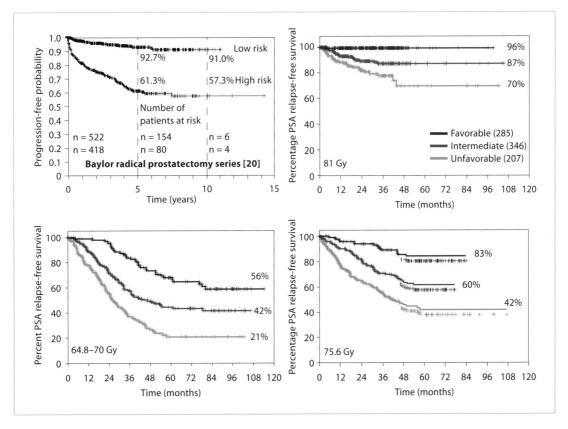

Fig. 13. Comparison of long-term outcome of radical prostatectomy with high-, intermediate- and low-dose 3DCRT/IMRT in prostate cancer.

Future Studies and Comments

After evaluating a series of 91.8-Gy IMRT treatment plans, it was concluded that 86.4 Gy represents the maximum dose feasible that can be delivered to the entire prostate PTV while maintaining acceptable toxicity outcomes. An alternative technique is to irradiate a portion of the prostate to a higher dose using a 'dose painting' approach, which simultaneously treats the more aggressive tumor-bearing areas to 90 Gy and the remaining PTV to 81 Gy. How could such areas be identified noninvasively for targeting? The term 'biologic target volume' describes a target area identified by any of several forms of biological and molecular imaging; areas of increased tumor burden or more aggressive/radioresistant tumor cells can be selectively treated. This is an important new direction of investigation.

Overall, there continue to be many research opportunities in areas that are of importance to this work: radiation and cancer biology, basic physics, target and normal tissue localization, treatment planning and delivery, reducing treatment uncertainties and new clinical applications. For those that may be beginning work in these areas, lessons can be offered from the evolution of conformal radiotherapy at MSKCC. This work, spanning more than a decade, benefited from a team of dedicated investigators that developed a testable hypothesis. This work indicates that it is important to define and defend the ongoing scientific programs to secure and maintain institutional resources. Also, it is important to collaborate with other investigators, seek advice (but do not *always* follow it) and follow one's principles and instincts. One must anticipate potential pitfalls, think outside the box and always focus on the vision of the end result.

Current Considerations in Prostate Cancer Radiotherapy – A Discussion

(M. Roach, S. Leibel, S. Vijayakumar)

Radiotherapy Target Volumes for Curative Treatment:
Prostate or Prostate + Pelvis

The results of RTOG 9413 demonstrate improvement of disease control by using target volumes that include the pelvis in addition to the prostate for patients at risk for nodal involvement. In achieving those results, the treatment techniques usually did not use daily target localization. Are the reported improvements due to better coverage of the prostate gland itself by the larger fields, rather than treatment of the regional lymph nodes? Could these same improvements be obtained more directly by better gland targeting through IMRT/IGRT?

Dr. Roach: The benefit of the 4-arm study reported above is that it shows that better treatment of the prostate gland could not be the explanation for the improvement of the results [3]. If one examines arms 3 and 4 of the randomized trial, arm 3 specified radiotherapy to the whole pelvis and arm 4 to the prostate only, both arms delivering hormone therapy after radiotherapy. There were more than 300 patients randomized in those 2 arms. In terms of outcome, their disease control curves were virtually identical. Therefore, in patients who receive hormone therapy after irradiation, there is no evidence that there is a better control rate when a larger field size is used. Therefore, better prostate coverage by using a larger field size could not explain the outcome improvements in the study. In the other 2 arms, hormonal therapy was used prior to radiotherapy. There was significant benefit in disease control when patients received initial hormone therapy then radiotherapy to the pelvis plus prostate rather than to the prostate alone. Thus, there is a sequence-dependent interaction between hormone therapy and pelvic nodal radiotherapy, and treatment of the nodal volumes is important. If better local control is achieved by better coverage of the prostate with modern technologies, I would expect that the benefit of elective nodal radiation would increase. This is because some of this benefit now has been obscured by the results of patients who failed because of inadequate local control. There is no reason to believe that better target localization of the prostate will answer the question of whether it is beneficial to treat the lymph nodes. The results I have presented show that the larger the field size, the better the control rate with initial hormone therapy.

Dr. Leibel: One must consider that as the radiation dose to the prostate increases, the local control of prostate tumor involvement will also increase. With prostate treatment to 81 Gy, radiotherapy results will likely improve over those achieved at 70 Gy with or without nodal irradiation. A study now needs to be undertaken that uses higher dose levels and addresses the same questions regarding hormonal therapy and nodal irradiation. In my discussion above, I make additional comments about this issue.

Dr. Vijayakumar: One must also consider that these studies are occurring over time, and that improvements in disease detection and staging also are occurring over these time periods. These improvements may cause stage migration of the patients being treated by each approach. While a prospective trial will hopefully avoid this problem, the problem will reappear when one attempts to compare the trial results with the results achieved at other institutions at differing times. It may also affect nonrandomized trials extending over long periods of time. We must be aware that several factors may be at work in these outcome results.

Radiation Total Dose and Dose Distribution

Given the above discussion of radiation dose and dose distribution, what final treatment doses are your institutions using, and how are those doses being prescribed? What dose variations are expected in your final dose specifications?

Dr. Roach: At UCSF, if the patient is not being treated with IMRT, our prescription dose is 72 Gy to the 92% isodose line, giving a central dose around 78 Gy. If we use IMRT, this involves using a static field, multileaf collimator form of IMRT, often with a forward planning procedure. When one uses IMRT, there is greater dose heterogeneity. So the treatment depends on where one is defining the dose. For our patients who are receiving IMRT, almost all are receiving in effect a concurrent boost because of this dose heterogeneity. For higher-risk patients, the dose is essentially the same to the prostate, though for some higher-risk patients, we may provide a boost using brachytherapy.

Dr. Leibel: I believe that one needs doses on the order of 81 Gy to cure prostate cancer. In more advanced cases, a higher dose is needed. In low-risk cases, the MD Anderson study showed that the outcomes at 70 and 78 Gy were identical whereas in the MGH (Massachusetts General Hospital) proton study, favorable-risk patients receiving 79.2 Gy did significantly better than those receiving 70 Gy. So, I think even low-risk patients need higher doses. Our analyses indicate that results improve with a final prescribed minimum dose of 81 Gy or greater. In the dose prescription, the IMRT doses are normalized so that the maximum dose in the PTV does not exceed 111% and the two rectal constraints are met (75.6 Gy to less than 30% of the rectal wall, 47 Gy to less than 53% of the rectal wall). The 100% isodose line covers 90–95% of the PTV for 81 Gy and 85–90% of the PTV for 86 Gy.

Dr. Vijayakumar: Outside of a protocol study we would prescribe 74 Gy to the PTV. This represents a tumor minimum dose prescription to the PTV. It is important to consider where the dose is prescribed. For instance, in the MD Anderson randomized study, the doses were specified to the isocenter and this is a large difference from our work and elsewhere.

Dr. Roach: Compared with the MSKCC work, the UCSF prescriptions may be using a larger dose gradient. When I specify the 92% isodose line, that line has a margin around the prostate. In addition, we should recognize that verification of dose delivery will be important in considering the dose prescribed. In most protocol studies, daily image guidance has not been performed and their results may reflect this in part. I might argue that the effective dose delivered with daily image guidance may be higher than without image guidance, and that this may be demonstrated in the results of future studies and the doses they define for curative therapy.

What doses are being delivered to the root of the seminal vesicles in higher-risk patients?

Dr. Roach: Our standard dose is 54–56 Gy for seminal vesicles that appear to be normal in a patient who is at risk for seminal vesicle involvement. If we are concerned about a particular portion of the seminal vesicles because the patient has disease that is limited to one part of the gland close to the seminal vesicle (for example, all the disease is on one side and mostly at the base), we will boost the proximal portion of that seminal vesicle to a higher dose. We might treat both seminal vesicles to 54–56 Gy, and then treat the ipsilateral length to 60 Gy and further boost the proximal portion to full dose, so that the seminal vesicle of concern may receive 78–80 Gy in its proximal part. If a patient has bilateral disease at the prostate bases and is considered to be stage T3, we are more likely to perform a boost using high-dose-rate brachytherapy.

Dr. Leibel: In T3 cases, we would not do any target size reductions. We would treat those patients to either 81 or 86 Gy but we would not perform a boost.

Dr. Vijayakumar: The seminal vesicle dose depends on the patient's treatment group – favorable, intermediate or unfavorable using the established criteria. For most favorable patients, one may treat the prostate alone. For intermediate-group patients, one probably needs to treat the proximal seminal vesicles, and prescribe about 50 Gy. If the seminal vesicles are involved, using clinical or other criteria, one needs a higher dose.

Does treatment to the pelvis limit the prescribed dose to the prostate?

Dr. Roach: No, and the UCSF group has many years of experience with treating the prostate to full dose and the pelvic nodes concurrently, in patients at risk for nodal disease. Whole-pelvic radiotherapy is delivered with full-dose therapy to the prostate, which might include an implant either with HDR (high-dose-rate brachytherapy) or permanent seeds, or IMRT. In our experience, it is possible to treat the prostate to the required dose as well as to treat the nodes, with careful attention to detail. This is made safer by IMRT, and I expect that one can deliver 50 Gy to the whole pelvis and even 81 Gy to the prostate with current technologies. In the recent RTOG trial, a dose of 50 Gy to the nodes reduced the risk of recurrence and this may be an adequate dose for these patients.

Use of IMRT Technology

Is the use of IMRT technology now expected or necessary practice in the modern treatment of prostate cancer?

Dr. Roach: I think that the most important role of IMRT is in the treatment of pelvic nodes. In patients who are in the intermediate- and high-risk groups, IMRT is very helpful in optimizing coverage of the nodes and primary, and in sparing normal tissues, as reflected in DVH analyses. For low-risk patients, I do not think that the doses commonly used for treatment give much advantage for IMRT over 3DCRT. In practice, it is often my preference to implant patients with low-risk disease rather than to treat them with external beam therapy in any case.

Dr. Leibel: For treatment volumes that include the regional nodes, IMRT is associated with minimal toxicity. It is much less than previously experienced with whole pelvic field treatment. In terms of using IMRT of the prostate, I believe that one needs doses of 81 Gy to cure prostate cancer. In more advanced cases, one needs a higher dose. If one is going to deliver these higher doses, then one needs better normal tissue sparing. This can be achieved with IMRT technology, proton beam irradiation or perhaps other approaches, but one needs some means of relatively protecting the normal tissues. Above 75 Gy, rectal toxicity escalates steeply if one does not further manage rectal dose. If one is to give curative doses to the prostate, then a precision dose delivery method that appropriately spares normal tissues must be used.

Dr. Vijayakumar: In our work, we have found that IMRT provides better dose distributions than 3DCRT in about 85% of patients. But in 15% of cases, the two methods had similar dose distributions to the critical structures. Therefore, not all patients may need to have IMRT. As reviewed in our chapter, we have found that the development of benchmark DVHs is useful in assessing whether a particular patient would benefit from IMRT. The use of IMRT requires sufficient physics, dosimetric and clinical quality assurance procedures to be in place. It is also important to have a consistent approach to the definition of target volumes and to the treatment planning procedures to treat those volumes. We have found it helpful to have a staff conference each week to review and evaluate the target volumes proposed for treatment, so that all of the department physicians and physicists participate in this process. Over time, consensus understandings of target delineations and treatment approaches develop, and these improve department efficiency, organization and quality assurance.

Use of Image Guidance

Is daily image guidance emerging as a standard of care for prostate cancer therapy? Is it as important as the use of IMRT technology itself?

Dr. Roach: For prostate cancer therapy, we image gold marker seeds on the treatment machine every day to correct for setup error and organ movement. We continue to perform daily imaging as we see clinical value in it. While these procedures are standard in our clinic, the standard of care for our profession is based on what most clinics are actually doing, not on what I or others think should be done. Other clinics may not as yet have the technical capability to perform guidance. However, common practice is moving quickly in this direction.

Dr. Leibel: One cannot impose professional guidelines until a practice becomes standardized in the profession. Certainly, some form of daily localization will help to immobilize the prostate within the actual treatment fields. However, good results are already achieved by institutions that do not perform daily image guidance, so it cannot be considered as a standard of care without further study and use.

Dr. Vijayakumar: It seems that we have consensus that some form of daily localization is highly encouraged.

When the lymph nodes of the pelvis are treated, the prostate will move independently from the lymph nodes. When daily image guidance is performed and a shift is required, how are the lymph node volumes to be managed?

Dr. Roach: At UCSF, the margin size for the lymph nodes is increased but not the margin for the prostate, when we are giving IMRT. For instance, if the prostate moves anteriorly then we move the field anteriorly, but we make sure that an anterior movement does not cause the lymph nodes to be missed by adding additional margin to those nodal volumes initially. Some limits on the amount of daily shift may be used, for example in patients who have pelvic kidneys or other unusual anatomy, or who have had prior radiotherapy in the area.

IMRT and IGRT following Prostatectomy

How are all of these recommendations to be applied to patients treated following prostatectomy?

Dr. Roach: We also use gold marker seeds for patients that have tumor recurrence or adverse pathologic features following prostatectomy for postoperative therapy. Even without biopsy confirmation, the surgical anastomosis may be the suspected area for target boosting and can be marked with gold seeds for daily electronic portal imaging. If the patient has adverse pathologic features that would have resulted in a recommendation for neoadjuvant hormonal therapy prior to nodal irradiation with definitive radiotherapy, then we treat their lymph nodes following prostatectomy in the same way. They receive neoadjuvant therapy, then pelvic radiotherapy. In fact, if they have positive pelvic nodes, we may treat para-aortic nodes. We have seen patients with pelvic failures after treatment to the prostate only, and we have seen patients with para-aortic failures after treatment to the pelvis only. In patients with rising PSA following implant or external radiotherapy to the prostate only, failure in pelvic nodes often can be observed with careful imaging evaluations, and it is not uncommon in our experience.

Dr. Leibel: I have consistently used IMRT in this setting, even though the prescribed dose is less. While one might consider using 3DCRT, the degree of sparing of the bladder and other normal tissues is much better with IMRT than with approaches that transect the normal tissues rather than conforming around them.

Dr. Vijayakumar: The issue in postprostatectomy radiotherapy remains the definition of the appropriate target volume. Even the most experienced radiotherapists differ in their recommendations regarding this. The rapid dose falloff characteristics of IMRT, together with the uncertainty of target volume definition, give considerable caution about how IMRT should be used following surgery. I have used ProstaScint scanning and image fusion in treatment planning to develop 2 or 3 separate targets, so that the uncertainties introduced with the rapid falloff of IMRT dose could be managed by having sequential CTV1, CTV2 and CTV3 volumes.

Future Directions

Dr. Roach: To improve the definition of lymph node involvement using MR imaging, supermagnetic nanoparticles are being developed as agents to evaluate the architecture of pelvic lymph nodes for metastatic involvement [21]. Called Combidex (ferumoxtran-10), it is a dextrose-coated ferrous material. This MRI contrast agent is now available in Europe and has received FDA evaluations in the United States. There are a number of groups who are investigating its use, and we are joining these efforts with studies at UCSF. We have also been evaluating the molecular profiles of prostate cancers. Preliminary data based on surgically staged patients treated at UCSF indicate that the molecular characteristics of cancers that metastasize to bone appear to be different than those that go to lymph nodes, and also appear to be different from those that do not metastasize. In the study RTOG 9413, only about 30% of patients are estimated to have actually been at risk for lymph node involvement. If such patients could be selected for regional nodal therapy, the benefit of this therapy could be improved. To investigate this, we are analyzing the RTOG 9413 specimens for their molecular profiling. Perhaps one day, patients may have prostate biopsy that includes such molecular analysis that would suggest the appropriate radiotherapy field volumes.

References

1 Roach M 3rd, Faillace-Akazawa P, Malfatti C: Prostate volumes and organ movement defined by serial computerized tomographic scans during three-dimensional conformal radiotherapy. Radiat Oncol Investig 1997;5:187–194.

2 Millender LE, Aubin M, Pouliot J, Shinohara K, Roach M 3rd: Daily electronic portal imaging for morbidly obese men undergoing radiotherapy for localized prostate cancer. Int J Radiat Oncol Biol Phys 2004;59:6–10.

3 Roach M 3rd, DeSilvio M, Lawton C, Uhl V, Machtay M, Seider MJ, Rotman M, Jones C, Asbell SO, Valicenti RK, Han S, Thomas CR Jr, Shipley WS: Phase III trial comparing whole-pelvic versus prostate-only radiotherapy and neoadjuvant versus adjuvant combined androgen suppression: Radiation Therapy Oncology Group 9413. J Clin Oncol 2003;21:1904–1911.

4 Roach M, DeSilvio M, Thomas CR, Valicenti R, Asbell SO, Lawton C, Shipley WS: Progression-free survival (PFS) after whole-pelvic (WP) vs mini-pelvic (MP) or prostate-only (PO) radiotherapy (RT): a subset analysis of RTOG 9413, a phase III prospective randomized trial using neoadjuvant and concurrent hormone therapy (N&CHT). Int J Radiat Oncol Biol Phys 2004;60: S264–S265.

5 Hanks GE, Hanlon AL, Schultheiss TE, Pinover WH, Movsas B, Epstein BE, Hunt MA: Dose escalation with 3D conformal treatment: five-year outcomes, treatment optimization, and future directions. Int J Radiat Oncol Biol Phys 1998;41:501–510.

6 Fisch BM, Pickett B, Weinberg V, Roach M 3rd: Dose of radiation received by the bulb of the penis correlates with risk of impotence after three-dimensional conformal radiotherapy for prostate cancer. Urology 2001;57:955–959.

7 Roach M, Winter K, Michalski JM, Cox JD, Purdy JA, Bosch W, Lin X, Shipley WS: Penile bulb dose and impotence after three-dimensional conformal radiotherapy for prostate cancer on RTOG 9406: findings from a prospective, multi-institutional, phase I/II dose-escalation study. Int J Radiat Oncol Biol Phys 2004;60:1351–1356.

8 Ryu J, Winter K, Michalski J, Purdy J, Markoe, A, Earle J, Perez, Roach M, Sandler H, Cox J, Pollack A: Preliminary report of toxicity following 3D conformal radiation therapy (3DCRT) for prostate cancer on 3DOG/RTOG 9406, level III (79.2 Gy). Int J Radiat Oncol Biol Phys 2001;51:136–137.

9 Kuban D, Pollack A, Huang E, Levy L, Dong L, Starkschall G, Rosen I: Hazards of dose escalation in prostate cancer radiotherapy. Int J Radiat Oncol Biol Phys 2003;57:1260–1268.

10 Koper PC, Jansen P, van Putten W, van Os M, Wijnmaalen AJ, Lebesque JV, Levendag PC: Gastro-intestinal and genito-urinary morbidity after 3D conformal radiotherapy of prostate cancer: observations of a randomized trial. Radiother Oncol 2004;73:1–9.

11 Michalski JM, Winter K, Purdy JA, Perez CA, Ryu JK, Parliament MB, Valicenti RK, Roach M 3rd, Sandler HM, Markoe AM, Cox JD: Toxicity after three-dimensional radiotherapy for prostate cancer with RTOG 9406 dose level IV. Int J Radiat Oncol Biol Phys 2004;58:735–742.

12 Zapatero A, Garcia-Vicente F, Modolell I, Alcantara P, Floriano A, Cruz-Conde A, Torres JJ, Perez-Torrubia A: Impact of mean rectal dose on late rectal bleeding after conformal radiotherapy for prostate cancer: dose-volume effect. Int J Radiat Oncol Biol Phys 2004;59:1343–1351.

13 Leibel SA, Kutcher GJ, Zelefsky MJ, Burman CM, Mohan R, Ling CC, Fuks Z: 3-D conformal radiotherapy for carcinoma of the prostate. Clinical experience at the Memorial Sloan-Kettering Cancer Center. Front Radiat Ther Oncol 1996;29:229–237.

14 Zelefsky JM, Fuks Z, Hunt M, Lee HJ, Lombardi D, Ling CC, Reuter VE, Venkatraman ES, Venkatraman ES, Leibel SA: High-dose radiation delivered by intensity-modulated conformal radiotherapy improves the outcome of localized prostate cancer. J Urol 2001;166:876–881.

15 Leibel SA, Fuks Z, Zelefsky MJ, Whitmore WF: The effects of local and regional treatment on the metastatic outcome in prostatic carcinoma with pelvic lymph node involvement. Int J Radiat Oncol Biol Phys 1994;28:7–16.

16 Brenner DJ: Fractionation and late rectal toxicity. Int J Radiat Oncol Biol Phys 2004;60:1013–1015.

17 Zelefsky MJ, Fuks Z, Happersett L, Lee L, Ling CC, Burman CM, Hunt M, Wolfe T, Venkatraman ES, Jackson A, Skwarchuk M, Leibel SA: Clinical experience with intensity-modulated radiation therapy (IMRT) in prostate cancer. Radiother Oncol 2000;55:241–249.

18 Zelefsky MJ, Fuks Z, Hunt M, Yamada Y, Marion C, Ling CC, Amoils H, Venkatraman ES, Leibel SA: High-dose intensity-modulated radiation therapy for prostate cancer: early toxicity and biochemical outcome in 772 patients. Int J Radiat Oncol Biol Phys 2002;53:1111–1118.

19 Levegrun S, Jackson A, Zelefsky MJ, Venkatraman ES, Skwarchuk MW, Schlegel W, Fuks Z, Leibel SA, Ling CC: Risk group dependence of dose-response for biopsy outcome after three-dimensional conformal radiation therapy of prostate cancer. Radiother Oncol 2002;63;11–26.

20 Vicini FA, Martinez A, Hanks G, Hanlon A, Miles B, Kernan K, Beyers D, Ragde H, Forman J, Fontanesi J, Kestin L, Kovacs G, Denis L, Slawin K, Scardino P: An interinstitutional and interspecialty comparison of treatment outcome data for patients with prostate carcinoma based on predefined prognostic categories and minimum follow-up. Cancer 2002:95:2126–2135.

21 Hahn PF, Deserno WM, Tabatabaei S, van de Kaa CH, de la Rosette J, Weissleder R: Noninvasive detection of clinically occult lymph-node metastases in prostate cancer. N Engl J Med 2003;348:2491–2499.

Dr. John L. Meyer
Department of Radiation Oncology
Saint Francis Memorial Hospital
900 Hyde Street
San Francisco, CA 94109 (USA)
Tel. +1 415 353 6420, Fax +1 415 353 6428
E-Mail JMeyerSF@aol.com

III. SBRT Concepts

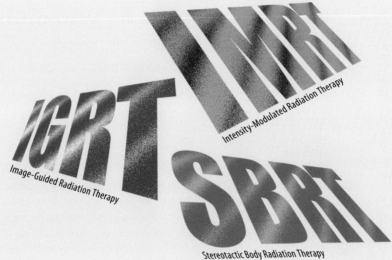

Meyer JL (ed): IMRT, IGRT, SBRT – Advances in the Treatment Planning and
Delivery of Radiotherapy. Front Radiat Ther Oncol. Basel, Karger, 2007, vol. 40, pp 340–351

The Promise of Stereotactic Body Radiation Therapy in a New Era of Oncology

Brian D. Kavanagh · Karen Kelly · Madeleine Kane

University of Colorado Comprehensive Cancer Center, Aurora, Colo., USA

Abstract

The fusion of state-of-the-art tumor imaging with precision radiation treatment delivery systems provides the technical platform from which stereotactic body radiation therapy (SBRT) has arisen. SBRT offers an opportunity to depart from classic radiation therapy paradigms involving many weeks of treatment toward more efficient and more potent treatment schedules in a variety of clinical settings. Here, the history of SBRT is briefly reviewed, and a projection of the anticipated role of SBRT within the context of multimodality cancer treatment regimens of the future is presented.

The scientific study and clinical practice of oncology have progressed remarkably in recent years. Insights into molecular interactions occurring within a cancer cell have been translated into novel medical treatments, and a variety of technological advances have allowed new surgical and radiotherapeutic techniques. Perhaps most importantly, multidisciplinary collaboration among cancer specialists has led to integrated, multimodality strategies that offer patients with a wide range of cancers a chance of longer survival with higher quality of life.

Within the discipline of radiation oncology in particular, the fusion of state-of-the-art tumor imaging with precision radiation treatment delivery systems has created an opportunity to shift from the classic radiation therapy paradigm of administering thirty or more individual low-dose treatments toward briefer, more intense, and more potent regimens in which a much higher dose per treatment is used for greater clinical effect. Figuring out how this new approach, known as stereotactic body radiation therapy (SBRT), will best be integrated into clinical oncology practice is a welcome challenge for investigators unafraid of departing from traditional mind-sets.

In this essay, we review the earliest investigations of SBRT, summarize briefly the major technical considerations of SBRT, and discuss the key radiobiological aspects of SBRT for tumor and normal tissues. We also offer a new interpretation of the Norton-Simon hypothesis as it relates to SBRT and present a case study to illustrate a vision of how SBRT might be incorporated into future cancer management strategies aimed at converting malignant diseases into chronic illnesses rather than catastrophic occurrences.

Historical Perspective

SBRT was pioneered on three continents by investigators in Europe, Asia, and North America. In the early 1990s at the Karolinska Institute in Stockholm, Ingmar Lax and Henric Blomgren collaborated to create a method of targeting extracranial tumors precisely by constructing a combined body frame-abdominal compression device that accomplished three goals: (1) comfortable patient immobilization, (2) minimization of respiratory motion via limitation of diaphragmatic excursion, and (3) placement of external fiducial markers that could be indexed to internal targets, thus allowing stereotactic localization [1]. The methodology was conceptually indebted to the landmark work of their compatriot, Lars Leksell, who had many years earlier developed a technique for high-dose, single-fraction stereotactic treatment of lesions within the brain [2]. The earliest report of the observations of Blomgren and Lax was very encouraging [3], and elsewhere in Europe other investigators soon followed their lead [4, 5].

Chronologically overlapping the early work in Sweden were the efforts led by Minoru Uematsu and colleagues at the National Defense Medical College of Japan, who were the first to juxtapose closely a CT scanner and linear accelerator into a synthesized 'FOCAL' unit (fusion of CT and linear accelerator). Their early observations included a group of 45 patients with 23 primary or 43 metastatic lung carcinomas treated to a dose of 30–75 Gy in 5–15 fractions, with or without additional conventional radiation therapy. After a median follow-up of 11 months, local progression occurred in only 2 of 66 treated lesions [6]. Also studying SBRT around that same time in Japan were groups at Hokkaido University and Kyoto University [7, 8].

In North America, Robert Timmerman, Lech Papiez, and colleagues initiated a phase I trial of SBRT for medically inoperable lung cancer at Indiana University in the late 1990s, the results of which have now been published [9]. Interest in tackling the medical physics and clinical challenges associated with SBRT spread quickly to investigators at the Medical College of Virginia [10], and active study is now under way at numerous centers throughout the United States. The historical background of SBRT has been described elsewhere in greater detail [11].

Stereotactic Body Radiation Therapy Equipment and Techniques

SBRT can be given using a wide variety of treatment devices and may incorporate specialized dose delivery methods such as intensity-modulated radiotherapy. Hypofractionated, high-dose-per-treatment radiation therapy may be applied in the form of either photons or protons. But to provide safe and effective SBRT, from a technical point of view, the sine qua non requirements are the following:
1. secure patient immobilization, typically accomplished by a customized body mold with or without an external frame with fiducial reference markers;
2. accurate tumor relocalization using one or more methods of image-guided radiotherapy involving near real-time CT verification, stereoscopic kilovoltage imaging, ultrasound, and/or other equivalent methods;
3. a solution to the problem of respiratory motion for liver and lung tumors – options include adequate expansion of the planning target volume to account for the motion, modified respiration (controlled breath hold or abdominal compression), or adaptive interaction (linear accelerator on-time gated with respiration or X-ray tumor tracking with real-time multileaf collimator adjustment).

In the first forays into the clinical territory now known as SBRT, investigators often had to construct homemade devices to adapt their treatment machines for safe and reliable performance. Now, however, there is an assortment of commercially available systems capable of facilitating accurate, efficient treatments. Some involve modular add-on components that can render almost any linear accelerator suitable for SBRT. For example, immobilization and repositioning devices include the Elekta Stereotactic Body Frame™ (Elekta, Norcross, Ga., USA), the Leibinger stereotactic body fixation system (Stryker, Kalamazoo, Mich., USA), and the Medical Intelligence Bodyfix™ system (Medical Intelligence, Schwabmuenchen, Germany). Relocalization systems include the Sonarray™ modular ultrasound unit (Zmed, Ashland, Mass., USA), Exactrac™ Ultrasound Localization (Brain-LAB, Inc., Westchester, Ill., USA), and the BAT™ system (Nomos, Sewickley, Pa., USA). Likewise, several systems provide one or another solution to the problem of respiratory motion. An example of a breath-hold device is the Active Breathing Coordinator™ (Elekta), which allows coordination of beam-on time during a fixed level of inspiration; an example of a respiratory gating system is the RPM™ (Varian, Palo Alto, Calif., USA), which tracks inspiration and expiration and turns the accelerator off when indicators predict that the tumor position is outside of an acceptable range of distance from baseline.

Also now available for purchase are specialized SBRT-ready linear accelerators that combine capacity for image-guided radiotherapy with compatibility with modern immobilization and respiratory motion solution technology. The Novalis™ (BrainLAB, Inc.), Elekta Synergy™, Varian Trilogy™, Siemens Primatom™ System, Tomotherapy HiArt™ System (TomoTherapy, Madison, Wisc., USA), and Cyberknife™ (Accuray, Sunnyvale, Calif., USA) are examples of linear accelerators well-suited for SBRT. A thorough description of the technical features and performance characteristics of these and other machines is beyond the scope of the present report.

Although the American Society for Therapeutic Radiology and Oncology and the American College of Radiology have issued certain general operational guidelines concerning the performance of SBRT [12], at different institutions there will certainly emerge stylistic variations in methodology, especially given the variety of different treatment delivery systems available for SBRT. While it is very likely possible to achieve similar results with a variety of technically different approaches, interinstitutional comparisons of clinical outcomes are not necessarily straightforward. For example, depending on the specific technique and approach utilized, there can be a variable amount of dose 'hotspots' within the target volume. The nominal prescription dose given to the periphery of the tumor might then be an inadequate representation of the true effective dose in that circumstance, and it has been argued that it would be better to describe the SBRT tumor dose with a composite index that accounts for dose heterogeneity within the target volume [13].

Fundamentals of Clinical Stereotactic Body Radiation Therapy Radiobiology

Normal Tissue Dose Constraints

For conventionally fractionated radiotherapy to the lung, the mean dose and percent of lung receiving more than 20 Gy are useful predictors of the risk of radiation pneumonitis, consistent with a view of lung architecture as a parallel structure. However, clinically apparent classic radiation pneumonitis is uncommon after SBRT [9]. Instead, the typical radiographic changes after high-dose SBRT are subsegmental or wedge-like fibrosis originating from the site of treatment and extending distally, consistent with the notion of a combined serial-parallel tissue architecture in the lungs [14], illustrated schematically in figure 1.

Concerns about normal tissue effects following SBRT for liver tumors have also been approached with a conceptually different strategy than has been applied for conventionally fractionated radiotherapy to the liver, where the mean dose to normal liver has been identified as a predictor for radiation hepatitis. In the University of Colorado phase I study of liver SBRT, Schefter et al. [15] applied an interpretation of the so-called critical volume model, initially proposed by Yaes and

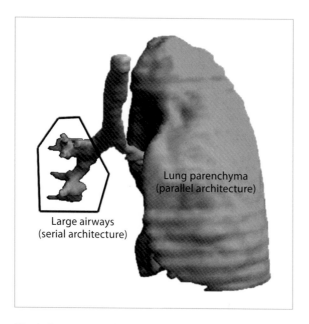

Fig. 1. Reconstructed three-dimensional representation of the trachea, proximal large airways, and left lung obtained from a planning CT scan image. Larger proximal airways are characterized as serial architecture because they are susceptible to stenosis or collapse if enough surrounding fibrosis develops. The lung parenchyma as a whole is arranged in microscopic functional subunits and may be considered to have parallel architecture on a macroscopic scale.

Kalend [16]. Based upon a conservative estimate of the minimum volume of normal liver that should be functionally preserved, it was specified that at least 700 cm³ of uninvolved normal liver had to receive a cumulative dose of less than 15 Gy during the entire course of treatment. Continued efforts to refine understanding of liver tolerance to SBRT are warranted, but with the use of this particular constraint, the SBRT dose was safely escalated to 60 Gy in 3 fractions without reaching a maximum tolerated dose.

Tumor Dose Objectives

In addition to the convenience for patients, who generally prefer to complete a course of therapy in three or so individual sessions rather than thirty or more treatments, there are two conditions in which an abbreviated, hypofractionated regimen is expected to be advantageous in terms of tumor cell kill compared with a protracted, conventionally fractionated course of therapy.

The first, more generally applicable condition is the scenario in which hypofractionated, high-dose-per-fraction radiotherapy is expected to convey a more cytotoxic effect as a result of basic principles of radiation dose response. The linear-quadratic (LQ) model is currently widely accepted as a very useful means of describing the biological impact of a given schedule of radiation treatments, taking into account the observed relationship between fraction size and expected logarithmic reduction in tumor cell survival. Fowler et al. [17] have applied LQ formalism to compare the relative biological effectiveness of various reported SBRT fractionation regimens with typical conventionally fractionated regimens for the example case of non-small-cell lung cancer. Compared with a conventional schedule of 60–70 Gy given in 30–35 fractions, SBRT schedules in the range of 45–69 Gy in 3–5 fractions are expected to have approximately twice the impact in terms of cytotoxicity.

The other condition for which an SBRT regimen would be expected to provide advantage is likewise predicated on aspects of LQ modeling, albeit with different emphasis. The parameters that describe the tumor-specific dose-response relationship are alpha and beta, which characterize the linear and quadratic aspects of the curve, respectively. Most tumors have an estimated alpha/beta ratio in the order of 10, and most normal tissue late effects are characterized by an alpha/beta ratio of approximately 3. The practical implication of these numbers is that in cases where a large volume of normal tissue will be exposed to radiation, small doses per fraction are used to maximize the therapeutic ratio, defined here as the degree of favorable effect on the tumor relative to unfavorable effects in normal tissues. One common notable exception to the rule is prostate cancer, for which the alpha/beta ratio is believed to be much lower than for most cancers, most likely in the range of 3 or less [18].

If the alpha/beta ratio of the tumor is equal or even lower than the alpha/beta ratio of surrounding normal tissue, the therapeutic ratio will be improved with larger doses per fraction. For example, if the tumor alpha/beta ratio is 2 Gy, an SBRT regimen of 37.3 Gy in 5 fractions would provide the same expected risk of complication to normal tissues as would a conventional regimen of 79 Gy in 39 fractions. However, the 5-fraction SBRT regimen would provide greater cytotoxicity to the tumor and would raise the estimated chance of tumor control from approximately 80% with the 39-fraction conventional regimen to 95% with the 5-fraction SBRT schedule [19].

One important caveat to all projected results based on LQ modeling is the question of whether the LQ model accurately describes the impact of the very high fraction sizes of SBRT, a point articulated by Guerrero and Li [20], who have reprised the Curtis lethal-potentially lethal model to address this issue [20, 21]. Also, another clinically important consideration is that different available techniques of SBRT deliver the radiation at different dose rates, over variable lengths of total time. The lesson from basic scientific study of the dose rate effect in an experimental model of cranial radiosurgery is that as a result of intrafractional repair processes, there can be a decrement in cytotoxicity when treatment time is excessively prolonged [22].

Stereotactic Body Radiation Therapy as Systemic Cytoreductive Intervention

While the prior section's discussion provides a rationale for SBRT in the primary management of certain cancers, the question of how SBRT might play a role in the management of patients with metastatic disease calls for a separate explanation. The hypothesis to be presented is effectively a complete reversal of the traditional understanding of the complementary role of radiotherapy, a fundamentally local therapy aimed at gross disease in the primary site, and adjuvant systemic therapy, conventionally given as a cytotoxic agent intended to prevent or delay the growth of occult metastatic disease. Here, we propose that in future oncology management strategies, these roles could be entirely reversed. New systemic agents targeting specific molecular signaling pathways in cancer cells and supporting stromal tissue would serve as the primary therapy intended to stifle cancer growth progression globally, and SBRT would be an adjuvant systemic cytoreductive intervention intended to lessen the total amount of cancer within the patient's body. The desired integrated effect is maximal prolongation of the time until a patient ultimately succumbs to a lethal burden of disease – or, better, prevention of such an ominous occurrence.

Norton-Simon Refocused

The notion of extending effort to prevent the development of a lethal burden of disease is rooted in the Norton-Simon hypothesis, which itself is derived in essence from the much earlier work of Benjamin Gompertz [22]. An early nineteenth century mathematician who worked as an actuary at an insurance company, among other professional activities, Gompertz is well remembered for a mathematical model of population growth as a function of an intrinsic growth rate, the number of individuals in the population at a given time, and the log of the ratio between the current population and the equilibrium value at steady state [22]. The net result is a prediction of population as a function of time that is approximately sigmoidal in shape: after an initial period of low values, there is a phase of accelerated growth followed by a later phase of reduced growth rate as the value reaches a plateau.

In 1976, Norton et al. [23] published a study in which they considered the rate of xenograft tumor growth within a host animal as a function of time and attempted to model it mathematically. Their key observation was that when their tumor growth data were plotted at time versus the log of cell tumor volume, the curve was well described by gompertzian kinetics. In other words, tumor growth entered a rapid exponential phase followed by slower growth near a plateau that eventually becomes a lethal burden for the host animal, resulting in death. In translating this observation into a testable clinical hypothesis in human patients, Norton and Simon [24] first recognized that traditional DNA-targeted chemotherapy is expected to render the greatest degree of cytotoxicity to cancer cells in a rapid phase of growth, when there is higher mitotic activity that renders DNA more susceptible to injury. Therefore, one articulation of the Norton-Simon hypothesis would be to propose that traditional cytotoxic chemotherapy should result in a rate of decrease in tumor volume that is proportional to the rate of growth in an untreated tumor of the same size [24].

One available means of exploiting this understanding to improve response and impact patient outcome favorably would be to increase the so-called 'dose density' of chemotherapy, shortening the interval between cycles of treatment to prevent a situation whereby a tumor might respond partially but then have time to regrow back into a relatively less sensitive, plateau level of volume with lower mitotic activity. More frequently repeated dosing would begin to capture tumors at relatively smaller volume, with consequently higher growth rates that render them even more sensitive to the next cycle of chemotherapy, and so on for subsequent cycles. The CALGB 97-41 randomized clinical trial compared dose-dense chemotherapy with conventionally sequenced chemotherapy in breast cancer patients. The demonstrated superiority of the dose-dense regimen supported the Norton-Simon hypothesis [25].

In relation to SBRT, the ramifications of the Norton-Simon hypothesis are twofold. First, and less importantly, in principle lesions treated by SBRT that are not eradicated would likely be at least debulked and rendered more sensitive to other cytotoxic agents. Secondly, and more importantly, when attention is refocused more broadly on the concept of the lethal burden of systemic disease, quite simply SBRT is an intervention that can eradicate large volumes of measurable gross disease, thus contributing to the overarching goal of preventing or delaying the time at which a patient succumbs to an overwhelming total-body burden of cancer. The following case study is offered as an example where this strategy was employed at times throughout the patient's management.

Case Study
Longitudinal Analysis of Systemic Disease Burden in a Patient Treated with SBRT
A 39-year-old woman, a nonsmoker, presented in early 2003 with severe left shoulder pain. An MRI revealed a destructive lesion in the left proximal humerus, and it was biopsy proven to be a metastasis of a poorly differentiated carcinoma. The workup also revealed a lung lesion consistent with a primary cancer, a liver metastasis, and a solitary brain metastasis.

The initial step in management was to give an expedient single-fraction palliative treatment to the left shoulder and radiosurgery to the cerebellar metastasis, allowing the patient to move quickly into a regimen of carboplatin and paclitaxel, which was given for 6 cycles.

In late 2003, the patient developed 3 new small brain metastases and was given whole-brain radiotherapy, 35 Gy in 14 fractions. The only other known sites of disease were the residual lesions in the liver and lung, and she was offered enrollment in an ongoing phase I study of liver SBRT [15]. In March, 2004, she received 48 Gy in 3 fractions to the liver lesion, and the same dose was also given to the lung lesion (fig. 2).

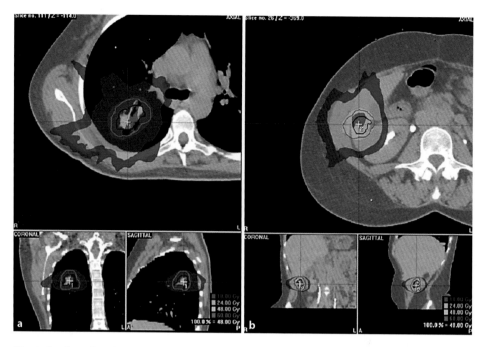

Fig. 2. Isodose distributions of lesions treated in March, 2004. **a** Lung lesion. **b** Liver lesion. In each side, the planning target volume is outlined in a light orange color.

The patient's management has continued since that time to include additional cycles of carboplatin in mid 2004 and, later, targeted therapy in the form of gefitinib followed by erlotinib. Overlapping those therapies have been numerous other radiotherapy treatments, including SBRT to a second liver lesion, a contralateral chest wall lesion, a sternal lesion, and a sacral lesion. Note that these bony sites were not only seen on PET scan but were also visible on CT as invasive masses extending into adjacent soft tissue, thus readily measurable. Doses given to these bony sites were typically in the order of 30 Gy in 3–5 fractions. All irradiated sites have been controlled to the date of this writing, though there is new measurable disease in the lung for which the patient is now receiving additional chemotherapy.

Figure 3 illustrates the patient's time course of disease plotted as calendar time versus the current volume of measurable disease and the cumulative volume of new disease up to that time point. Also indicated along the x-axis are all instances in which radiotherapy, given via SBRT or another technique, was applied aggressively with the intention of eradicating all treated gross disease, not just palliation. It is, of course, impossible to gauge the comparative contributions of SBRT and the systemic therapies selectively administered in terms of their contribution toward eliminating the various measurable deposits of cancer around the body. Almost certainly, the systemic agents have played a role in suppressing or delaying the emergence of disease sites in scattered other parts of the body. Nevertheless, it should be appreciated that SBRT was only applied to sites of tumor that persisted or emerged following the systemic therapy and that these sites have remained controlled.

Kavanagh · Kelly · Kane

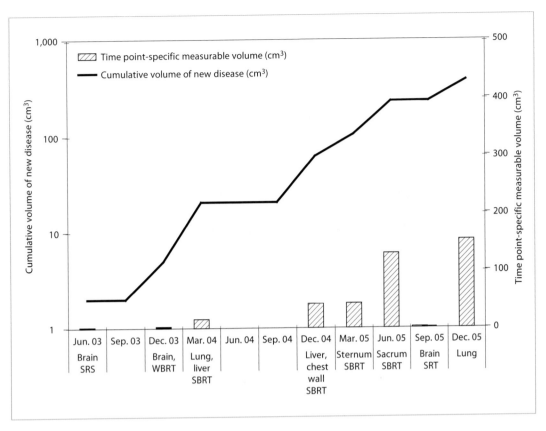

Fig. 3. Time versus time point-specific measurable disease volume (hatched columns, right y-axis) and cumulative volume of new disease (solid line, left y-axis). The left y-axis is a logarithmic scale, while the right y-axis is linear. In September, 2005, the patient had 3 small brain lesions and was given 18 Gy in 3 fractions using a reusable head immobilization device. SRS = Stereotactic radiation surgery; WBRT = whole-brain radiation therapy.

Not depicted in any way in figure 3 is the projected total-body burden of disease that would be present and measurable if all of the irradiated sites had continued to progress. As of December, 2005, the cumulative volume of measurable disease that had emerged to date was 390 cm³. If the irradiated extracranial sites had continued to increase at a doubling time of 12, 6, or 3 months, then the December 2005 burden of disease would be approximately 550, 890, or 3,720 cm³, respectively. Although it is not known with certainty whether these amounts are a lethal burden for the patient, they represent a substantial amount of tumor. Further study is needed to determine whether there really is a typical lethal burden of disease as projected by the Norton-Simon hypothesis that is clinically relevant, and structured prospective clinical trials will be required to determine whether SBRT can achieve meaningful and durable impact on the systemic disease burden when administered as adjuvant cytoreductive therapy.

Conclusions

The emergence of SBRT in the field of radiation oncology has temporally coincided with the dawn of a new era in all of oncology. SBRT has a potentially curative role in the primary management of lung, prostate, and selected other extracranial malignancies. Additionally, SBRT might serve well as a focally cytoreductive agent applied to sites of gross disease in concert with novel systemic agents that target key signal transduction pathways in cancer cells and thus inhibit cancer cell proliferation in widespread parts of the body.

It is now the responsibility of the radiation oncology community to approach the investigation of SBRT with discipline and integrity. Among the major attractive features of SBRT are the fact that it is entirely noninvasive and the fact that it is much more convenient and potent than conventionally fractionated external beam radiotherapy. There are numerous invasive strategies that have the potential to achieve clinical results similar to SBRT: radio frequency ablation, cryosurgery, video-assisted thoracoscopic surgery, and chemoembolization, to name a few. SBRT will be seen as superior whenever it can achieve equal or better clinical outcome for the same or better overall cost-effectiveness.

References

1 Lax I, Blomgren H, Naslund I, Svanstrom R: Stereotactic radiotherapy of extracranial targets. Z Med Phys 1994;4:112–113.

2 Leksell L: The stereotaxic method and radiosurgery of the brain. Acta Chir Scand 1951;102:316–319.

3 Blomgren H, Lax I, Naslund I, Svanstrom R: Stereotactic high dose fraction radiation therapy of extracranial tumors using an accelerator. Acta Oncol 1995;34:861–870.

4 Herfarth KK, Debus J, Lohr F, Bahner ML, Rhein B, Fritz P, Hoss A, Schlegel W, Wannenmacher MF: Stereotactic single-dose radiation therapy of liver tumors: results of a phase I/II trial. J Clin Oncol 2001;19:164–70.

5 Wulf J, Hadinger U, Oppitz U, Thiele W, Ness-Dourdoumas R, Flentje M: Stereotactic radiotherapy of targets in the lung and liver. Strahlenther Onkol 2001;177:645–655.

6 Uematsu M, Shioda A, Tahara K, Fukui T, Yamamoto F, Tsumatori G, Ozeki Y, Aoki T, Watanabe M, Kusano S: Focal, high dose, and fractionated modified stereotactic radiation therapy for lung carcinoma patients: a preliminary experience. Cancer 1998;82:1062–1070.

7 Shirato, H, Shimizu, S, Tadashi, S, Nishioka T, Miyasaka, K: Real time tumour-tracking radiotherapy. Lancet 1999;353:1331–1332.

8 Nagata Y, Negoro Y, Aoki T, Mizowaki T, Takayama K, Kokubo M, Araki N, Mitsumori M, Sasai K, Shibamoto Y, Koga S, Yano S, Hiraoka M: Clinical outcomes of 3D conformal hypofractionated single high-dose radiotherapy for one or two lung tumors using a stereotactic body frame. Int J Radiat Oncol Biol Phys 2002;52:1041–1046.

9 Timmerman R, Papiez L, McGarry R, Likes L, DesRosiers C, Frost S, Williams M: Extracranial stereotactic radioablation: results of a phase I study in medically inoperable stage I non-small cell lung cancer. Chest 2003;124:1946–1955.

10 Cardinale RM, Wu Q, Benedict SH, Kavanagh BD, Bump E, Mohan R: Determining the optimal block margin on the planning target volume for extracranial stereotactic radiotherapy. Int J Radiat Oncol Biol Phys 1999;45:515–520.

11 Timmerman RD, Kavanagh BD: Stereotactic body radiation therapy. Curr Probl Cancer 2005;29:120–157.

12 Potters L, Steinberg M, Rose C, Timmerman R, Ryu S, Hevezi JM, Welsh J, Mehta M, Larson DA, Janjan NA; American Society for Therapeutic Radiology and Oncology; American College of Radiology: American Society for Therapeutic Radiology and Oncology and American College of Radiology practice guideline for the performance of stereotactic body radiation therapy. Int J Radiat Oncol Biol Phys 2004;60:1026–1032.

13 Kavanagh BD, Timmerman RD, Benedict SH, Wu Q, Schefter TE, Stuhr K, McCourt S, Newman F, Cardinale RM, Gaspar LE: How should we describe the radiobiologic effect of extracranial stereotactic radiosurgery: equivalent uniform dose or tumor control probability? Med Phys 2003;30:321–324.

14 Timmerman RD, Lohr F: Normal tissue dose constraints applied in lung stereotactic body radiation therapy; in Kavanagh BD, Timmerman RD (eds): Stereotactic Body Radiation Therapy. Philadelphia, Lippincott, Williams & Wilkins, 2005.

15 Schefter TE, Kavanagh BD, Timmerman RD, Cardenes HR, Baron A, Gaspar LE: A phase I trial of stereotactic body radiation therapy (SBRT) for liver metastases. Int J Radiat Oncol Biol Phys 2005;62:1371–1378.

16 Yaes RJ, Kalend A: Local stem cell depletion model for radiation myelitis. Int J Radiat Oncol Biol Phys 1988;14:1247–1259.

17 Fowler JF, Tome WA, Welsh JS: On the estimation of required doses in stereotactic body radiation therapy; in Kavanagh BD, Timmerman RD (eds): Stereotactic Body Radiation Therapy. Philadelphia, Lippincott, Williams & Wilkins, 2005.

18 Brenner DJ: Hypofractionation for prostate cancer radiotherapy – What are the issues? Int J Radiat Oncol Biol Phys 2003;57:912–914.

19 Fowler JF, Ritter MA, Chappell RJ, Brenner DJ: What hypofractionated protocols should be tested for prostate cancer? Int J Radiat Oncol Biol Phys 2003;56:1093–1104.

20 Guerrero M, Li X: Extending the linear-quadratic model for large fraction doses pertinent to stereotactic radiotherapy. Phys Med Biol 2004;49:4825–4835.

21 Benedict SH, Lin PS, Zwicker RD, Huang DT, Schmidt-Ullrich RK: The biological effectiveness of intermittent irradiation as a function of overall treatment time: development of correction factors for linac-based stereotactic radiotherapy. Int J Radiat Oncol Biol Phys 1997;37:765–769.

22 Gompertz B: On the nature of the function expressive of the law of human mortality, and on a new mode of determining the value of life contingencies. Phil Trans R Soc Lond B Biol Sci 1825;123:513–585.

23 Norton L, Simon R, Brereton HD, Bogden AE: Predicting the course of Gompertzian growth. Nature 1976;264:542–545.

24 Norton L, Simon R: The Norton-Simon hypothesis revisited. Cancer Treat Rep 1986;70:163–169.

25 Fornier M, Norton L: Dose-dense adjuvant chemotherapy for primary breast cancer. Breast Cancer Res 2005;7:64–69.

Dr. Brian D. Kavanagh
Department of Radiation Oncology
Anschutz Cancer Pavilion
1665 N. Ursula St., Suite 1032, PO Box 6510
Mail Stop F706
Aurora, CO 80045 (USA)
Tel. +1 720 848 0156, Fax +1 720 848 0222
E-Mail Brian.Kavanagh@uchsc.edu

Meyer JL (ed): IMRT, IGRT, SBRT – Advances in the Treatment Planning and
Delivery of Radiotherapy. Front Radiat Ther Oncol. Basel, Karger, 2007, vol. 40, pp 352–365

Optimizing Dose and Fractionation for Stereotactic Body Radiation Therapy

Normal Tissue and Tumor Control Effects with Large Dose per Fraction

Robert Timmerman · Michael Bastasch · Debabrata Saha · Ramzi Abdulrahman · William Hittson · Michael Story

Department of Radiation Oncology, University of Texas Southwestern Medical Center, Dallas, Tex., USA

Abstract

Stereotactic body radiation therapy (SBRT) is a potent noninvasive means of administering high-dose radiation to demarcated tumor deposits in extracranial locations. The treatments use image guidance and related treatment delivery technology for the purpose of escalating the radiation dose to the tumor itself with as little radiation dose to the surrounding normal tissue as possible. The local tumor control for SBRT has been higher than anything previously published for radiotherapy in treating typical carcinomas. In addition, the pattern, timing and severity of toxicity have been very different than what was seen with conventional radiotherapy. In this review, the clinical characteristics and outcomes of SBRT are presented in the context of their underlying mechanisms. While much of the material is unproven and speculative, it at least qualitatively searches for understanding as to the biological basis for the observed clinical effects. Hopefully, it will serve as a motivation for more sophisticated biological research into the effects of SBRT.

Stereotactic body radiation therapy (SBRT) is a potent yet noninvasive means of administering high-dose radiation dose to demarcated tumor deposits in extracranial locations. The treatments use image guidance and related treatment delivery technology for the purpose of escalating the radiation dose to the tumor itself with as little radiation dose to the surrounding normal tissue as possible. The local tumor control for SBRT has been higher than anything previously published for radiotherapy in treating typical carcinomas. In addition, the pattern, timing and severity of toxicity have been very different than what was seen with conventional radiotherapy. In this review, the clinical characteristics and outcomes of SBRT are presented in the context of their underlying mechanisms. While much of the material is unproven and speculative, it at least qualitatively searches for understanding as to the biological basis for the observed clinical effects. Hopefully, it will serve as a motivation for more sophisticated biological research into the effects of SBRT.

SBRT is defined by its conduct. It employs a limited number of very large dose per fraction treatments (with a biologically equivalent dose of at least 75–100 as a minimum or even higher), fields only slightly larger than gross tumor targets, high confidence in precision even for moving targets (with 95% probability of including the entire target with margins of 0.5–1.0 cm), and dosimetry constructed to be very conformal with sharp gradients from high- to low-dose areas [1]. At the completion of the delivery of this very potent and biologically damaging dose, dramatic tissue effects may occur, both in normal tissues and within the intended tumor target. Irrespective of the dose and fractionation, tissue responses are dependant on three basic characteristics: dose delivered (including dose per fraction), volume exposed, and inherent tissue radiosensitivity. To some degree, these characteristics are not independent, but rather, interdependent. For example, at a constant level of dose, volume effects in normal tissue may demonstrate a spectrum from no noticeable effect to dramatic dysfunction. Furthermore, the type of toxicity and its manifestations in the person may change throughout this spectrum. We know that radiosensitivity varies among various tumor types, even within the same patient. It also varies with age, getting less sensitive as the host matures and organ volumes enlarge. Throughout the history of radiation oncology, biologists have attempted to understand these processes and discover their underlying mechanisms. They have done this mostly in the context of the delivering the only type of radiation generally available called conventionally fractionated radiotherapy (CFRT). With the advent of technology facilitating SBRT, the lessons learned with CFRT investigation may or may not apply.

Traditional Radiobiology

Traditional radiobiology generally describes survival curves and tries to define models that would account for the observed data. As demonstrated in figure 1a, these curves initially have a curving portion then become more linear, in plots of log of surviving fraction versus dose. The initial curving portion of the curve is called the 'shoulder' and is said to represent a damage/repair process called 'sublethal' damage. With CFRT, a typical daily dose of around 2 Gy per fraction is given, which for most tissues would not reach the linear portion, and we repeat

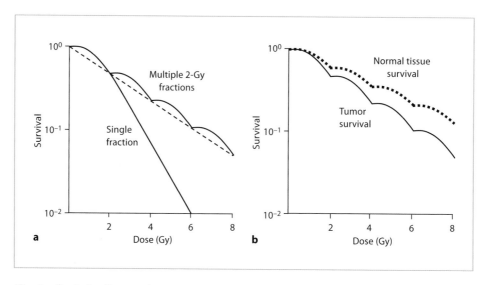

Fig. 1. a Typical cell survival curve shape comparing single-dose and multiple-dose radiation exposure. **b** Cell survival differs between normal tissues and tumor tissues for multiple-fraction exposure.

that fraction many times as shown in figure 1. Each time we give this rather small daily dose, the cumulative dose is never as potent as an equivalent single-fraction dose. This is still potentially beneficial as there often is a difference in the survival characteristics of the tumor on that curvy portion versus the normal tissues resulting in a therapeutic ratio that may be positive for CFRT as shown in figure 1b.

The shoulder, or the curvy portion of the survival curve, exists because of the 4 'Rs' of radiobiology that have been engrained into radiation oncology residency training for decades. There is *repair* of sublethal damage, which is beneficial for dose spilling to normal tissues. The normal tissues will *repopulate* during the course of a CFRT. Since CFRT is protracted in time, tumor cells will proceed through their cell cycle. Through this process of *reassortment,* tumor cells initially in a resistant phase will proceed eventually into a sensitive phase when exposed to damaging radiation. Finally, as tumors shrink, the central necrotic core becomes closer to the peripheral blood supply allowing *reoxygenation* which makes all cells more sensitive. If the story stopped here, we would conclude that CFRT is always better and not explore SBRT type dose fractionation schemes. However, the 4 Rs realistically also work against ideal therapeutic outcome. In other words, tumors can *repair* and may *repopulate* as well during the course of protracted CFRT resulting in local tumor progression. Also, normal tissues may become more sensitive during a protracted course of radiation, leading to more toxicity.

Timmerman · Bastasch · Saha · Abdulrahman · Hittson · Story

So why do we fractionate? Many would casually convey that it is simply the right thing to do based on long experience (tradition) within the field of radiation oncology. Indeed, when hypofractionated schedules similar to what are now being used for SBRT were explored 100 years ago during the advent of radiotherapy, toxicity was prohibitive. Others have gone even further and said that hypofractionated radiation is simply not as effective as fractionated radiation at controlling tumors, and have cited historical clinical comparisons [2–4]. Overall, the dogma championing CFRT has mostly been justified by implying better tumor control. Survival curves should promptly dismiss this notion as tumor kill, total dose for total dose, shows hypofractionation is always more effective for any tumor cells that have a shoulder. The real reason we use CFRT is in fact because of the normal tissues, not the tumor. Because of our lack of dose delivery technology capable of limiting normal tissue exposure, normal tissue volumes in classic CFRT delivery have been typically much larger than the tumor volume itself. In such a scenario, the only option for delivering high tumor dose is to use CFRT. Therefore, the use of CFRT during the past 80 years in the field of radiation oncology draws from a compromise, not an inherent advantage.

The survival curve also shows us that for CFRT small increments in dose per fraction really do not change the surviving fraction very much. The arithmetic slope of the curve within the shoulder is small, such that for any increase in dose or the 'run', you get a modest decrease in tissue survival or the 'rise'. CFRT operates in this shoulder region. But at large doses per fraction, for a small increment in dose you get a rather dramatic increase in effect. That effect may be improved tumor kill, which would be favorable. However, this is a double-edged sword. The dramatic change in effect with modest increase in dose may also be enhanced toxicity, particularly if radiation is spilled to the uninvolved normal tissues.

Modeling the Survival Curve

Mathematicians can easily show that any real function (i.e., one that only has one y-value for each x-value) can be characterized by a geometric power series. A power series has a progression of terms starting with a constant, then a linear term, then a quadratic term, then a cubic term, and so forth as depicted in figure 2a. Now, if the series goes out to infinity, it will perfectly match the shape of any real function, in our case the survival curve. If we truncate that power series, say after 3 terms, it may approximate the curve, particularly in a certain range, but it will not perfectly match. In the case of the radiation survival curve, the constant is theoretically zero, because at zero doses there is 100% survival, and the log of one is zero. So for a truncated power series with 3 terms, we end up with the linear term and the quadratic term. If we call the coefficients *alpha* and *beta,* here is the

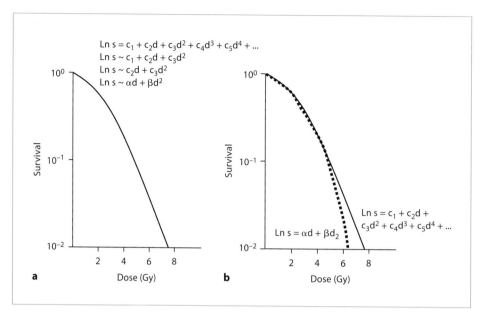

Fig. 2. a Real functions such as the shape of the cell survival curve can be expressed as a power series. A theoretical perfect match can be obtained when the number of terms is taken to infinity; however, approximate correlation can be obtained with truncated series such as the linear-quadratic model where the coefficients correspond to alpha and beta. **b** While the data may fit the truncated series well over a low dose range where most measurements are taken, the truncated linear-quadratic series overpredicts cell kill compared with the full series and actual results due to dominance by the quadratic term constantly curving the slope downward.

'linear-quadratic' model [5]. The physical meanings of the linear and quadratic terms have been linked to single-strand or double-strand DNA breaks. While this may be partly true, the most precise definition is that they are mathematical coefficients describing physical data.

Since the alpha-beta model describing the survival curve is not the entire power series, it is not exactly fitting the curve. When fitting data to a truncated power series to determine the coefficients, the goodness of fit will be best in the range of the measured input data. In the case of CFRT and the application of the alpha-beta model, most of the data have been collected, appropriately, in the range of the shoulder where actual clinical practice is carried out. Since very large dose per fraction treatments historically could not be carried out, due to prohibitive toxicity, there was no compelling reason to fit the data well after 6 to 10 Gy per fraction. At very low dose per fraction, even below what is used in CFRT, the alpha-beta model's survival values are dominated by the alpha (linear) term because its coefficient is larger than that of the beta (quadratic) term. At higher doses per fraction within the shoulder, the beta term dominates since it is applied to the dose

Timmerman · Bastasch · Saha · Abdulrahman · Hittson · Story

squared. The quadratic term changes the slope of the survival curve, giving the shoulder portion its characteristic shape. Eventually, however, the quadratic term would overwhelmingly dominate the representation of the curve by constantly curving downward, implying greater fractions of cell kill as shown in figure 2b. In reality, though, the actually measured curve becomes linear after the shoulder (not quadratic), which is a fact not handled well by the linear-quadratic formalism. In effect, the alpha-beta model overpredicts cell kill at large doses per fraction.

Biologically Equivalent Dose

Professor Fowler helped us use the alpha-beta or linear-quadratic model prudently for CFRT [5]. He derived the formalism of biologically equivalent dose, allowing us to compare the potency of various fractionation regimens so long as we had reliable information about survival characteristics for the applied range (e.g. alpha-beta ratios). In the preceding paragraphs, we argued that the alpha-beta formalism breaks down when applied to treatment schedules with very large dose per fraction. While we maintain this position, it is still convenient and cautiously useful to apply this formalism in these extrapolated circumstances. It might be useful, for example, in assigning the starting dose for a phase I study or making estimates of normal tissue tolerance for protocols. However, do not forget the limitations of the linear-quadratic model. At large doses, it becomes a poor fit, with overestimation of the effect of the treatment. Furthermore, it does not account for the duration of the treatment, for the variation in the tissue architecture or function (e.g. lung vs. spinal cord), nor look at the impact of nonchromosomal mechanisms of radiation damage like apoptosis or vascular injury. The net effect and most important observation is that the tumor control conversion will be overstated and the normal tissue conversion will be understated. By using the alpha/beta conversion without reservation, clinicians will think that SBRT at a given dose is both more effective at controlling tumor as well as safer than it is in reality. This can be a very dangerous fallacy for the patient.

Organ/Tissue Function and Microscopic Architecture

Prof. Wolbarst et al. [6] described the concept of functional subunits in a model of cell structure. They said that there were two types of functional subunits, structurally defined and structurally undefined. The structurally defined subunits had a very demarcated architecture, the undefined subunits were monotonous. They stated that organ damage would result from constituent damage to the functional subunits composing the organ.

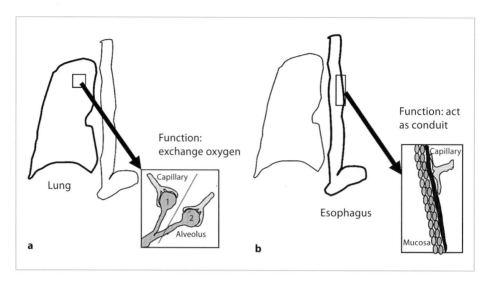

Fig. 3. a Structurally defined normal tissues like the peripheral lung exhibit a distinct demarcation between functional subunits 1 and 2. The functional subunits independently perform the tissue function, exchanging oxygen. **b** Structurally undefined normal tissues like the mucosa of the esophagus show no distinct separation between functional subunits, which in the esophagus act in concert to perform the overall function of acting as a conduit for passage of food to the stomach.

In order to understand this model, it is convenient to consider some simplified examples. Start with the lung which is structurally defined at the level of the alveolus and capillary since there is a clear distinction between each adjacent capillary/alveolus complex capable of exchanging gases as shown in figure 3a. In contrast, there is the structurally undefined esophagus where we have a monotonous tube which functions as a conduit as shown in figure 3b. However, both cases are similar in that a cellular layer including a population of stem cells (capable of repopulating this layer) lies over a basement membrane. Consider a dose of irradiation capable of eradicating all the mucosal cells and their stem cells in a given volume. For the tissue to 'heal', stem cells from somewhere beyond the volume irradiated must migrate into the functional subunit to 'rescue' by way of repopulation of the mucosa. In the case of the structurally defined lung, if you irradiate a specific alveolus/capillary functional subunit to the point where all stem cells within the subunit are eradicated, neighboring adjacent subunits cannot serve to rescue that affected subunit because stem cell migration is blocked by the intervening basement membranes. Even though there may be numerous stem cell clonogens in a neighboring alveolus, they cannot physically help their neighbor as shown in figure 4a. For the structurally undefined tissue of the esophagus, however, stem cells are free to migrate to help repair damage. Structurally undefined

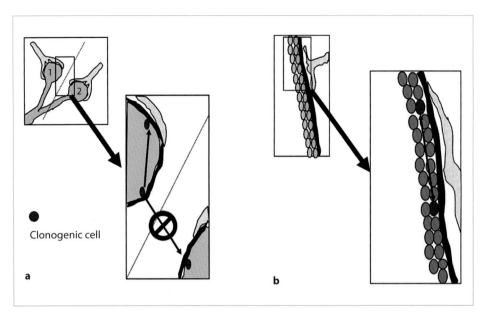

Fig. 4. a Migration of clonogenic stem cells within structurally defined tissues is unhindered within a particular functional subunit (e.g. within a specific alveolus). However, clonogenic cells even adjacent to another functional subunit cannot rescue a damaged neighbor since they cannot migrate across basement membranes. **b** Migration of clonogenic stem cells within structurally undefined tissues is unhindered by the basement membrane and is only limited by practical distance for stem cell movement. As such, adjacent functional subunits can be rescued from injury given time and the ability of neighboring stem cells to migrate.

stem cell migration is only limited by a reasonable distance, nothing anatomical as indicated in figure 4b. This would explain the observation that the radiation tolerance per cubic centimeter of the lung is significantly lower than that of the esophagus.

Tissues that are made up mostly of structurally defined subunits like the peripheral lung are called *parallel functioning* tissues. Tissues that are made up of the monotonous undefined subunits are called *serially functioning* tissues. The parallel tissues are in the peripheral lung, the peripheral liver, the peripheral kidney, and in the acini regions of glands. The serial tissues would include the body's more linear or hollow structures like the spinal cord, the esophagus, bowels, and ducts. Parallel functioning tissues are typically very large and have inherent functional redundancy or reserve. After radiation dose injury to the parallel tissues, which may occur at quite low levels, the toxicity will be mostly related to volume. That is why for things like pneumonitis, we talk about the 'V20' (volume receiving more than 20 Gy) rather than a toxic dose. For serially functioning tissues, it is the dose that is the more important predictor of toxicity. We use metrics like

'TD 5/5' (tolerance dose that causes 5% of patients to have radiation injury within 5 years) for spinal tolerance or esophageal tolerance. The trouble with these models is that most organs are actually a mixture of parallel and serially functioning tissues.

In the 1980s, Yeas and Kalend [7] came up with the notion of the *critical volume model*. The critical volume defined the organ volume exceeding the threshold dose to wipe out all stem cells within all irradiated functional subunits. For tumors near serially functioning tissues, radiation tolerance would be relatively high and even higher with protracted radiation. In order to give tumoricidal dose while still maintaining the possibility to rescue adjacent functional subunits, it made sense to fractionate the dose, more like conventional treatments, or to use radiosensitizers. For tumors near parallel functioning tissues, even small doses would eliminate the functional subunits with little chance of rescue. As such, it would be best in terms of tumor kill to give the dose all at once, and then do a lot of measures to exclude volume because volume was the problem with toxicity. So, for these structures, it was most important to find radiation methods to limit moderate- and high-dose irradiation of normal tissues. Finally, we introduced our need for the techniques of SBRT. Now we have many vendors that offer the technologies to help us do these SBRT treatments. Indeed this technology is very useful if you are in parallel functioning tissues to improve the dose distribution and minimize the high-dose regions. But for treatments next to a serially functioning tissue, these technologies will only be of limited benefit.

Serially Functioning Tissue Macroscopic Architecture

Our bodies have two basic types of linearly arranged serially functioning hollow lumen tissues as indicated in figure 5. One is a *linear tubular* structure like the esophagus or the gastrointestinal tract. The other is the *branching tubular* structure like the hepatic ducts and the bronchus of the lungs, extending out toward the parallel functioning tissues in the periphery [8].

The function of a linear tubular organ is to just transmit something downstream. The 'something' may include nutrients, secretions, electrical signals, or waste products. Within the walls or channels of linear tubular structures, specialized structures may aid this process. In the case of the hollow viscus or bowels, for instance, the clonogens are monotonously layered on a basement membrane throughout the lumen. They have a vascular supply that starts from two main arterial feeders following the tube longitudinally. These vessels are connected to arcades of vessels that go around providing vascular supply to the circumference of the walls.

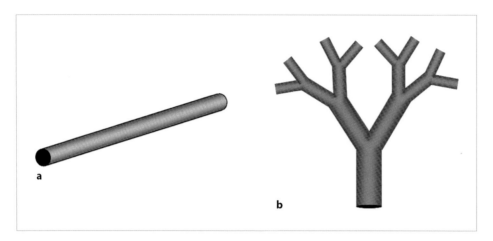

Fig. 5. a Serially functioning tissue arranged as a straight or curved line without branch points is referred to as a linear structure. Ablative injury to the circumference of a linear tubular structure at any point along its length will eventually totally disrupt the function of the organ. In the case of the linear tubular small intestine, such an injury would result in a bowel obstruction. **b** Serially functioning tissue arranged akin to a tree or bush with a larger trunk dividing into major limbs and finally smaller limbs and branches is referred to as a branching structure. Ablative injury to a branch will primarily cause dysfunction downstream from the injury, not the organ as a whole unless the major trunk itself is damaged. The airways in the lung and duct in the liver follow a branching tubular structure.

In contrast, while branching tubular organs function for the same reasons, they have branching conduits that split akin to the branches of a tree or bush. Their blood supply follows along those same branches out to the periphery from the central trunk. In this arrangement, conduits beyond a split point are no longer transmitting the same material even though the structure of two adjacent branches may be identical.

Severe damage to any segment of a linear tubular structure like the small intestine (as might be caused by SBRT) results in total and catastrophic dysfunction of the organ. This might include a bowel obstruction that totally disrupts effective digestion. In contrast, with severe damage to a branching tubular structure like the pulmonary airways, the severity of the dysfunction depends to a great degree on the position of the damage within the branching structure. If the damage occurs at a distal branch, only the relatively small volume of tissue supplied by that particular branch will become dysfunctional. However, if the damage occurs in the larger more proximal trunks, a severer dysfunction will occur as many downstream branches are cut off. In either case, damage to tubular structures tends to manifest in the patient as 'late' toxicity often not appearing for 4–6 months after therapy.

Stereotactic Body Radiation Therapy and Ablation

The main objective of therapeutic radiation is to disrupt clonogenicity, and there are many genes involved with clonogenicity. Stem cells are typically fairly radio-sensitive, so often it does not take much dose to affect them. Cellular division or clonogenicity is a very complicated process regulated by a multitude of genes. The entire process can be stymied by radiation damage to any one of these genes, which may occur at relatively modest doses. Cellular function, like the secretion of a hormone, is usually only coded for by one gene or a few genes, and therefore radiation must damage every one of those genes in every functioning cell to disrupt the function. As such, it takes a very high dose of radiation to disrupt cellular function. As an illustration, growth control of a pituitary adenoma is achieved at a relatively modest dose, but to stop the secretion of a hormone from a hormone-secreting pituitary adenoma takes a much higher dose. Another example can be borrowed from the use of radioactive iodine to treat thyroid cancer. The therapy is so well targeted that massive doses reach both the thyroid cancer and the residual functioning thyroid gland. These doses both disrupt clonogenicity and cellular function. Such a treatment has been termed *ablative*. In turn, typical dose regimens used with SBRT are also often ablative to the tissues seeing dose levels near the target dose.

The assumptions with SBRT, at least in the region of the planning target volume, are that we will destroy clonogenicity and that tumors will be totally disrupted. More than likely, we will also destroy tissue function (e.g. transmitting air through an involved bronchus). In the shell of normal tissue just outside of the planning target volume, the dose is so high that it will effectively disable all of the clonogenicity and function of that portion of the organ. So in that regard, SBRT is almost like a surgeon's knife, effectively cutting the tissues and leaving them totally disabled both at the point of contact and downstream. Nonetheless, from a tumor control point of view, ablative dose levels are still desirable since in this range the likelihood of disrupting clonogenicity in every tumor cell is very high.

Normal Tissue Consequences of Ablative Dose Delivery

With SBRT, radiotherapy can act almost like a knife. As such, lessons can be learned from surgeons. The surgeon must achieve homeostasis, remove all devascularized tissues, and restore continuity of a hollow viscus. If a surgeon removes a tumor of the esophagus, he/she has to reconnect the ends or the patient would suffer. If a surgeon removes a lung tumor, he/she does not just enucleate the tumor. Instead, the surgeon must take out all downstream lung which otherwise would necrose and lead to postoperative complications. So if we use SBRT in these same

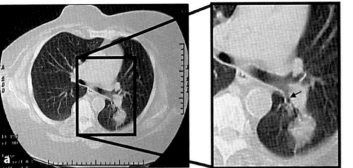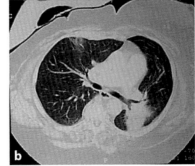

Fig. 6. a Early-stage lung cancer patient prior to ablative dose SBRT. There is a small branching bronchus designated by the arrow oriented toward the tumor. This airway was situated inside the planning target volume and received the ablative dose. **b** Two-year posttreatment CT scan showing dense consolidation distal to the small airway indicated in **a**. The consolidation was not avid on PET and is most consistent with postradiation atelectasis.

examples and we treat a tumor of a hollow viscus like an esophageal cancer, what we can expect is that the function of that structure, that is the tubular function, will be destroyed. If we do not restore it, the patient will have a severe problem. It would be dangerous to treat esophageal tumors with ablative doses using SBRT, because you will end up with a debilitating stenosis. In the case of the branching tubular structures like the lung, SBRT will affect all tissues downstream from airways exposed to ablative dose. We will end up with a collapsed, atelectatic tissue downstream. The overall posttreatment function of the organ depends heavily on the volume of downstream lung. Obviously, lesions treated in the lung periphery will be less prone to problems as compared with lesions near the main stem bronchus.

For the branching tubular organs, the lung has been the most prominently treated site. Downstream collapse from bronchial injury is commonly observed as shown in figure 6 [9–14]. The liver has a similar architecture to the lung but it has the capacity to regenerate [15]. This capacity will make little difference, however, if the draining bile ducts are obliterated. Whether stenting can prevent the effects of radiation-induced biliary sclerosis is yet unclear. So as long as we do not set the patient back too far during the course of an SBRT treatment, liver will likely be a preferred site to treat.

The normal tissue tolerances to SBRT remain unclear. Large doses per fraction are associated with increased late effects. Late effects take more time to observe. Therefore, we must collect toxicity data years after therapy to quantify risk and define tolerance. The Radiation Therapy Oncology Group has included tolerances in its 0236 protocol for SBRT in medically inoperable lung cancer. These were agreed upon by extrapolation, limited data, and committee discussions. In all likelihood, they will have to be modified over time with more adequate follow-up.

Tumor Control Dose

SBRT uses anything from 1 to 5 fractions. Different centers have used different dose levels. Some have argued that they have found adequate dose levels, but typically based on retrospective testing. Prospective testing is now ongoing, but results are still immature. At any rate, it is clear that better tumor control is achieved when using ablative dose ranges. This would require at least 10 Gy per fraction for 3–5 fractions. The only prospective dose escalation study testing multiple levels up to a maximum tolerated dose was carried out at Indiana University. It showed that 20 Gy per fraction times 3 (60 Gy total) was tolerable in most patients with early-stage medically inoperable lung cancer. It also showed that doses of 16 Gy times 3 or less had higher rates of local tumor progression [9]. In a previous section, we made an argument that alpha/beta conversions overpredict dose potency in this range. At any rate, in cancer therapy development, the first objective of clinical studies is to determine a potent dose in phase I studies. That way, the therapy will be in its most potent form for phase II and III trials for testing. It would be feasible, if needed, to reduce the dose because of excessive toxicity with late follow-up. Again, ideally the therapy should afford tumor control probabilities near 90%. Such probabilities are attainable with SBRT so long as adequate dose is delivered.

Conclusions

What are the true dose-response characteristics of SBRT? What are the mechanisms of both tumor and normal tissue injury? To date, the answers to these questions are unclear. It can already be appreciated, however, that lessons learned from the long history of CFRT do not necessarily apply to SBRT. The biggest obstacle to delivering SBRT surrounds the treatment of tumors near serially functioning tissues. Technology cannot solve this problem. The future of SBRT will require a considerable amount of work to be done in the realm of classic radiobiology. The encouraging results in parallel functioning organs may very well change the patterns of care for many diseases, including early-stage lung cancer, as trials mature. However, the true potential of SBRT will not be realized until chemical modifiers or dose schedules can be developed to use this same ablative therapy in and about serially functioning tissue. This challenge should be viewed as a true opportunity.

References

1 Potters L, Steinberg M, Rose C, Timmerman R, Ryu S, Hevezi JM, Welsh J, Mehta M, Larson DA, Janjan NA; American Society for Therapeutic Radiology and Oncology; American College of Radiology: American Society for Therapeutic Radiology and Oncology and American College of Radiology practice guideline for the performance of stereotactic body radiation therapy. Int J Radiat Oncol Biol Phys 2004;60:1026–1032.

2 Rosenthal DI, Glatstein E: We've got a treatment, but what's the disease? Or a brief history of hypofractionation and its relationship to stereotactic radiosurgery. Oncologist 1996;1:1–7.

3 Glatstein E: Personal thoughts on normal tissue tolerance, or, what the textbooks don't tell you. Int J Radiat Oncol Biol Phys 2001;51:1185–1189.

4 Goffman TE, Glatstein E: Hypofractionation redux? J Clin Oncol 2004;22:589–591.

5 Douglas BG, Fowler JF: The effects of multiple small doses of X-rays on skin reactions in the mouse and a basic interpretation. Radiat Res 1976;66:401–426.

6 Wolbarst, AB, Chin, LM, Svensson, GK: Optimization of radiation therapy: integral-response of a model biological system. Int J Radiat Oncol Biol Phys 1982;8:1761–1769.

7 Yeas RJ, Kalend A: Local stem cell depletion model for radiation myelitis. Int J Radiat Oncol Biol Phys 1988;14:1247–1259.

8 Timmerman RD, Kavanagh BD: Stereotactic body radiation therapy. Curr Probl Cancer 2005; 29:120–157.

9 Timmerman R, Papiez L, McGarry R, Likes L, DesRosiers C, Frost S, Williams M: Extracranial stereotactic radioablation: results of a phase I study in medically inoperable stage I non-small cell lung cancer. Chest 2003;124:1946–1955.

10 Aoki T, Nagata Y, Negoro Y, Takayama K, Mizowaki T, Kokubo M, Oya N, Mitsumori M, Hiraoka M: Evaluation of lung injury after three-dimensional conformal stereotactic radiation therapy for solitary lung tumors: CT appearance. Radiology 2004;230:101–108.

11 Takeda T, Takeda A, Kunieda E, Ishizaka A, Takemasa K, Shimada K, Yamamoto S, Shigematsu N, Kawaguchi O, Fukada J, Ohashi T, Kuribayashi S, Kubo A: Radiation injury after hypofractionated stereotactic radiotherapy for peripheral small lung tumors: serial changes on CT. AJR Am J Roentgenol 2004;182:1123–1128.

12 Yamada Y, Shiomi H, Sumida I, Suzuki O, Isohashi F, Oh RJ, Tanaka E, Inoue T, Nakamura H: Quantitative evaluation of changes in irradiated lung fields after stereotactic irradiation by the Polygon Method. Radiat Med 2004;22:98–105.

13 Slotman BJ, Solberg T (eds): Extracranial Stereotactic Radiosurgery and Radiotherapy, ed 1. Hamilton, BC Decker, Inc, in press.

14 Kavanagh B, Timmerman RD (eds): Stereotactic Body Radiation Therapy. Baltimore, Lippincott, Williams, and Wilkins, 2005.

15 Herfarth KK, Hof H, Bahner ML, Lohr F, Hoss A, van Kaick G, Wannenmacher M, Debus J: Assessment of focal liver reaction by multiphasic CT after stereotactic single-dose radiotherapy of liver tumors. Int J Radiat Oncol Biol Phys 2003; 57:444–451.

Dr. Robert Timmerman
Department of Radiation Oncology
University of Texas Southwestern Medical Center
5801 Forest Park Road
Dallas, TX 75390-9183 (USA)
Tel. +1 214 645 7651, Fax +1 214 645 7622
E-Mail
Robert.Timmerman@UTSouthwestern.edu

IV. SBRT Clinical Treatment Programs

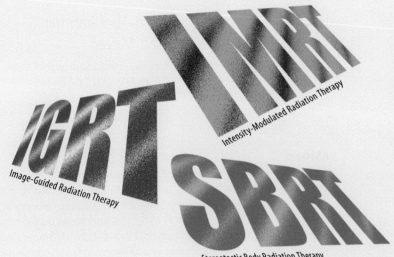

Meyer JL (ed): IMRT, IGRT, SBRT – Advances in the Treatment Planning and
Delivery of Radiotherapy. Front Radiat Ther Oncol. Basel, Karger, 2007, vol. 40, pp 368–385

Lung Cancer: A Model for Implementing Stereotactic Body Radiation Therapy into Practice

Robert Timmerman[a] · Ramzi Abdulrahman[a] ·
Brian D. Kavanagh[b] · John L. Meyer[c]

Departments of Radiation Oncology, [a]University of Texas Southwestern Medical Center,
Dallas, Tex., [b]University of Colorado Health Sciences Center, Aurora, Colo., [c]Saint Francis
Memorial Hospital, San Francisco, Calif., USA

Abstract

Primary and metastatic tumors to the lung have been principle targets for the noninvasive high-dose-per-fraction treatment programs now officially called stereotactic body radiation therapy (SBRT). Highly focused treatment delivery to moving lung targets requires accurate assessment of tumor position throughout the respiratory cycle. Measures to account for this motion, either by tracking (chasing), gating, or inhibition (breath hold and abdominal compression) must be employed in order to avoid large margins of error that would expose uninvolved normal tissues. The treatments use image guidance and related treatment delivery technology for the purpose of escalating the radiation dose to the tumor itself with as little radiation dose to the surrounding normal tissues as possible. Clinical trials have demonstrated superior local control with SBRT as compared with conventionally fractionated radiotherapy. While late toxicity requires further careful assessment, acute and subacute toxicity are remarkably infrequent. Radiographic and local tissue effects consistent with bronchial damage and downstream collapse with fibrosis are common, especially with adequate doses capable of ablating tumor targets. As such, great care must be taken when employing SBRT near the serially functioning central chest structures including the esophagus and major airways. While mechanisms of this injury remain elusive, ongoing prospective trials offer the hope of finding the ideal application for SBRT in treating pulmonary targets.   Copyright © 2007 S. Karger AG, Basel

The primary treatment for early-stage non-small-cell lung cancer (NSCLC) is surgery. Surgical therapy, especially lobectomy or pneumonectomy, is associated with 3- to 5-year survival rates (effective cure) of 60–80% of patients [1–4]. Lesser surgical therapies, such as wedge resection and segmentectomy, have been shown to be inferior surgical procedures due to local recurrence and decreased survival

Table 1. Local control and survival in early-stage NSCLC

Stage	Treatment	Survival, %	Local control, %
I	surgery	60–80	60–80
I[1]	conventional radiotherapy	15–45	15–45
II	surgery	30–50	30–50
II[1]	conventional radiotherapy	10–30	10–30

[1] Predominantly medically inoperable patients.

as compared with anatomical resections [5]. Alternate therapies, such as conventionally fractionated radiotherapy (CFRT), are much less effective with 3- to 5-year survival rates of only 15–45% [6–12]. However, the patients treated with CFRT are by no means the same patients that are treated surgically, and a direct comparison of survival rates cannot be made. Generally, radiotherapy-treated patients have a host of medical problems that would make a lobectomy or pneumonectomy intolerable, including severe pulmonary disease, heart disease, diabetes or vascular disease. These patients are called 'medically inoperable' and have competing causes of death in the 3- to 5-year period after cancer diagnosis; survival is inherently greatly compromised. Nonetheless, with such a disparity in survival between surgery and CFRT, there is an obvious need for improvement that beckons for translational research programs and controlled clinical trials.

Metastases to the lungs are primarily treated with chemotherapy, because these lesions are unlikely to represent the only organ of involvement for most cancers. As a systemic treatment, chemotherapy has the most optimal bioavailability at the site of tumor progression. Unfortunately, chemotherapy has been relatively ineffective at achieving long-term control, especially of gross disease, for the majority of common cancers. Surgical metastectomy and other ablative procedures have been increasingly used in selected patients with lung metastases [13–17]. Occasionally, these interventions render the patient truly free of disease. Coupled with more effective systemic therapy, surgical and ablative treatments for lung cancer will likely be increasingly utilized in upcoming years.

Local Control in Primary Lung Cancer

As noted in table 1, the local control rates in NSCLC are about the same as the survival rates, both with surgery and radiotherapy. This does not mean that all patients die of local recurrence, but it is interesting to note that local control is a surrogate measure for survival. Certainly, a cure can never be attained without local control. It makes one hypothesize that improvements in local control in lung cancer might lead to improvements in survival. In the case of radiotherapy, there is certainly room for improvement.

Strategies for Improving Local Control with Radiotherapy

There are three basic strategies for improving local control with radiotherapy: to increase the total dose, the radiosensitivity, or the dose per fraction. All of these strategies have been studied in prospective trials. All modern strategies employ some form of image guidance to improve the confidence in targeting (minimizing margins without missing disease at margins) and to avoid toxicity. Trials using all of these methods are described below, with emphasis on the large-dose-per-fraction ablative schedules common to stereotactic body radiation therapy (SBRT).

Trials with Higher Total Dose

Three trials in North America have examined the effects of increasing doses of CFRT. Each was originally designed in a period prior to the widespread use of concurrent chemotherapy, and each trial tested the use of increasing doses of irradiation delivered by three-dimensional conformal techniques. All stages of local/regional disease were included in these trials; however, because of the dose escalation design, the majority of patients treated at the highest doses had early-stage disease.

In a published phase I trial, Rosenzweig et al. [18], from the Memorial Sloan-Kettering Cancer Center, reported that doses of up to 84 Gy in total were tolerable as long as a normal tissue complication probability constraint was kept below 25%. Their data suggested that survival was improved in patients receiving 80 Gy or more. In a similarly designed study of dose escalation based on normal tissue toxicity predictions, Hayman et al. [19] from the University of Michigan escalated doses up to 102.9 Gy using three-dimensional conformal techniques and conventional fractionation. Local failures were significant; however, isolated regional failures in clinically uninvolved and untreated lymph node groups were uncommon. Finally, the Radiation Therapy Oncology Group (RTOG) carried out a multicenter dose escalation study of radiotherapy either alone or with induction chemotherapy, and found that 83.8 Gy was tolerated in patients when their treatment plans limited the volume of lung receiving 20 Gy or more to under 25% [20]. No dose-response relationship was observed, and locoregional failure was observed in 50–78% of patients.

While these trials continue to mature, it is clear that very high doses (up to 100 Gy) of CFRT can be delivered with three-dimensional conformal techniques. Although these trials do not constitute a formal comparison, it appears that the highest doses achieved result in better local control than the standard 60 Gy in 30 fractions commonly used in practice. Still, in the dose range of 80 Gy and higher, there is no convincing evidence that higher doses result in improved local control.

Furthermore, local failures continue to occur even at the highest dose levels, possibly owing to the very protracted overall treatment times. In separate analyses, Mehta et al. [21] and Machtay et al. [22] showed that prolongation of treatment time in lung cancer resulted in poorer survival rates. For treatment prolongation beyond 5–6 weeks in total, patients lose 1–2% survival per day as a group owing to accelerated tumor clonogen repopulation. This problem is the impetus for dramatically accelerated treatment regimens including the continuous hyperfractionated accelerated radiation therapy regimen from Europe [23].

Radiosensitizing Agents with CFRT

The current standard of care for treating stage III NSCLC involves giving radiotherapy concurrently with chemotherapy. This strategy exploits the radiosensitization afforded by chemotherapy agents like platinum-based drugs when given concurrently with radiotherapy. An ideal radiosensitizer would preferentially sensitize tumor tissues more than normal tissues. While chemotherapy is not ideal in this sense, it does afford more tumor kill at a given dose of irradiation as compared with radiation alone at the same dose. Unfortunately, normal tissues like the esophagus are damaged relatively more with concurrent therapy. Still, with proper supportive care, this strategy is viable. In stage I NSCLC, the concurrent administration of chemotherapy with radiation therapy is considered in fitter patients, but there is no high-level evidence supporting its use. In medically inoperable patients, concurrent chemotherapy with radiation therapy may even be detrimental, depending on patient tolerance.

Increasing the Dose per Fraction

Increasing the dose per fraction would theoretically result in more tumor cell inactivation by allowing the therapy to avoid the 'shoulder' region of the survival curve common to lung cancers, as shown in figure 1. This strategy has taken two forms, including traditional hypofractionation and ablative fractionation. Traditional hypofractionation involves using daily doses of more than 2.5–3 Gy but less than 6–7 Gy per fraction. In a recently completed trial by the Cancer and Leukemia Group B (CALGB 39904), the total dose of CFRT was fixed at 70 Gy. The number of treatments was successively lowered such that the dose per fraction increased. Results of this trial with traditional hypofractionation are pending [Bogart, J., pers. commun., December 2005].

SBRT is a modern therapy that utilizes such high doses per fraction that it is unlikely that cellular proliferative capacity or even function remains after only a few fractions. A treatment that disrupts both cell division and cell function is called 'ablative', as originally related to the administration of radioactive iodine for well-differentiated thyroid cancer. The remainder of this paper will focus on this mode of treatment delivery.

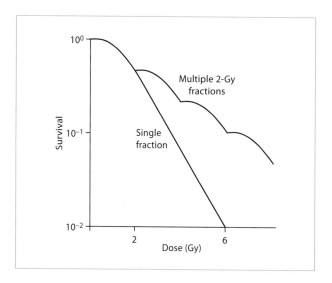

Fig. 1. Clonogenic survival for single-fraction radiation delivery versus conventional fractionation demonstrates that single fractions are much more potent at a given total dose.

Stereotactic Body Radiation Therapy

Ablative fractionation is a double-edged sword. A large total dose of irradiation is profoundly more potent in eradicating tumor if given in a single fraction (as opposed to multiple smaller fractions), but is also much more damaging to normal tissues. Feared consequences of very-large-dose-per-fraction treatments are known as toxic 'late' effects, including devascularization, fibrosis, ulceration and necrosis, and these may not become manifest for years after therapy. The tissues that form conduits or linear 'electrical' circuits are referred to as serially functioning tissues and include the bowel, blood vessels and nerves [24, 25]. Nerves and blood vessels are thought to be particularly prone to such late effects. These serially functioning tissues are of greatest concern clinically. They may function with irreparable damage for many months, even years, after radiation insult and then undergo catastrophic failure.

The current strategy for SBRT to avoid such late effects is simply to treat the tumor while employing state-of-the-art technology to avoid the uninvolved normal tissues. This rational exclusion of normal tissue volumes requires that four important steps be taken: that patients are selected who do not require prophylactic (adjuvant) radiotherapy, tumor motion is prudently accounted for, treatment dosimetry provides rapid dose falloff to normal tissues, and targeting accuracy is very high. Methods to achieve these first three goals will be discussed initially, and the fourth will be dealt with in greater detail in the following section.

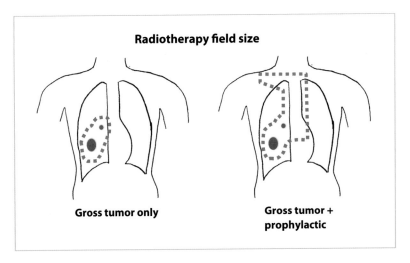

Fig. 2. The effect of including (or omitting) areas at risk for lymph node metastases in NSCLC. Gross tumor only portals treat substantially less normal tissue.

The Rational Exclusion of Normal Tissue Volumes in SBRT

Generally, it is assumed that the ablative doses delivered within the tumor target itself are nontoxic. This notion could be erroneous when normal-functioning tissue traverses the target (e.g. an acoustic schwannoma in the skull base), but in general it is a reasonable position. As such, toxicity is related to the dose outside of the target. For ablative fractionation, this toxicity is generally related to the doses delivered within a radius of 0–3 cm beyond the margin of the target volume, where the doses are still quite high in the steep falloff gradients. One might envision a sort of a shell or peel around the tumor that constitutes the damaged normal tissue area and results in toxicity. The goal of avoiding toxicity would be to limit the volume of this high-dose shell.

Limiting Prophylactic Treatment

Based on a fair amount of retrospective data on NSCLC, it is reasonable to omit the irradiation of tissues that are radiographically uninvolved [26–28]. Granted, there is a known risk of microscopic tumor involvement in various adjacent lymph node chains. However, in CFRT studies the primary tumor was rarely controlled, making it difficult to rationalize increasing normal tissue volumes to treat only areas at risk for involvement. The avoidance of elective nodal irradiation constitutes the most dramatic reduction of all in normal tissue volume avoidance, as demonstrated in figure 2. Similarly, based on the local control data on SBRT, it is reasonable to avoid large clinical target volume (CTV) expansions around the gross tumor volume (GTV) that might target microscopic tentacles extending

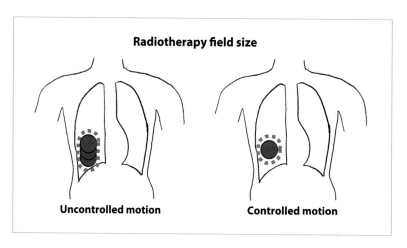

Fig. 3. Uncontrolled tumor motion requires enlargement of a beam's eye view radiation portal in order to avoid target inaccuracy. Careful assessment and control of motion dramatically decreases normal tissue exposure.

from the tumor. In our SBRT experience, we equate the GTV to the CTV. While it is known from histopathological specimens that such microscopic disease does emit from the gross tumor in lung cancer [29–31], it may be effectively dealt with first by carefully defining the GTV using appropriate pulmonary CT windows and then by delivering adequately high doses to the GTV margin. In that way, the falloff dose using photons is high enough to eradicate such extensions, as validated by the high rates of local control. Large expansions of GTV to CTV, as are commonly done in CFRT, result in dramatically higher normal tissue doses that can limit the delivery of high target doses or increase toxicity.

Addressing Target Motion

In brain radiosurgery, once the skull is immobilized and referenced to the treatment device, the issue of intrafraction motion is not burdensome. Such is not the case when performing SBRT. It is neither practical nor prudent to artificially stop organ motion in the body. Ideally, patients' hearts will continue to beat, they will breath, and their bowels will sustain peristalsis. Of course, such motion may dramatically affect targeting accuracy. Insisting that the tumor be included in the radiation portal throughout the entire course of a treatment (which may last hours in some cases) would therefore require that the aperture be significantly enlarged compared with a nonmoving target, as shown in figure 3.

Prior to accounting for motion, the tumor must first be monitored and quantified. Image guidance has been very helpful in this regard. Generally, a surrogate is identified to help quantify the actual tumor position. In the case of lung cancers,

Timmerman · Abdulrahman · Kavanagh · Meyer

the tumor outline itself may be recognized on fluoroscopy or computed imaging. A motion map showing the target position during all phases of the respiratory cycle can be determined. Modern four-dimensional scanners can be very helpful for accurate assessment of these motion maps, but are not absolutely essential. Caution should be maintained when using systems that force the patient to breath in an 'artificial' fashion during simulation that is different from treatment. Maximum inspiration/expiration CT-scanning-generated motion maps may dramatically and unnecessarily increase the subsequent volume to be irradiated during free breathing at treatment, resulting in toxicity. When the tumor cannot be visualized on fluoroscopy, the diaphragm is commonly used as a motion surrogate. This practice can be problematic if the correlation between tumor motion and diaphragm motion is poor. In any case, simply measuring the motion, even if done very carefully with a four-dimensional CT scan, is not sufficient. The typical motion of a lung tumor near the diaphragm involves 2–3 cm of excursion. Adding a 2- to 3-cm margin would limit dose delivery or increase toxicity, which is unacceptable for SBRT. An effective accounting of the tumor motion is required that ultimately allows portal margins of not greater than 1 cm, as described in the following paragraphs.

To decrease the volume irradiated, three general categories of respiratory motion control have been employed in SBRT, and include tumor tracking or chasing, gating, and respiratory inhibition.

Tracking. Tracking first requires a tumor motion surrogate correlated to all phases of the respiratory cycle. The surrogate, such as a point on the chest wall or a breathing flow detector, drives the position of the radiation beam. In the case of the Cyberknife, the entire linear accelerator moves with the tumor movement. Other strategies involve moving the collimators of a conventional linear accelerator within a beam's eye view.

Respiratory Gating. Respiratory gating is a commonly practiced approach to motion control. Like tracking, it also requires knowledge of the tumor position within a respiratory cycle. If the tumor is confidently identified at a specific phase of respiration, then the treatment can be limited to only that respiratory phase and the tumor treated with a small margin. Generally, gating occurs at the end of expiration, which is a longer phase and relatively stable.

Respiratory Inhibition. The final category of motion control is respiratory inhibition, where the respiratory cycle is artificially manipulated to facilitate minimizing margins. Two techniques within this category have been used. 'Forced breath hold' effectively restricts the tumor to a stable position that is correlated with the treatment beams. Both inspiration and expiration breath holding have been described. At a known tidal volume, patients hold their breath until uncomfortable, and the beam is only activated while the breath is held with the proper tidal volume. Finally, the most commonly utilized method of motion control for SBRT

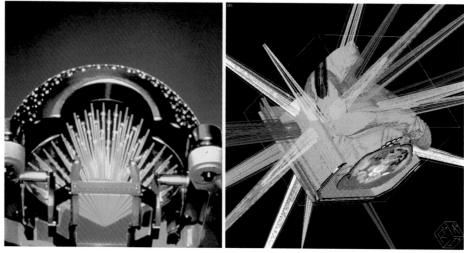

Intracranial   Extracranial

Fig. 4. Similarities between intracranial radiosurgery and SBRT include the use of multiple beams to limit entry dose and achieve high conformality.

is 'abdominal compression'. This is a simple method where diaphragmatic excursion, the biggest component of respiratory motion, is limited by pressing uniformly on the abdomen with an external device. Limiting diaphragmatic breathing forces the patient to employ chest wall breathing (expanding the chest wall by using the intercostal muscles). While motion is never completely controlled by this method, the relative increase in chest wall breathing to diaphragmatic breathing dampens tumor motion, thus permitting margin reduction.

Of the various methods described, both gating and breath-hold techniques require a period where the beam is on and off. This duty cycle results in increased treatment time that may be problematic, especially if the beam output on the radiation device is low. Furthermore, some methods are difficult to tolerate for some patients. The choice of motion control must be individualized to facilitate small target volume yet accurate treatment.

Dosimetry

Finally, as a means of normal tissue volume avoidance, there is a need to construct dosimetry that is of very high quality. The potent dose must only hit the target, but must also have very sharp falloff dose gradients outside the region of the tumor. Generally this is accomplished by using multiple fields (often 10 or more), multiple degrees of arc rotations, noncoplanar fields, and nonopposing fields. As shown in figure 4, this type of dosimetry construction effectively mimics radiosurgery in the brain. For treatment in the brain (an organ both poorly tolerant and less effec-

                                     Timmerman · Abdulrahman · Kavanagh · Meyer

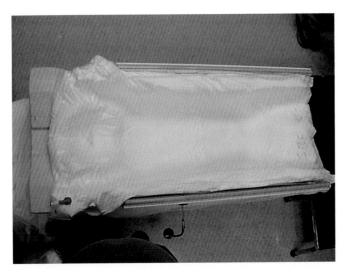

Fig. 5. The vacuum pillow integrated into the frame-based SBRT system forms a cast of the patient's contours facilitating relocalization and comfortable treatment sessions.

tive at repair of irradiation), high entrance doses are avoided to reduce global effects like memory problems, while high doses outside of the target are avoided to reduce radionecrosis. SBRT is a logical extension of brain radiosurgery much more than of CFRT or intensity-modulated radiation therapy. Mimicking brain radiosurgery, with the added charge of accounting for inherent organ motion, is the best approach to delivering prudent SBRT.

SBRT Treatment Logistics
Frame-Based versus Frameless
The logistics of SBRT vary from center to center. At the University of Texas Southwestern Medical Center, the process starts with immobilization and simulation on day 1. At our center, and at most centers with published results, a body frame for SBRT treatment is used. At one time, this 'frame-based' approach was necessary for stereotactic treatment delivery based on external fiducials. With modern image guidance, including four-dimensional CT scanning and cone beam scanning on the treatment couch (both of which are available at our center), such external fiducial targeting is not absolutely essential. Still, we utilize the frame-based system because of other important benefits. Foremost among these is the fact that a properly designed frame system comfortably immobilizes the patient from simulation to treatment. The large vacuum bag surrounding the patient on three sides creates a cast providing uniform support for the treatments that last longer than with CFRT, as shown in figure 5. The frame fiducials, once essential for accurate

targeting, now become a valuable quality assurance check for positioning. Finally, our commitment to use abdominal compression, either as the sole motion control method or in combination with other methods including gating, is facilitated by the use of a frame. In fact, when patients are too large to fit into the available commercial frames, we construct larger frames in our fabrication shop to facilitate the SBRT treatment. In the end, we reject the use of frameless SBRT. There is a misconception that frameless systems constitute a higher level of technological sophistication. In reality, technologies that facilitate relocalization without a frame actually compliment the frame-based approach. Despite our access to the most modern technologies, we continue to use the frame-based approach (as well as the simple but elegant abdominal compression techniques).

Target Volumes for SBRT in the Lung

As noted above, at our center targets are defined based on pulmonary window CT scans. The GTV is not expanded to a CTV that is based on microscopic extension. The treatment dose used might be high enough to treat possible extension, by fall-off of dose around the GTV. Centers that prefer lower doses for perceived safety reasons might ironically need larger margins, thereby increasing toxicity, in order to adequately treat such tumor extensions. We only include tissues that have obvious tumor involvement, because the approach of adding additional tissue 'when in doubt' (a practice common in the teaching of CFRT delivery) may dramatically increase risk with SBRT. If in doubt about target delineation, it is prudent to fuse in other imaging platforms such as PET or MRI to better define the tumor. The motivation in SBRT is to find ways to confidently exclude uninvolved tissues and make the target as compact as possible.

Example Dosimetry

The GTV is expanded to the planning target volume based on a specific assessment of motion for each tumor treated. From 10 to 15 beams are then defined, from multiple noncoplanar and nonopposing directions, to create dose distributions, as shown in figure 6. In this case, a small tumor is surrounded by the prescription dose, i.e. 60 Gy. The dose falls off quickly in all directions both in the axial and coronal planes. Proper treatment planning creates a cloud of radiation dose that allows the tumor to modestly move within the volume. In striking distinction from CFRT, there is no effort in planning SBRT to construct a uniform dose distribution within the target. Instead, the dosimetrist should require that the target be adequately covered by the prescription dose, but concentrate on optimizing the dose falloff outside the target and respecting normal tissue dose constraints.

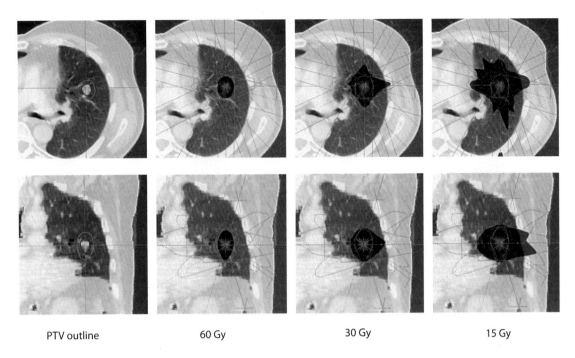

| PTV outline | 60 Gy | 30 Gy | 15 Gy |

Fig. 6. Typical dosimetry for an early-stage NSCLC SBRT treatment. PTV = Planning target volume.

Early-Stage Medically Inoperable Lung Cancer: A Model for Implementing SBRT into Practice

Phase I Dose Escalation Study

Using the treatment process described above, a formal phase I dose escalation toxicity study of 47 patients with medically inoperable lung cancers was performed at Indiana University [32]. The starting dose was 8 Gy per fraction times 3 (24 Gy in total). All patients were treated with 3 fractions at all dose levels. Patients were stratified into 3 groups based on target volume: T1 tumors, T2 tumors <5 cm, and T2 tumors that were 5–7 cm. There was no restriction regarding the location of the tumor in the lung; both central and peripheral tumors were treated. Waiting periods were built into the protocol design so that toxicity could be observed after the acute phase. A total of 7 dose levels were tested. The maximum tolerated dose was never reached for T1 tumors and T2 tumors less than 5 cm, despite reaching 60–66 Gy in 3 fractions. For the largest tumors, dose was escalated to 72 Gy in 3 fractions but this proved to be too toxic; dose-limiting toxicity included pneumonia and pericardial effusion. Classic radiation pneumonitis (fever, chest pain, shortness of breath, and dry cough), which we thought would constitute the dose-limiting toxicity, only occurred sporadically. It did occur, but no more frequently after high doses than low doses.

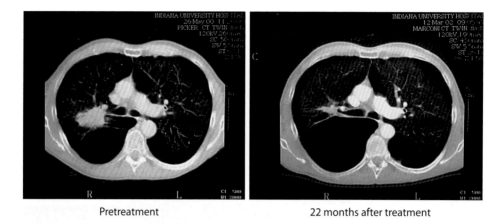

| Pretreatment | 22 months after treatment |

Fig. 7. Tumor and normal tissue response after low- to moderate-dose SBRT in lung cancer.

At the lower doses (e.g. 12 Gy × 3), very impressive tumor responses and few normal tissue effects were observed by 3 months, as shown in figure 7. Unfortunately, many of these patients ultimately had tumor recurrence.

As the dose was escalated beyond 48 Gy, striking imaging changes began to appear near the treated tumor by around 6–12 months, as shown in figure 8. These seemed to be related to a bronchial toxicity that is not commonly observed after CFRT. In defining the optimal treatment dose, radiographic changes by themselves were not considered dose limiting without concurrent symptoms in the patients. In many cases, radiographic changes could mimic tumor recurrence. However, with no salvage therapy available in this population, patients were followed without further treatment and their disease responses defined later. Repeat PET scans and biopsies showed no evidence of tumor recurrence in the large majority of patients treated at the higher dose levels. In the end, doses of 60–66 Gy in 3 fractions were determined to be generally safe for medically inoperable NSCLC patients.

Indiana University Phase II Study

Upon completion of the phase I study finding a clearly potent dose for SBRT, the Indiana group embarked on a 70-patient phase II study in the same population. The study was aimed at validating toxicity in a larger patient population and determining efficacy, as measured by local control or survival, using the defined dose of 60 Gy for the smaller tumors and 66 Gy for the larger ones. The target control rate for the statistical power calculation was 80%, dramatically higher than the typical 30–45% control seen with CFRT. As part of the phase II study, ventilation/perfusion scans and PET scans were performed in some patients to try to understand how the tumor and the normal tissues responded metabolically, over time in the posttreatment period.

Timmerman · Abdulrahman · Kavanagh · Meyer

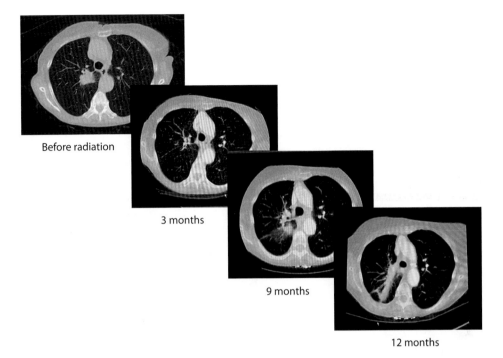

Before radiation

3 months

9 months

12 months

Fig. 8. Tumor and normal tissue response after high-dose SBRT in lung cancer demonstrates posttreatment bronchial injury with downstream effects.

The results of this phase II trial are maturing and yet to be published. However, an important observation was reported in an oral presentation at the American Society for Therapeutic Radiology and Oncology meeting in October, 2005: interim analysis showed that severe toxicity (grades 3–5) was significantly more likely in patients treated for tumors in the regions around the proximal bronchial tree or central chest region, as shown in figure 9. In fact, the risk of severe toxicity was 11 times greater after treatment of central tumors as compared with peripheral tumors.

To date, 3 of the 70 patients (4.3%) have had local recurrence. The Kaplan-Meier 2-year local control rate is 95%. When local failures occurred, they tended to appear 1–2 years after completion of therapy, and other studies of SBRT for lung tumors will require at least this much time or longer to assess the rates of local failure. After a wedge resection, the median time to local failure is about 9 months, indicating that SBRT may be better than wedge resection in relation to local control. Whether SBRT is as effective as lobectomy remains to be seen.

Ongoing Protocols
Several phase I and II prospective trials are ongoing for treating lung neoplasms with SBRT. The willingness of investigators to carry out prospective clinical test-

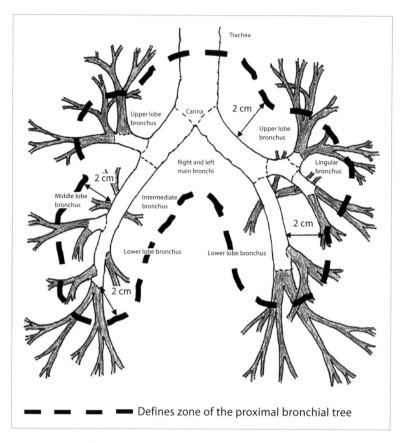

Labels within figure:
- Trachea
- 2 cm
- Upper lobe bronchus
- Carina
- Upper lobe bronchus
- Right and left main bronchi
- Lingular bronchus
- 2 cm
- Middle lobe bronchus
- Intermediate bronchus
- Lower lobe bronchus
- Lower lobe bronchus
- 2 cm
- 2 cm

— — — — — Defines zone of the proximal bronchial tree

Fig. 9. Ablative fractionation is potentially more dangerous in the zone of the proximal bronchial tree, defined by the dashed lines.

ing is rapidly allowing SBRT to find its place in the cancer arsenal. Historically, intracranial radiosurgery has been adopted clinically despite few prospective trials. Even centers with large volumes of patients have entered few of these patients on prospective clinical trials. Unfortunately, this mind-set of relying on retrospective reports, common in the intracranial radiosurgery realm, has limited its acceptance and made it difficult to determine its suitability for specific cases. From a scientific point of view, carefully conducted medium-sized prospective trials are profoundly more valuable than retrospective reports on the treatment of large or even massive populations.

In the RTOG, several trials are ongoing or in development. RTOG 0236 using SBRT for medically inoperable lung cancer in patients with peripherally situated tumors (i.e., those outside of the dashed line in fig. 9) is nearing completion of accrual. This trial restricts tumor size to ≤5 cm. It will likely be replaced by a trial giving systemic therapy adjuvantly along with SBRT in patients at higher risk of systemic relapse. Another trial in patients with centrally situated tumors is being planned that will use a more gentle fractionation scheme for medically inoperable patients. RTOG 0618 is in the finalization process for patients with operable NSCLC. This trial, patterned after RTOG 0236, will include an early assessment for surgical salvage in people with less than ideal response. As such, SBRT is being studied in broader indications for NSCLC by building on the results of careful prospective testing.

A consortium of centers headed by the University of Colorado is studying the use of SBRT in treating patients with lung metastases. A phase I study for up to 3 lesions has been completed and is awaiting publication. In that study, a dose of 60 Gy in 3 fractions was reached without observing dose-limiting toxicities. A phase II trial is under way at the dose level of 60 Gy in 3 fractions. The proper implementation of SBRT for metastatic disease remains controversial. However, the prognostic factors used for employing surgical metastectomy allow a reasonable common ground for selecting SBRT. The use of SBRT for metastatic lesions brings additional clinical concerns, since the effects of treating multiple lesions may not equate to the simple sum of individual treatments. More study is needed to optimize SBRT programs for metastatic disease.

Conclusions

Very little basic science or translational investigation into ablative fractionation or SBRT is described in the literature. For the most part, technological innovation is helpful when treating in so-called parallel functioning tissues. However, when treating adjacent to serially functioning tissues, technological innovation is only partially helpful. More collaboration between physicians, physicists, and radiobiology scientists is needed to move the field forward. Indeed, the roadblocks encountered when treating near the spinal cord, esophagus, trachea and intestines will only be solved by biological innovation.

In conclusion, failure to control the primary tumor is the largest problem in the radiotherapy of lung cancer. There continues to be a sizeable population of frail patients who have localized lung cancers appropriately treated nonsurgically. This group can only increase in number with the wider acceptance of CT screening. Toxicity from SBRT occurs quite late after therapy and is mostly related to serially functioning tissues like hollow tubular organs. With our early reports, we have observed impressive rates of local control. Like toxicity, local failure occurs long after therapy, sometimes years, such that adequate follow-up is necessary to form conclusions about dose and dose response. Finally, more prospective clinical testing and more biological investigation are necessary in order to move SBRT forward as a noninvasive local therapy for lung cancer.

References

1 Mountain CF: A new international staging system for lung cancer. Chest 1986;89:225S–233S.

2 Naruke T, Goya T, Tsuchiya R, et al: Prognosis and survival in resected lung carcinoma based on the new international staging system. J Thorac Cardiovasc Surg 1988;96:440–447.

3 Adebonojo SA, Bowser AN, Moritz DM, et al: Impact of revised stage classification of lung cancer on survival: a military experience. Chest 1999; 115:1507–1513.

4 Arriagada R, Bergman B, Dunant A, et al; International Adjuvant Lung Cancer Trial Collaborative Group: Cisplatin-based adjuvant chemotherapy in patients with completely resected non-small-cell lung cancer. N Engl J Med 2004; 350:351–360.

5 Ginsberg, RJ, Rubinstein LV: Randomized trial of lobectomy versus limited resection for T1 N0 non-small cell lung cancer. Ann Thorac Surg 1995;60:615–623.

6 Armstrong JG, Minsky BD: Radiation therapy for medically inoperable stage I and II non-small cell lung cancer. Cancer Treat Rev 1989;16:247.

7 Haffty BG, Goldberg NB, Gerstley J, et al: Results of radical radiation therapy in clinical stage I, technically operable non-small cell lung cancer. Int J Radiat Oncol Biol Phys 1988;15:69–73.

8 Kaskowitz L, Graham MV, Emami B, et al: Radiation therapy alone for stage I non-small cell lung cancer. Int J Radiat Oncol Biol Phys 1993;27:517.

9 Dosoretz DE, Katin MJ, Blitzer PH, et al: Radiation therapy in the management of medically inoperable carcinoma of the lung: results and implications for future treatment strategies. Int J Radiat Oncol Biol Phys 1992;24:3.

10 Dosoretz DE, Katin MJ, Blitzer PH, et al: Medically inoperable lung carcinoma: the role of radiation therapy. Semin Radiat Oncol 1996;6:98–104.

11 Sibley GS, Jamieson TA, Marks LB, et al: Radiotherapy alone for medically inoperable stage I non-small cell lung cancer: the Duke experience. Int J Radiat Oncol Biol Phys 1998;40:149–154.

12 Dosoretz DE, Galmarini D, Rubenstein JH, et al: Local control in medically inoperable lung cancer: an analysis of its importance in outcome and factors determining the probability of tumor eradication. Int J Radiat Oncol Biol Phys 1993;27: 507–516.

13 Downey RJ: Surgical treatment of pulmonary metastases. Surg Oncol Clin N Am 1999;8:341.

14 Watanabe M, Deguchi H, Sato M, et al: Midterm results of thoracoscopic surgery for pulmonary metastases especially from colorectal cancers. J Laparoendosc Adv Surg Tech A 1998;8:195–200.

15 VanderMeer TJ, Callery MP, Meyers WC: The approach to the patient with single and multiple liver metastases, pulmonary metastases, and intra-abdominal metastases from colorectal carcinoma. Hematol Oncol Clin North Am 1997;11: 759–777.

16 Todd TR: Pulmonary metastectomy. Current indications for removing lung metastases. Chest 1993;103(4 suppl):401S–403S.

17 Ris HB, Vorburger T, Noce R, et al: Surgery and chemotherapy for pulmonary metastases: long-term results from a combined modality approach. Thorac Cardiovasc Surg 1991;39:224–227.

18 Rosenzweig KE, Fox JL, Yorke E, et al: Results of a phase I dose-escalation study using three-dimensional conformal radiotherapy in the treatment of inoperable nonsmall cell lung carcinoma. Cancer 2005;103:2118–2127.

19 Hayman JA, Martel MK, Ten Haken RK, et al: Dose escalation in non-small-cell lung cancer using three-dimensional conformal radiation therapy: update of a phase I trial. J Clin Oncol 2001;19:127–136.

20 Bradley J, Graham MV, Winter K, et al: Toxicity and outcome results of RTOG 9311: a phase I–II dose-escalation study using three-dimensional conformal radiotherapy in patients with inoperable non-small-cell lung carcinoma. Int J Radiat Oncol Biol Phys 2005;61:318–328.

21 Mehta M, Scrimger R, Mackie R, et al: A new approach to dose escalation in non-small-cell lung cancer. Int J Radiat Oncol Biol Phys 2001;49:23–33.

22 Machtay M, Hsu C, Komaki R, et al: Effect of overall treatment time on outcomes after concurrent chemoradiation or locally advanced non-small-cell lung carcinoma: analysis of the Radiation Therapy Oncology Group (RTOG) experience. Int J Radiat Oncol Biol Phys 2005;63: 667–671.

23 Saunders M, Dische S, Barrett A, et al: Continuous hyperfractionated accelerated radiotherapy (CHART) versus conventional radiotherapy in non-small-cell lung cancer: a randomized multicentre trial. CHART Steering Committee. Lancet 1997;350:161–165.

24 Wolbarst AB, Chin LM, Svensson GK: Optimization of radiation therapy: integral-response of a model biological system. Int J Radiat Oncol Biol Phys 1982;8:1761–1769.

25 Yeas RJ, Kalend A: Local stem cell depletion model for radiation myelitis. Int J Radiat Oncol Biol Phys 1988;14:1247–1259.

26 Curran WJ, Moldofsky PJ, Solin LJ: Analysis of the influence of elective nodal irradiation on postirradiation pulmonary function. Cancer 1990;65:2488–2493.

27 Krol AD, Aussems P, Noordijk EM, et al: Local irradiation alone for peripheral stage I lung cancer: could we omit the elective regional nodal irradiation? Int J Radiat Oncol Biol Phys 1996;34: 297–302.

28 Williams TE, Thomas CR Jr, Turrisi AT 3rd: Counterpoint: better radiation treatment of non-small cell lung cancer using new techniques without elective nodal irradiation. Semin Radiat Oncol 2000;10:308–314.

29 Shah RM, Edmonds P, Wechsler RJ, et al: Adjacent parenchymal abnormalities in peripheral bronchogenic carcinoma: correlation of thin-section CT with histology. J Thorac Imaging 2004;19:87–92.

30 Goldstein NS, Ferkowicz M, Kestin L, et al: Wedge resection margin distances and residual adenocarcinoma in lobectomy specimens. Am J Clin Pathol 2003;120:720–724.

31 Giraud P, Antoine M, Larrouy A, et al: Evaluation of microscopic tumor extension in non-small-cell lung cancer for three-dimensional conformal radiotherapy planning. Int J Radiat Oncol Biol Phys 2000;48:1015–1024.

32 Timmerman R, Papiez L, McGarry R, et al: Extracranial stereotactic radioablation: results of a phase I study in medically inoperable stage I non-small cell lung cancer. Chest 2003;124:1946–1955.

Dr. Robert Timmerman
Department of Radiation Oncology, University of Texas Southwestern Medical Center
5801 Forest Park Road
Dallas, TX 75390-9183 (USA)
Tel. +1 214 645 7651, Fax +1 214 645 7622
E-Mail
Robert.Timmerman@UTSouthwestern.edu

Meyer JL (ed): IMRT, IGRT, SBRT – Advances in the Treatment Planning and
Delivery of Radiotherapy. Front Radiat Ther Oncol. Basel, Karger, 2007, vol. 40, pp 386–394

Stereotactic Body Radiotherapy for Unresectable Pancreatic Cancer

Stephanie T. Chang · Karyn A. Goodman · George P. Yang · Albert C. Koong

Department of Radiation Oncology, Stanford University School of Medicine, Stanford, Calif., USA

Abstract

Pancreatic cancer is a devastating disease with few effective treatment modalities. Recent techno-logical advances have made possible the delivery of single-fraction stereotactic body radiotherapy (SBRT) to patients with locally advanced pancreatic tumors. This paper presents experience at Stan-ford University with SBRT for patients with unresectable pancreatic cancer. Pancreatic tumors of up to 100 cm^3 could be treated. Patients achieved greater than 90% local control for the remainder of their lives. Currently, the standard dose for pancreatic tumors treated at this institution is 25 Gy given in a single fraction. Four-dimensional CT and PET scans have been essential for optimal treatment planning. PET-CT scanning may be a more effective method for evaluating tumor response than conventional CT scanning. Adjuvant systemic therapies could be administered in coordination with SBRT. SBRT is an effective method of treating patients resulting in excellent local control. Current re-search is aimed at defining the optimal method of combining this treatment with other cancer therapies.

The low survival rates associated with pancreatic cancer underscore the need for improved treatment strategies. More than 32,000 new cases of pancreatic cancer are diagnosed annually in the USA, and a similar number of deaths due to pancreatic cancer occur each year, indicating that most patients diagnosed with pancreatic cancer eventually succumb to this disease. Overall, the 5-year survival rate for this entire group of patients is less than 5% [1]. Better therapies are clearly needed for this disease. Although there is a TMN staging system for pancreatic cancer, most investigators differentiate patients into three groups: resectable (median survival, 13–20 months), locally advanced (median survival, 9–13 months), and metastatic (median survival, 3–6 months).

At presentation, the majority of patients have either locally advanced or metastatic disease. Since surgical resection is not indicated in these cases, investigators in this field have pursued a strategy of combining chemotherapy and radiation therapy. The Gastrointestinal Tumor Study Group completed a landmark study on 194 patients with unresectable pancreatic adenocarcinoma. They reported that patients treated with a combination of radiotherapy and 5-FU chemotherapy had an improvement in survival compared to patients treated with radiation alone [2]. Another Gastrointestinal Tumor Study Group study revealed improved survival in pancreatic cancer patients treated with chemoradiation compared to chemotherapy alone [3]. These studies established the efficacy of combined modality therapy for the treatment of locally advanced pancreatic cancer.

Because of the high local failure rate reported in these studies (nearly 50%), investigators from Massachusetts General Hospital combined an intraoperative radiotherapy approach with external beam radiotherapy as a strategy to increase the dose intensity of the treatment [4]. In this somewhat heterogeneously treated group of unresectable pancreatic cancer patients (150 patients over 25 years), there was a 15% rate of long-term gastrointestinal complications, primarily in the form of duodenal ulcers. The 5-year overall survival (OS) rate was 4%. However, patients with smaller tumors had an even higher 5-year OS. These results demonstrate that long-term survival in unresectable pancreatic cancer is possible with intensive local therapy.

Investigators at Stanford University have pursued a strategy of stereotactic body radiotherapy (SBRT) as a method of radiation dose intensification. These authors have recently completed a phase I and phase II study using Cyberknife® (Accuray, Sunnyvale, Calif., USA) to deliver a single fraction of radiation for the treatment of unresectable pancreatic cancer [5, 6]. Achieving local control of pancreatic tumors in this population is important to prevent pain, gastric outlet obstruction, and biliary obstruction. The application of SBRT in this patient population is ideal for a number of reasons. First, survival for patients with locally advanced pancreatic cancer is poor, so the duration of any proposed treatment may represent a significant fraction of a patient's remaining life. In patients who have an expected survival of 6 months, it is a significant advantage to compress a typical 5- to 6-week course of conventional radiation into a 1-day SBRT treatment. Furthermore, the likely toxicities associated with any treatment impact a patient's quality of life and represent another important consideration. Finally, since OS is determined by the control of systemic metastases, a rapid course of radiotherapy allows for the administration of more intensive systemic chemotherapy.

Stereotactic Body Radiotherapy Treatment Program

Pancreatic Tumor Fiducial Seed Movement during Respiration
For each Cyberknife treatment, 3–5 gold fiducial seeds are implanted in a patient's tumor. Typically, this procedure is performed on an outpatient basis by interventional radiologists using CT guidance. With normal respiration, pancreatic tumors can move as much as 2–3 cm from inspiration to expiration. During SBRT, it is essential to account for this respiratory-associated movement. The movement is complex and can occur in any dimension. Arbitrary expansion of the treatment margin to account for this movement will result in treating larger volumes, perhaps unnecessarily, which may lead to increased normal tissue toxicity. Conversely, inadequate margins may result in 'marginal misses' and lead to increased local failures. Recognizing the extent of tumor movement allows clinicians to place an 'intelligent' nonuniform margin around the tumor volume. This approach decreases the risk of normal tissue toxicity and minimizes the risk of a 'marginal miss'.

Treatment Planning
During the planning process, a custom immobilization device is constructed for each patient and treatment planning scans are performed using a respiratory-gated or four-dimensional CT approach. The planning scan is a pancreatic protocol CT scan consisting of biphasic imaging and 1.25-mm cuts through the area of interest. In addition, an FDG-PET scan is performed simultaneously. These studies are fused together to define the tumor location with respect to nearby normal tissues in the most optimal manner.

Figure 1a is an example of a typical treatment planning scan for a patient treated by Cyberknife. The red line shows the pancreatic tumor. The densities within this volume are the implanted fiducials. Radiation dose is prescribed to the isodose line that completely surrounds the tumor. In this case, radiation was prescribed to the 70% isodose line represented by the green line. Also shown is the 50% isodose line delineated in purple.

Figure 1b shows the same patient in a different plane, and the 10% isodose line is represented in blue. From these examples, it is evident that there is a rapid drop-off in dose as a function of distance from the isocenter. Since the duodenum is the most sensitive structure in the upper abdomen, every attempt is made to limit the 50% isodose line to one wall of the duodenum. Figure 2 represents a different patient with a tumor in the head of the pancreas. Because of the proximity of the tumor to the duodenum, it is impossible to avoid treating part of the duodenum to a high dose. However, with the use of tuning/avoidance structures, the dose to the contralateral duodenal wall is minimized. Specifically, in this case, only one wall of the duodenum receives 50% of the dose.

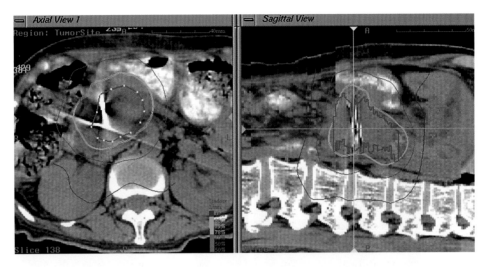

Fig. 1. Isodose curves for a patient with locally advanced pancreatic cancer treated with Cyberknife SBRT. The red line represents the tumor volume. The green line is the 79% isodose line, the purple line is the 50% isodose line, and the blue line is the 10% isodose line. This technique is highly conformal and results in a sharp radiation dose gradient.

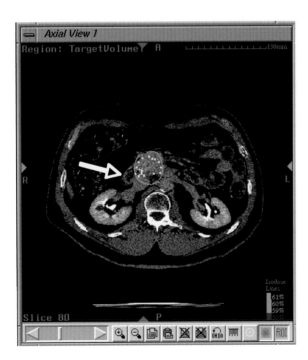

Fig. 2. Relative sparing of the duodenum in this Cyberknife SBRT-treated patient. During the radiation treatment planning, a tuning structure was used to protect the duodenum from the high-dose region. The arrow points to the duodenum.

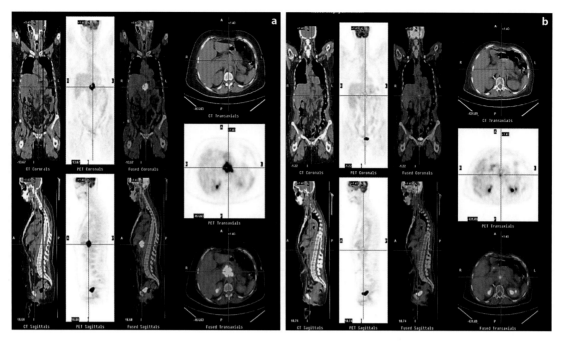

Fig. 3. Example of FDG-PET response in a locally advanced pancreatic cancer patient before (**a**) and after (**b**) Cyberknife SBRT.

Case Study

Patient. A 48-year-old man presented with moderate abdominal pain radiating to the back and weight loss. A CT revealed a mass in the head of the pancreas extending into adjacent soft tissues that measured 4 × 3 × 3 cm.

Treatment. 25 Gy was delivered in a single fraction.

Result. 6 weeks after SBRT, the patient had complete relief of pain and complete resolution of metabolic activity was shown by PET-CT scanning (fig. 3).

Phase I Results

In this dose escalation study, Koong et al. [5] treated 15 patients with locally advanced pancreatic cancer with single fractions of 15, 20 or 25 Gy. Table 1 summarizes the characteristics of the patients enrolled onto this study. The investigators observed minimal acute toxicity, and the maximum tolerated dose was not reached. The study was stopped at 25 Gy because the clinical objective of local control was met. All of the patients treated with this fractionation scheme had their tumors locally controlled or showed lack of local progression from the time of treatment until death [5].

Chang · Goodman · Yang · Koong

Table 1. Characteristics of the patients enrolled on the phase I dose escalation Cyberknife SBRT study

Patient	Age	Location	Previous Tx
1	65	body	none
2	81	head	none
3	57	body	none
4	68	body	none
5	62	body	none
6	80	head	none
7	64	head	none
8	81	head	none
9	50	head	none
10	82	head	gemcitabine, Taxotere
11	43	tail	5-FU/XRT, gemcitabine
12	51	head	none
13	60	head	gastrojejunostomy
14	55	head	5-FU/XRT
15	61	head	gastrojejunostomy

Tx = Treatment; XRT = external beam radiotherapy.

Table 2. The mean dose to abdominal organs in the cohort of pancreatic cancer patients treated at 25 Gy in the phase I study

Structure	Mean dose to 50% Gy	Mean dose to 5% Gy
Duodenum	14.5	22.5
Bowel	1.1	12.3
Liver	0.7	7.0
Left kidney	1.5	5.0
Right kidney	2.0	5.8

Table 2 records the mean dose to different structures in the upper abdomen for patients receiving 25 Gy in the phase I study. Many of the tumors treated were pancreatic head tumors in which the pancreatic head abuts the duodenum, resulting in a portion of the duodenum receiving a high radiation dose. In these patients, half of the duodenum received 14.5 Gy in a single fraction and 5% of the duodenum received 22.5 Gy or higher. The rest of the organs in the upper abdomen received a significantly lower dose.

Table 3. Summary of the patient and radiation treatment parameters for patients from the phase II (IMRT + Cyberknife) study

Patient	Gender	Age	Tumor location	Target volume, ml	D_{max}, Gy
1	M	59	head	64.8	34.86
2	F	50	head	60.4	39.06
3	M	64	head	34.1	35.71
4	M	61	head	n/a	n/a
5	F	82	body	n/a	n/a
6	M	69	head	58.6	43.85
7	F	61	head	49.4	35.71
8	F	54	body	57.2	39.06
9	M	59	body	92.2	36.23
10	F	51	body	32.4	37.31
11	F	78	body	45.7	37.32
12	M	53	head	57.2	35.70
13	F	78	head	50.6	38.45
14	M	52	head	74.1	32.46
15	F	81	head	13.9	35.22
16	F	51	head	61.6	32.04
17	M	79	head	n/a	n/a
18	M	79	head	34.0	39.06
19	F	76	body	28.4	38.46

D_{max} = Maximum dose.

Phase II Study

In 2005, Koong et al. [6] reported a phase II study combining the use of conventionally fractionated radiotherapy using an intensity-modulated radiation therapy (IMRT) technique with a Cyberknife SBRT boost to the primary tumor. The primary tumor and regional lymph nodes were treated using a standard IMRT technique to 45 Gy with concurrent 5-FU. Within 1 month of completing standard chemoradiation therapy, the primary tumor received a 25-Gy single-fraction boost using Cyberknife. Table 3 describes the patient and SBRT treatment parameters for this study. The 3 patients for whom the volume of treatment and the maximum dosage were not recorded were patients who had systemic progression of their disease prior to Cyberknife therapy, and therefore received only conventionally fractionated IMRT followed by gemcitabine-based chemotherapy.

Toxicity
When combining standard chemoradiotherapy with Cyberknife SBRT, there were a larger number of reported toxicities as shown in table 4. Most of the grade 1 toxicities were mild nausea that was self-limited. A larger number of patients experi-

Table 4. Gastrointestinal toxicities as defined by the RTOG Acute Toxicity Scale from patients treated with 45 Gy (concurrent 5-FU, conventionally fractionated IMRT, pancreatic tumor + regional lymph nodes) followed by 25-Gy single-fraction Cyberknife SBRT

Toxicity grade	No.
Grade 0	3
Grade 1	7
Grade 2	3
Grade 3	2
Grade 4	1

enced grade 2 and 3 toxicities. The most clinically significant toxicities occurred in 2 patients who developed duodenal ulcers 4–6 months following therapy. These toxicities were all medically managed.

Phase II Results

A total of 19 patients were enrolled in the phase II study. Three patients progressed systemically after the 5-week course of IMRT prior to SBRT and thus continued onto gemcitabine-based chemotherapy without receiving Cyberknife SBRT. Sixteen patients completed all of the planned therapy, resulting in a median OS of 33 weeks with a median follow-up time of 23 weeks [6].

Fifteen of 16 patients achieved local control of their tumors until death. One patient developed dyspepsia and underwent an endoscopy. The endoscopist described seeing a small duodenal ulcer and a tumor invading into the duodenum, but when the lesion was biopsied, there was no viable tumor. Although it is unclear whether or not this event indeed represents a true local progression, the patient was scored as experiencing a local failure nonetheless [6].

Because it was difficult to assess tumor response by conventional CT criteria (in fact, none of these patients responded by standard CT criteria, they simply had disease stability), the investigators performed functional imaging studies using FDG-PET scans prior to and following radiotherapy as another means of assessing response. In the last 4 consecutive patients enrolled onto this study, the metabolic imaging characteristics of the tumors were used to assess response following SBRT. The treated tumors of all 4 patients demonstrated a significant reduction in FDG-PET activity after radiotherapy.

Figure 3 is an example of a pancreatic cancer patient imaged with FDG-PET before and after SBRT. Prior to Cyberknife treatment (fig. 3a), there was intense hypermetabolic activity in the pancreatic tumor corresponding to the mass seen on the CT scan. Four weeks following treatment (fig. 3b), the metabolic activity from this region was significantly decreased. However, in the corresponding CT scan, there was no significant change in the size of the pancreatic mass. Similar results were found in the last 4 consecutive patients treated on this study. These findings suggest that FDG-PET scans may be a complementary imaging modality in assessing treatment response following high-dose radiotherapy. Additional studies are ongoing to determine the utility of FDG-PET scans in this setting.

Conclusions from the Phase II Study

Overall, the combination of 45 Gy (IMRT, primary tumor and regional lymph nodes) with concurrent 5-FU followed by a 25-Gy SBRT boost to the primary tumor resulted in increased gastrointestinal toxicity. However, over 90% of the evaluable patients did not demonstrate any radiographic evidence of progression until death. Compared to historical controls, OS was not significantly improved due to the rapid progression of systemic disease. More effective systemic therapies are needed to significantly impact OS. Finally, the use of FDG-PET scans to assess treatment response is a promising imaging modality following high-dose radiotherapy for pancreatic tumors.

In addition to the use of Cyberknife SBRT for locally advanced pancreatic cancer, investigators at Stanford University are also conducting studies using a respiratory-gated linear accelerator-based method of SBRT (Trilogy™, Varian Medical Systems, Palo Alto, Calif., USA. In these studies, both Cyberknife- and Trilogy-based SBRT treatment techniques are integrated with systemic gemcitabine-based chemotherapy.

References

1 Jemal A, Murray T, Ward E, et al: Cancer statistics. CA Cancer J Clin 2005;55:10–30.
2 Kalser MH, Ellenberg SS: Pancreatic cancer. Adjuvant combined radiation and chemotherapy following curative resection. Arch Surg 1985; 120:899–903.
3 Gastrointestinal Tumor Study Group: Treatment of locally unresectable carcinoma of the pancreas: comparison of combined modality therapy (chemotherapy plus radiotherapy) to chemotherapy alone. J Natl Cancer Inst 1988;80:751–755.
4 Willett CG, Del Castillo CF, Shih HA, et al: Long-term results of intraoperative electron beam irradiation (IOERT) for patients with unresectable pancreatic cancer. Ann Surg 2005;241:295–299.
5 Koong AC, Le QT, Ho A, et al: Phase I study of stereotactic radiosurgery in patients with locally advanced pancreatic cancer. Int J Radiat Oncol Biol Phys 2004;58:1017–1021.
6 Koong AC, Christofferson E, Le QT, et al: Phase II study to assess the efficacy of conventionally fractionated radiotherapy followed by a stereotactic radiosurgery boost in patients with locally advanced pancreatic cancer. Int J Radiat Oncol Biol Phys 2005;63:320–323.

Dr. Albert C. Koong
Stanford University School of Medicine,
Department of Radiation Oncology
875 Blake Wilbur Dr., MC 5847
Stanford, CA 94305 (USA)
Tel. +1 650 498 7703, Fax +1 650 725 8231
E-Mail akoong@stanford.edu

Meyer JL (ed): IMRT, IGRT, SBRT – Advances in the Treatment Planning and
Delivery of Radiotherapy. Front Radiat Ther Oncol. Basel, Karger, 2007, vol. 40, pp 395–406

Prostate Cancer Therapy with Stereotactic Body Radiation Therapy

Todd Pawlicki · Cristian Cotrutz · Christopher King

Department of Radiation Oncology, Stanford University School of Medicine,
Stanford, Calif., USA

Abstract

The purpose of this work is to provide background and current directions of image guidance for localized prostate cancer treatments. We will describe the external beam hypofractionation protocol for localized prostate cancer currently in progress at Stanford University and the biological bases for large fractions in an abbreviated treatment course for prostate cancer. The need for image guidance in external beam prostate cancer treatments will be discussed. Our experience with two image-guided implementations of hypofractionated radiotherapy for localized prostate cancer will be presented. These are the Cyberknife System (Accuray, Inc.) and the Trilogy System (Varian Medical Systems, Inc.).

In this work, we describe a hypofractionation protocol for stereotactic body radiotherapy for prostate cancer. This protocol, initiated by one of the authors (C.K.), has received institutional review board (IRB) approval from our institution. We will discuss the justification for a prostate hypofractionation protocol, its implementation, and our early clinical results. Future methods of radiation delivery and imaging for prostate hypofractionation will also be presented.

Patients enrolled in this protocol are treated on the Cyberknife (Accuray Inc., Sunnyvale, Calif., USA). Previous articles by Dr. Timmerman et al. [this vol., pp. 368–385] and by Dr. Kavanagh et al. [this vol., pp. 340–351] have given discussions on the pertinent radiobiology, and together with Dr. Smith's paper [this vol., pp. 143–161] on the Cyberknife technology provide excellent background for this report.

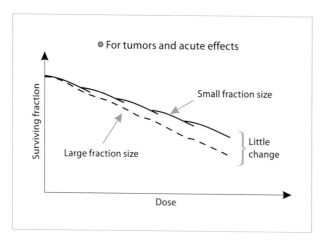

Fig. 1. Schematic of the fractionated effect of radiation for tumors and acute effects.

Radiotherapy Fractionation and Prostate Cancer

It is well known that the curve for the single dose-response cell survival relationship can be described by a linear-quadratic (LQ) model [1] of the form $\exp(-\alpha d - \beta d^2)$. The surviving fraction for a multifraction regimen is given by $[\exp(-\alpha d - \beta d^2)]^n$. As shown in figure 1, the LQ model illustrates that a smaller fraction size will have a relatively small benefit in reducing acute effects. Unfortunately, a smaller fraction size also gives a component of tumor sparing. For late effects, on the other hand, smaller radiation doses per fraction result in comparatively greater tissue sparing (fig. 2). This is due to the 'steeper curvature' of the curve for late effects compared with tumor or acute effects (i.e., a smaller α/β ratio for late effects). The net benefit of fractionation is that we can increase the therapeutic ratio (tumor control/complications). One can say that by fractionating radiotherapy we are increasing this therapeutic ratio not by increasing the effectiveness of dose to the tumor, but rather by reducing the late effects in normal tissues. To summarize, fraction size is the dominant factor in determining normal tissue late effects. To some extent, a smaller fraction size allows a reduction of acute effects as well.

α/β for Prostate Cancer and the Rationale for Hypofractionation
The α/β ratio is a measure of tissue sensitivity to dose fraction size, which comes from the LQ model of cell survival discussed previously. The uniqueness of prostate cancer can be found in the α/β ratio. It has been suggested that the α/β ratio for prostate cancer is approximately 1.5, and that it is significantly lower than for all other cancers [2–5] (fig. 3). This encourages us to consider treating prostate

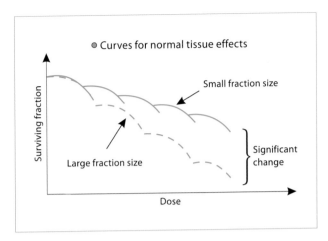

Fig. 2. Schematic showing the fractionation effect of radiation for normal tissue late effects.

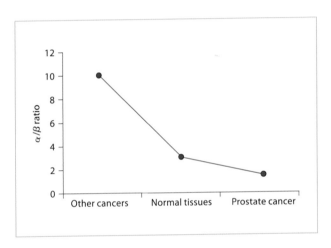

Fig. 3. The α/β ratio of prostate cancer compared to normal tissues and other cancers.

cancer on a fractionation scheme different from those used for other cancers. The biologically effective dose (BED) is given by

$$BED = nd \cdot \left(1 + \frac{d}{\alpha/\beta}\right),$$

which relates the total dose *(nd)* to the relative effectiveness of a radiotherapy regimen.

Table 1 shows the total dose, dose per fraction, and number of fractions in the leftmost column. These data are used to determine the BEDs for the different radiotherapy regimens. For conventional fractionations, e.g. 74 Gy at 2 Gy per

Table 1. Different fractionation regimens for prostate cancer: the BEDs for acute effects, late effects and tumor control are compared

D/d/n[1]	BED – prostate ($\alpha/\beta = 1.5$)	BED – NTLE ($\alpha/\beta = 3$)	BED – acute effects ($\alpha/\beta = 10$)
74 Gy/2 Gy/37	172.6	123.3	88.8
36.15 Gy/7.23 Gy/5	211.5	123.3	62.5
90 Gy/2 Gy/45	210.0	150	108

NTLE = Normal tissue late effects.
[1] Total dose/dose per fraction/number of fractions.

fraction for 37 fractions, if we use the BED to determine the same normal tissue late effects (i.e., 123.3), we see that a hypofractionated schedule (i.e., 7.23 Gy × 5 = 36.15 Gy) provides a greater effective dose to the tumor and, at the same time, a lower effective dose for acute effects.

In fact, the same BED to the prostate as in our protocol (211.5) would result in entirely unacceptable levels of normal tissue late effects and acute effects if it came from a regimen of 2.0 Gy per fraction.

In developing our program of hypofractionation for prostate cancer, our biologic analysis has added an insightful basis for our work. However, other factors come into play in selecting this regimen of hypofractionation for clinical use. These include the clinical evidence that hypofractionation is an acceptable treatment regimen for prostate cancer from experience with high-dose-rate brachytherapy, as well as from experience with an external beam regimen of 6 Gy × 6 fractions [6].

Stanford's Hypofractionation Protocol for Prostate Cancer

Patients eligible for entry on the hypofractionation protocol are at a low risk [T1c or T2a, initial prostate-specific antigen (PSA) level ≤10 ng/ml, biopsy Gleason score ≤3 + 3]. The dose schedule is 7.25 Gy per fraction for 5 fractions to a total dose of 36.25 Gy. Radiotherapy is given every other day. This protocol has received IRB approval prior to commencement [7]. All patients are currently treated on the Cyberknife. However, the IRB protocol was written without restriction concerning the radiation delivery device used; the only constraint was to have proper accounting of the prostate motion, and conformal isodoses.

Prostate Motion

Throughout this volume, there are many excellent discussions on inter- and intrafraction organ motion. For the prostate, the dominant uncertainty in its position is due to interfraction motion, that is, the day-to-day setup uncertainty of the patient. In general, intrafraction motion can be accounted for with an acceptably sized planning target volume. Another important point is that the magnitude of prostate motion is not correlated with respiration in any significant way. The prostate can experience large (>1.0 cm) stochastic motion during a radiotherapy fraction.

At our institution, we have already implanted 3 gold fiducials into the prostate for its daily localization in patients treated with conventional fractionation intensity-modulated radiation therapy (IMRT). This is standard procedure at many centers. Prior to delivery of every fraction, the therapists acquire an anterior-posterior (AP) and lateral image set and localize the detected fiducials, then they overlay the set onto the planning digitally reconstructed radiographs (DRRs). The patient is then shifted by the amount specified in the image overlay. Two additional images are acquired to verify that the shift has been done correctly. However, at the time of the second set of images, we have found that sometimes the fiducials have shifted again (assuming that the therapists have made the correct table movements). This means that the fiducials in the DRRs do not overlay with the fiducials in the acquired AP and lateral images for the patient shift verification. Therefore, the therapists are sometimes required to make more than one shift on a given treatment day. This can be interpreted as prostate motion during the time needed to acquire an AP and lateral image set, match the fiducials between the DRRs and acquired images, shift the patient, and acquire a second AP and lateral image set to verify that the table movements are correct. Thus, there is a certain degree of intrafraction prostate motion. Many investigators have determined that this can be due to effects such as gas passing through the rectum or relaxing of the pelvic muscle by the patient. Figure 4 shows just such a situation for one of our conventionally treated prostate cases with fiducials. Intrafraction prostate motion is stochastic, and prostate motion cannot be predicted with a mathematical model or tracked using external markers. Together, these findings suggest that one must track the prostate in real time for optimal localization during therapy.

Why Use the Cyberknife for a Hypofractionated Prostate Protocol?
The primary reason to use the Cyberknife for the prostate protocol is image guidance. One can place fiducials inside of a target and the Cyberknife has the ability to automatically track the motion of the fiducials. At this time, no other commercially available external radiation delivery system has the ability to automatically track fiducial markers by orthogonal kilovoltage (kV) imaging. This tracking is done in 'real time'. Localization of the prostate (acquired approximately every 30–90 s) is determined by the three gold fiducial seeds placed into the prostate, and the position of the robot is automatically adjusted based on detected changes of the prostate position.

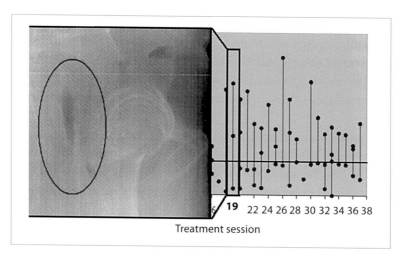

Fig. 4. Serial localization and repositioning of the prostate (using fiducials as a surrogate) during the fraction because of stochastic prostate motion due to rectal gas.

Treatment Planning

We have previously mentioned that three gold fiducials are placed by the urologists on an outpatient basis. About 1 week following these implants, CT image sets are acquired at 1.25 mm slice thickness. Treatment planning is done using the Cyberknife system. Our planning target volume is 5 mm around the prostate except for 3 mm posteriorly. Each patient is given the Expanded Prostate Cancer Index Composite and the International Prostate Symptom Score validated questionnaires, and PSA levels are obtained every 3 months after therapy.

Treatment Delivery

The Cyberknife is shown in figure 5a. Also shown is a typical set of beam orientations for a single prostate treatment (fig. 5b). Typical treatments consist of about 100–120 individual beams for each patient. Patients are immobilized with a Vac-Loc bag. We do not use additional external immobilization devices to fix the external surface of the patient. The goal in using the Cyberknife is to track the prostate movement, which is due to internal organ motion and is not necessarily affected by the external body positioning of the patient. Planning time on the Cyberknife system takes about 1 h for the initial plan. Two to four iterations are typically required, depending on the experience of the treatment planner. Total treatment time is about 40 min from the moment that the patient is first moved onto the table until the last beam. Imaging is done every 5–7 beams, which corresponds to about every 30–90 s.

The dose distributions produced by the Cyberknife are similar to those of a conventional IMRT planning and delivery system. Later in this article, we will

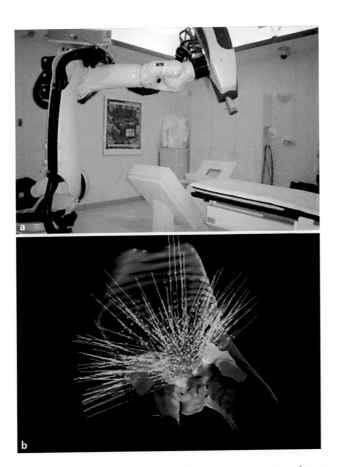

Fig. 5. a The Cyberknife. **b** The typical beam orientations for prostate cancer treatment.

show a dose-volume histogram (DVH) comparison of treatment delivered by the Cyberknife and by linear accelerator multileaf collimator-based IMRT. There are subtle differences in the dose distributions produced by each system, but a detailed investigation of those differences is outside the scope of this presentation.

Cases and Early Prostate-Specific Antigen Responses
The first patient was treated on this protocol in December of 2003. At the time of this writing, 23 patients had been treated. Their average age was 65 years (range, 48–73). All had experienced grade 1 genitourinary toxicity and an average gastrointestinal toxicity score of 1.3 (range, 1–2). The average follow-up thus far is only 6 months (range, 2–15). Since this is short, one cannot draw definitive conclusions, but certainly the treatments so far have been well tolerated. Figure 6 shows a plot of the relative PSA values declining with months following radiotherapy. The fall-off in these values is similar to that seen following conventional radiotherapy.

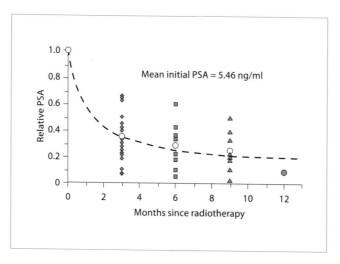

Fig. 6. Relative falloff of PSA since radiotherapy.

A Possible Linear Accelerator-Based Solution for Stereotactic Therapy of Prostate Cancer

The Varian Trilogy System (Varian Medical Systems Inc., Palo Alto, Calif., USA) is now installed at Stanford, and we are considering this option to treat our prostate patients on our hypofractionated protocol. The main question that we are interested in is: can we do 'real-time' fiducial tracking with the Trilogy System? The onboard imaging (OBI) system from Varian is similar to the solutions developed by other vendors. The Trilogy System (shown schematically in fig. 7) consists of a kV X-ray tube, flat panel detector, amorphous silicon detector, and software for two-dimensional image matching. A cone beam CT reconstruction module is also available. A conventional IMRT plan can deliver an adequate dose distribution. Figure 8 shows a 7-field, 15-MV IMRT dose distribution DVH compared with the 6-MV Cyberknife dose distribution DVH for a patient. One can obtain conformal target coverage just the same as with the Cyberknife. In this particular patient, we were able to obtain slightly better dose distributions with IMRT planning, shown with solid lines, compared with the Cyberknife DVHs shown with circles. However, the main point is that the dose distribu-tions produced by these two systems are roughly equivalent. There are other techniques to be evaluated, such as conformal arcs or other optimization procedures, that may give one system a benefit over the other. Now, in terms of conventional IMRT treatment planning, the two systems are fairly equivalent.

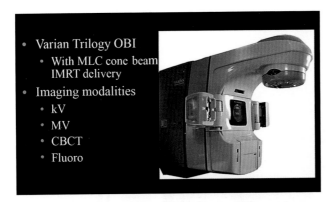

Fig. 7. Varian Trilogy with OBI shown attached to the gantry as 'arms'. One side is the kV X-ray source and the other is the kV amorphous silicon detector. The MV imager is distal to the treatment beam. MLC = Multileaf collimator; CBCT = cone beam CT.

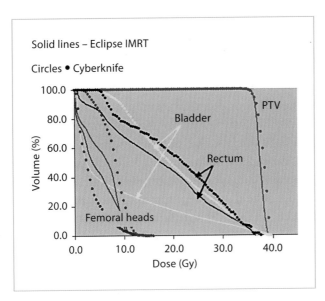

Fig. 8. DVH comparison for a single patient of the Cyberknife versus linear accelerator multileaf collimator-based IMRT. PTV = Planning target volume.

Linear Accelerator-Based Treatment and Digitally Reconstructed Radiograph and Megavoltage-Kilovoltage Image Matching

To perform 'real-time' imaging on the Trilogy, we consider imaging the fiducials and shifting the patient if necessary prior to each treatment beam angle. Because the megavoltage (MV) and kV imagers are orthogonal to one another, at each beam angle an orthogonal image set can easily be acquired. The OBI software

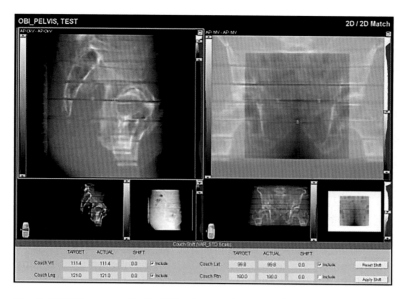

OBI_PELVIS, TEST   2D / 2D Match

	TARGET	ACTUAL	SHIFT			TARGET	ACTUAL	SHIFT		
Couch Vrt	111.4	111.4	0.0	☑ Include	Couch Lat	99.8	99.8	0.0	☑ Include	Reset Shift
Couch Lng	121.0	121.0	0.0	☑ Include	Couch Rtn	100.0	100.0	0.0	☐ Include	Apply Shift

Fig. 9. MV-kV image set in the OBI software showing information about table positions.

will allow you to either manually or automatically fuse the images that are acquired on the accelerator to either DRR or other kV image sets. At this time, the
manual image match is used because it is fairly easy for the operator to determine
when a match has been made using fiducials. The table is translated if necessary
based on those images, and then for each beam angle this process is repeated. The
steps are as follows: (1) move gantry to next treatment beam angle, (2) acquire
MV/kV orthogonal image set, (3) use manual image match to determine fiducial
position, (4) translate the table if necessary, (5) return to step 1 until treatment is
completed.

   Figure 9 shows the Varian OBI user interface, with the DRR and the kV images
acquired. In the Varian implementation of this system, orthogonal images are
linked together along their common axis. Conventionally, an AP image is acquired as well as a lateral image. Any patient shift identified on one image is not
reflected in the orthogonal image. On the new OBI system, however, any patient
shift that is identified along the common axis is immediately reflected in the
orthogonal image.

Linear Accelerator Treatment and Imaging Time
Until now, we have used phantom studies to become familiar with the software
and overcome any difficulties encountered in learning to use the new software
and new technologies. We found that putting a patient (or our phantom) on the
table took about 4 min. We know that on a day-to-day basis, the first shift to

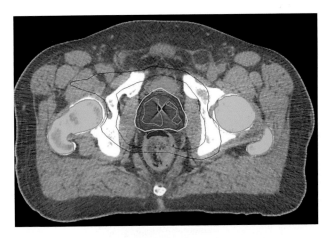

Fig. 10. The patient's axial CT scan through the prostate with Cyberknife treatment isodose overlay. The plan is normalized to the global dose maximum and the isodose lines shown are 97, 90, 70, 50, and 30% of the maximum.

resolve interfraction prostate motion is going to be the largest shift. For each subsequent field, the time spent acquiring the MV-kV image set and moving or evaluating those images using the software takes about 1 min per field. This will be slightly longer if one actually has to make a shift for each individual field. The total treatment time in terms of gantry motion, mode up, beam on, and moving to the next gantry angle takes about 1.4 min. Thus, the total treatment time, if we add all of these things together, is around 16 min for a 5-field IMRT plan. Five fields may not be enough to achieve an adequate dose distribution, due to excessive peripheral dose in the patient or need for better rectal sparing. Furthermore, real patient treatments always require additional time, compared with phantom studies. What these preliminary data do show – at least in terms of the Cyberknife with 'real-time' imaging – is that treatments can be duplicated in a similar time frame with MV-kV image matching using the Varian Trilogy System.

Case Study, Cyberknife

Patient. A 65-year-old man with clinical stage T1c prostate cancer, initial PSA level of 7.2 ng/ml and a biopsy Gleason score of 3 + 3 present in 3 out of 12 cores. His prostate measured 42 cm^3 on TRUS. A bone scan was not done. Options offered to the patient were radical prostatectomy, permanent brachytherapy, IMRT or participation in a clinical trial using hypofractionated stereotactic radiotherapy.

Treatment. Hypofractionated stereotactic radiotherapy, total dose 3,625 cGy in 5 fractions of 725 cGy each delivered every other day using the Cyberknife.

Early Results. Acute rectal and urinary irritative side effects were well tolerated, and by 4 months were nearly completely resolved. By 18 months, his PSA level had steadily declined to a value of 0.7 ng/ml (fig. 10).

References

1 Hall EJ: Radiobiology for the Radiologist, ed 4. Philadelphia, Lippincott Company, 1994.
2 Brenner DJ, Hall EJ: Fractionation and protraction for radiotherapy of prostate carcinoma. Int J Radiat Oncol Biol Phys 1999;43:1095–1101.
3 King CR, Fowler JF: A simple analytic derivation suggests that prostate cancer alpha/beta ratio is low. Int J Radiat Oncol Biol Phys 2001;51:213–214.
4 Fowler J, Chappell R, Ritter M: Is alpha/beta for prostate tumors really low? Int J Radiat Oncol Biol Phys 2001;50:1021–1031.
5 Brenner DJ, et al: Direct evidence that prostate tumors show high sensitivity to fractionation (low alpha/beta ratio), similar to late-responding normal tissue. Int J Radiat Oncol Biol Phys 2002; 52:6–13.
6 Lloyd-Davis RW, Collins CD, Swan AV: Carcinoma of prostate treated by a radical external beam radiotherapy using hypofractionation: 22 years' experience (1962–1984). Urology 1990;36: 107–111.
7 King CR, et al: Hypofractionated Radiotherapy for Localized Prostate Cancer. Stanford, Stanford University IRB Panel, 2004.

Dr. Todd Pawlicki
Department of Radiation Oncology
Stanford University School of Medicine
875 Blake Wilbur Dr., MC 5847
Stanford, CA 94305 (USA)
Tel. +1 650 498 7898, Fax +1 650 498 4015
E-Mail tpaw@reyes.stanford.edu

Meyer JL (ed): IMRT, IGRT, SBRT – Advances in the Treatment Planning and
Delivery of Radiotherapy. Front Radiat Ther Oncol. Basel, Karger, 2007, vol. 40, pp 407–414

Spinal and Paraspinal Lesions: The Role of Stereotactic Body Radiotherapy

Iris C. Gibbs

Department of Radiation Oncology, Stanford University, Stanford, Calif., USA

Abstract

Stanford University has a long legacy of contributions to the field of radiation therapy. The Cyberknife image-guided robotic radiosurgery is the latest in a series of radiation advancements that allows for improved treatment of tumors. Here we present a decade of experience in using robotic radiosurgery to treat 295 spinal and paraspinal lesions including spinal metastases, benign intradural tumors, and arteriovenous malformations. Our analysis of clinical outcomes confirms the promise of this technology in terms of efficacy and safety.

Stanford University and the Cyberknife

In 1994, the first prototype robotic image-guided radiosurgery system known as Cyberknife was introduced at Stanford University Medical Center [1]. Since then, over 2,000 patients and nearly 2,500 lesions have been treated. The introduction of this image-guided therapy device continues a long legacy of contributions to the fields of imaging and radiation therapy from this institution, from the early adoption of diagnostic X-rays to the development and use of the first megavoltage medical linear accelerator in the Northern hemisphere [2].

In a collaborative effort during the 1990s, Dr. John Adler of Stanford's Department of Neurosurgery worked alongside physicists and robotics experts to create the concept of a frameless radiosurgery machine that would eliminate the need for rigid skeletal fixation used in other radiosurgery systems. After several years of development, the prototype Cyberknife (then the 'Neurotron 100') was installed in 1994. Stanford's clinical experience has contributed to the appreciation of the accuracy of the Cyberknife and to the 2001 FDA clearance approval of the device for treatment of tumors 'anywhere in the body where radiation treatment is indicated'.

From 1994 to 2005, a total of 2,071 patients with 2,473 lesions were treated. This experience began gradually; during the first 5 years, only 92 patients were treated. After the FDA clearance in 2001, the volume of patients more than doubled, and since 2004 approximately 500 patients have been treated annually.

Because the Cyberknife system does not rely on rigid patient fixation from a stereotactic frame, tumors outside of the intracranial compartment can be treated with an approach similar to intracranial lesions. Since the first patient was treated on Stanford's Cyberknife, radiosurgery has been redefined to include the highly accurate treatment of not only brain tumors but also extracranial tumors including those that move with respiration. Over the past 5 years, the most rapid increase in our use of Cyberknife has been in treatment of spine, lung, pancreas, and prostate lesions. Here we review our Cyberknife experience (1994–2005) for the treatment of spinal and paraspinal lesions.

Spine Lesions 1995–2005

Spinal treatments present a significant challenge due to the proximity of the spinal cord and its sensitivity to radiation. We used hypofractionated courses of treatment to meet this challenge. As pioneers of image-guided spinal radiosurgery, we had only our clinical judgment and our knowledge of alpha/beta estimates for the spinal cord and normal tissues to devise individualized treatment schedules. In general, hypofractionation over 2–5 days was used when the single-fraction maximum dose to the spinal cord would have exceeded 10 Gy.

From 1994 to 2005, a total of 295 benign and malignant spinal lesions were treated on an institutional review board-approved registry protocol. These consisted of meningiomas, nerve sheath tumors, metastatic tumors, chordomas, arteriovenous malformations (AVMs), hemangioblastomas, and other lesions.

Prior to September 2004, spinal lesions above the level of C3 were treated with the skull tracking system used for brain tumors, while the fiducial-based image tracking was used for spinal lesions below the level of C3. In this second approach, patients first underwent percutaneous placement of 3–5 stainless steel, screw-shaped fiducials (Accuray, Inc.) into the posterior elements of adjacent vertebrae under fluoroscopic guidance. This minor outpatient procedure was typically done 2–5 days prior to treatment. After September 2004, when the XSight™ hierarchical mesh tracking system was introduced, fiducials were no longer required for targeting. With this software, the imaging system correlates images of bone anatomy rather than implanted fiducials.

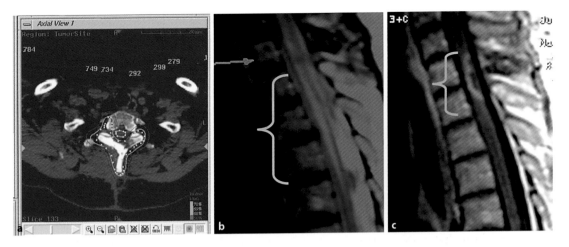

Fig. 1. Spinal cord injury after Cyberknife 21.5 Gy in 2 fractions for T1 spinous process breast metastasis. **a** Radiosurgery treatment plan where the target lesion is shown in red and the prescription isodose in green. **b** Edema within the spinal cord. **c** Contrast-enhancing spinal cord abnormality.

Spinal Metastases

Of the metastatic spinal tumors, a cohort of 74 patients with 102 lesions and a mean follow-up of 9 months has recently been reviewed. There were 77 vertebral column lesions, 11 intramedullary lesions, and 14 extramedullary lesions. Most of the lesions emanated from breast, lung, renal cell or gastrointestinal primary sites. Fifty patients had received prior radiotherapy within or adjacent to the treatment site. Patients were treated to 16–25 Gy in 1–5 fractions and were followed clinically every 1–3 months. Pain relief was assessed by a visual analog scale. Fifty-four of the 62 symptomatic patients had pain as a component of their symptoms. Fifty-two (84%) of the patients who presented with symptoms reported improvement or resolution of them after treatment. Over half of the patients experienced further systemic disease progression. No patient required further radiation or surgical intervention; although 2 patients experienced worsened symptoms.

Three patients developed new spinal cord complications. The first patient to develop a spinal complication was a 60-year-old woman with breast cancer who had received prior radiation therapy to the breast and an adjacent left supraclavicular field approximately 6 years before presenting with an isolated spinous process metastasis at T1 (fig. 1). This lesion was treated with 21.5 Gy over 2 fractions. Approximately 6 months after the treatment, the patient started having abnormal spinal cord symptoms, initially sensory, and MRI showed significant cord edema at the level of the treatment site. At 6 months, the MRI scan showed enhancement in the spinal cord overlying that area. At 2 years, the contrast-enhancing abnormality as well as the spinal cord edema completely resolved, leaving myelomalacia at that level of the spinal cord. The patient has regained some strength, but remains with limited mobility.

The other 2 patients who developed complications had T5 metastatic breast cancer and T6 metastatic renal cell carcinoma, respectively. Each showed clinical and radiographic signs of myelopathy at 6 months and 10 months, respectively. Both patients had received antiangiogenic or epidermal growth factor inhibitor-targeted therapy within 2 months of developing clinical myelopathy. The degree to which this may have contributed to the myelopathy is unknown.

When we analyzed the potential spinal cord dose-volume relationships that might predict complications, we determined no significant relation of total dose or average dose. However, we observed that no complication occurred when the volume of the spinal cord receiving a biologically equivalent dose of 12 Gy in a single fraction (i.e. BED_3 of 58 Gy) was less than 0.15 cm^3. Therefore, our current goals in treatment planning are to minimize the volume of the spinal cord receiving a dose of 10 Gy to approximately 0.3 cm^3.

Case Study 1
Patient. A 55-year-old man with metastatic lung cancer, previously treated with neoadjuvant chemotherapy followed by lobectomy, presented with a persistent, isolated T11 vertebral body spinal metastasis causing pain.

Treatment. 20 Gy was prescribed to the 82% isodose surface in 2 fractions to the T11 vertebral body lesion of a volume of 6.67 cm^3 (modified conformity index = 1.53; maximum dose = 24.4 Gy; maximum point dose to the spinal cord = 17.9 Gy in 2 fractions). The volume of the spinal cord receiving a biologically equivalent dose of 10 Gy in a single fraction was <0.004 cm^3.

Result. The patient is alive at 15 months after treatment with complete back pain relief, though he has other areas of systemic metastases (fig. 2).

Benign Tumors

A cohort of 51 patients with 55 benign extra-axial, intradural tumors that we treated and followed for at least 6 months has recently been reviewed [3]. These cases included 30 schwannomas, 9 neurofibromas, and 16 meningiomas. A dose of 16–30 Gy, given over 1–5 consecutive daily radiosurgical treatments, was delivered to tumors ranging in size from 0.136 to 24.6 cm^3. The 9 neurofibromas were in 7 patients with neurofibromatosis type 1. Ten patients with neurofibromatosis type 2 had 12 schwannomas.

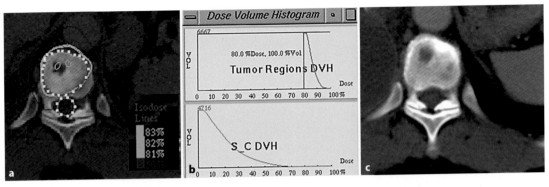

Fig. 2. a Axial slice from the radiosurgery treatment plan with superimposed prescription isodose line (green) and 50% isodose line (purple) showing the rapid falloff of dose. **b** The dose-volume histograms for the target and spinal cord. **c** A posttreatment axial CT slice at 15 months shows the stability of the bone.

Although 40% of the schwannomas were in neurofibromatosis type 2 patients, 82% were symptomatically stable or improved overall. In the neurofibroma patients, the response rate was not as high. Half of these patients developed worsening symptoms. In patients with meningiomas, most achieved stable to improved symptoms. Two lesions in this series showed transient radiographic increase in size that required no intervention. Three other tumors required surgical intervention because of radiographic (1 patient) or symptomatic (2 patients) progression. One patient had a lamina fracture as a complication of the fiducial placement. One patient with a cervicothoracic meningioma developed new myelopathy after receiving a maximum dose of 18 Gy in 3 fractions.

The typical response after spinal radiosurgery for benign lesions is illustrated in figure 3. A cervical schwannoma shows central hypointensity 1 year after receiving 19 Gy in 2 fractions.

Case Study 2
Patient. A 55-year-old man with left C4–5 schwannoma.

Treatment. 18 Gy was prescribed to the 80% isodose surface in a single fraction to the extramedullary tumor of a volume of 2.178 cm^3 (modified conformity index = 1.46; maximum dose = 22.5 Gy; maximum point dose to the spinal cord = 18 Gy). The volume of the spinal cord receiving a biologically equivalent dose of 10 Gy in a single fraction was <0.3 cm^3.

Result. The patient remains asymptomatic 3 years after treatment. Follow-up MRI shows a moderate decrease in tumor size (fig. 4).

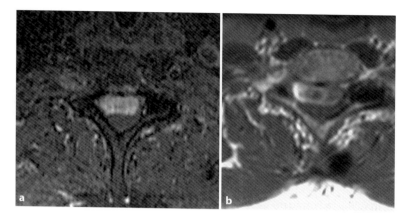

Fig. 3. C7-T1 spinal schwannoma. **a** Pretreatment MRI scan illustrating a homogeneous contrast-enhancing tumor ventral to the spinal cord. **b** One year after treatment, a central hypointensity is seen on MRI. This radiographic change is characteristically seen in the meningiomas, schwannomas, and neurofibromas as soon as 6 months after treatment with Cyberknife.

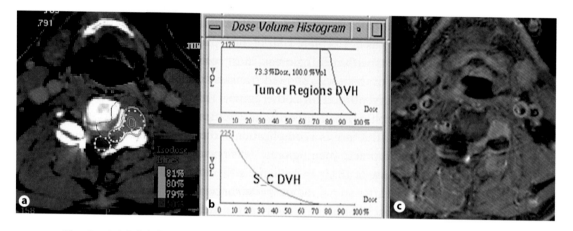

Fig. 4. a Axial slice from the radiosurgery treatment plan with superimposed prescription isodose line (green) and 50% isodose line (purple). **b** The dose-volume histograms for the target and spinal cord. **c** A posttreatment axial MRI slice at 2 years is stable.

Spinal Arteriovenous Malformation

Based on the favorable impact of radiosurgery in the management of cerebral AVMs, the first intramedullary spinal cord AVM was treated in 1997. When microsurgery or embolization was no longer a viable option, radiosurgery was offered. A cohort of 15 intramedullary spinal cord AVMs, treated from 1997 to 2005, has recently been reviewed [4]. There were 9 cervical, 3 thoracic, and 3 conus medullaris lesions. The target lesion was identified on the treatment planning contrast CT as correlated with diagnostic angiography. Because of the intramedullary location, the radiosurgical treatment was hypofractionated in 2–5 daily sessions. The mean prescription dose was 20 Gy. The radiosurgery treatment schedule evolved over time, favoring a fewer number of sessions. In this way, the relative biologically equivalent dose gradually escalated over the course of this study. Patients were followed annually by MRI, and spinal angiography was repeated at 3 years after treatment. After a mean follow-up of 28 months (range, 3–59 months), 8 lesions had completed the 3-year follow-up with angiography, and only 1 of the 8 showed complete obliteration. It is noteworthy that while more than two thirds of patients initially presented with hemorrhage (some with multiple hemorrhages), there were no further hemorrhages or neurological deteriorations after the Cyberknife procedure. One patient was retreated after 3 years, and 4 years later (now 7 years after initial treatment), there remains a small nidus. This patient remains neurologically intact without further hemorrhage. Among the intramedullary spinal cord AVMs, there have been no spinal complications of therapy.

Conclusion

Though much will be gained by further follow-up, these data suggest that image-guided radiosurgery for spinal tumors and lesions is feasible and relatively safe overall. Our results, along with emerging data from other institutions, will add to the understanding of the radiation response of the spinal cord and the factors that may augment that response. In the series presented here, a total of 4 patients developed myelopathy. Two of these had prior irradiation and 2 were exposed to agents that might alter the local vasculature. These factors may be important in determining the radiation tolerance of the spinal cord. Interestingly, however, within the cohort of patients with intramedullary spinal cord AVMs, which were treated with quite aggressive courses of hypofractionated radiosurgery, no myelopathy developed. Since many of these lesions were small (<1.5 cm^3), these findings might also suggest a dose-volume response of the spinal cord. We await longer follow-up and more detailed analyses to confirm these assertions.

Guidelines for Clinical Practice

- Spinal tumors that cause symptomatic spinal cord compression should not be treated by radiosurgery.

- Radiosurgery can be used to treat previously irradiated patients. It is advisable to avoid reirradiation within 6 months of prior radiation unless radiosurgery is being used as a boost, in which case the prescription dose should be lowered.

- Until further evidence emerges, care should be taken to avoid spinal radiosurgery when targeted antiangiogenic therapy is planned within 2 months of the procedure.

- Though dose schedules continue to evolve, any treatment schedule should limit the volume of spinal cord that receives the biologic equivalent dose of 10 Gy in a single fraction to less than 0.3 cm^3 when treating extramedullary tumors.

- Though no complications occurred among intramedullary tumors or arteriovenous malformations of up to 5 cm^3, intramedullary lesions >1.5 cm^3 in volume should be routinely avoided.

References

1 Adler JR Jr, Murphy MJ, Chang SD, et al: Image-guided robotic radiosurgery. Neurosurgery 1999; 44:1299–1306.
2 Jones H, Illes J, Northway W: A history of the Department of Radiology at Stanford University. AJR Am J Roentgenol 1995;164:753–760.
3 Dodd RL, Ryu M, Kamnerdsupaphon P, Gibbs IC, Chang SD, Adler JR Jr: CyberKnife radiosurgery for benign intradural extramedullary spinal tumors. Neurosurgery 2006;58:674–685.
4 Sinclair J, Chang SD, Gibbs IC, Adler JR Jr: Multisession CyberKnife radiosurgery for intramedullary spinal cord arteriovenous malformations. Neurosurgery 2006;58:1081–1089.

Dr. Iris C. Gibbs
Department of Radiation Oncology
Stanford University School of Medicine
875 Blake Wilbur Drive, Room G222A
Stanford, CA 94305-5847 (USA)
Tel. +1 650 736 1480, Fax +1 650 725 8231
E-Mail iris.gibbs@stanford.edu

Meyer JL (ed): IMRT, IGRT, SBRT – Advances in the Treatment Planning and
Delivery of Radiotherapy. Front Radiat Ther Oncol. Basel, Karger, 2007, vol. 40, pp 415–426

Liver, Renal, and Retroperitoneal Tumors: Stereotactic Radiotherapy

Brian D. Kavanagh[a] · Tracey E. Schefter[a] · Peter J. Wersäll[b]

[a]University of Colorado Comprehensive Cancer Center, Aurora, Colo., USA;
[b]Karolinska Hospital and Tumor Institute, Stockholm, Sweden

Abstract

Stereotactic body radiation therapy (SBRT) is currently under active study at numerous centers for clinical application in the management of patients with primary or metastatic tumors of the liver, primary or metastatic tumors of the kidney, and selected other retroperitoneal tumors. Accurate patient positioning and tumor relocalization are essential for SBRT use in the liver and other abdominal and retroperitoneal sites, as at other tumor sites. In a phase I clinical trial at the University of Colorado, patients with liver metastases have received SBRT. Eligible patients had 1–3 discrete liver metastases and no prior radiotherapy to the liver. The aggregate tumor diameter (sum of diameters) was <6 cm. Respiratory control was used. Normal liver volume to be preserved was determined prior to therapy. Dose was prescribed to a planning target volume that included the gross tumor volume plus at least a 5-mm radial and 10-mm superior-inferior margin. SBRT was administered with 6- to 15-MV beams through either dynamic conformal arcs or a combination of multiple noncoplanar static beams. The dose was safely escalated to 60 Gy in 3 fractions. After SBRT to hepatic lesions, it is extremely difficult to radiographically evaluate tumor response within the first few months, and radiographic response analysis may require 4–6 months after SBRT. Care must be taken to avoid focal high-dose therapy to the gastrointestinal mucosa, where the maximum point dose is likely to be the major limitation rather than the mean dose. SBRT has a potential role in the management of renal cell carcinoma, either as an alternative to surgery to the primary site or as cytoreductive therapy directed toward metastatic sites, and in the management of selected retroperitoneal tumors.

Stereotactic body radiation therapy (SBRT) is a therapeutic option in selected cases of primary or metastatic liver tumors, primary or metastatic kidney cancer, and certain tumors involving other retroperitoneal sites. In each case, there are special technical and clinical considerations to be considered. Here we present an overview of published literature, with a description of key applied concepts and illustrative case studies.

Stereotactic Body Radiation Therapy for Liver Tumors

Target Volume Definition and Respiratory Motion Adaptation
A fundamental issue in all of clinical radiation oncology is the question of whether the perceived target volume to be treated is the true target volume. When non-invasive external beam therapy is guided by noninvasive imaging studies, it is valuable to establish the reliability of the imaging studies in terms of how well they represent the lesion volume and location. Kelsey et al. [1] at the University of Colorado approached this topic for hepatocellular carcinoma (HCC) by means of a clinicopathologic correlative study. For 18 patients with 27 tumors treated surgically for HCC, the preoperative imaging studies were correlated with tumor volume identified on gross pathologic examination. The radiographic and pathologic sizes were closely correlated with either CT or MRI imaging. In most cases (81%), the imaging study overestimated the true gross pathologic size of the HCC. The authors concluded that SBRT utilizing a 0.5- or 1.0-cm margin around the radiographically evident tumor would have encompassed the gross pathologic tumor in 93 and 100% of cases, respectively.

Accurate patient positioning and tumor relocalization are essential for liver SBRT. Dawson et al. [2] reported the setup accuracy of a system of active breathing control supplemented with daily megavoltage imaging for liver SBRT. The average breath-hold time was 12 s. With this combination of techniques, the average motion of the diaphragm during treatment was observed to be less than 1 mm. Fuss et al. [3] at the University of Texas San Antonio used daily ultrasound-based image to reposition patients to upper abdominal target volumes. A combination of adjacent vascular and ductal structures (the portal vein, hepatic artery, bile ducts, aorta, celiac trunk, and superior mesenteric artery) were used as internal reference fiducials to facilitate anatomic localization. The authors found the technique reliable more than 95% of the time, with occasional difficulty resulting from excess gastrointestinal gas that limited visibility. CT scan verification of ultrasound-directed setup guidance confirmed a statistically significant improvement in setup error using this system, with an observed mean magnitude of residual setup error of less than 5 mm.

Stereotactic Body Radiation Therapy for Hepatocellular Carcinoma
Evidence supporting the utility of high-dose, hypofractionated radiation therapy in the management of HCC includes the observations from the University Tsukuba and Loma Linda University involving the application of proton beam treatment. Chiba et al. [4] from Tsukuba reported an experience of 162 patients with medically or surgically inoperable HCC treated by proton beam therapy with or without transarterial embolization and percutaneous ethanol injection. The median total radiation dose was 72 Gy in 16 fractions. The overall survival rate for

all of the 162 patients was 23.5% at 5 years, and the actuarial local control rate at 5 years was 87% for the 192 discrete tumors treated. Adverse prognostic factors in their experience included worse baseline hepatic function and greater number of tumors in the liver. Bush et al. [5] at Loma Linda University reported a similar experience with the use of proton irradiation for patients with unresectable HCC. The total dose given was 63 Gy (calculated as cobalt gray equivalents) in 15 fractions. Among 34 patients with a median follow-up of 20 months, the 2-year actuarial local control and overall survival rates were 75 and 55%, respectively. Subsequent liver transplantation was performed in 6 patients, 2 of whom had no residual carcinoma on histopathologic analysis of the specimen removed.

Regarding the use of photon irradiation, a recently reported French phase II trial assessed the efficacy and tolerance of conventionally fractionated external beam radiotherapy for HCC in cirrhotic patients [6]. A dose of 66 Gy was given to 27 patients with HCC, 15 of whom had previously been treated. Among 23 evaluable patients, nearly 80% (18 patients) experienced a complete response, and another 3 achieved partial response. The experience of Shim et al. [7] was similarly encouraging insofar as it strongly suggested a clinical benefit for conventionally fractionated radiotherapy after transcatheter arterial chemoembolization, a commonly applied therapy.

Among the first group of patients who received SBRT at the Karolinska Institute were 9 patients with HCC and 2 with other primary intrahepatic cancers [8]. Twenty separate tumors were treated in the 11 patients; the doses given ranged from 14 to 45 Gy in 1–3 fractions. Partial or complete response was observed in 60 and 10% of lesions, respectively. Patients commonly developed a low-grade elevation in body temperature and nausea a few hours after treatment, usually prevented with antibiotics. Most patients had only mild symptoms, but 1 patient died 2 days after a single 30-Gy dose to a large HCC in the left lobe of the liver. In an ongoing multicenter prospective pilot trial of SBRT for HCC (H. Cardenes, Indiana University, principal investigator), the initial part of the study is a phase I lead-in to a phase II study. The initial dose cohort was 36 Gy in 3 fractions, and the plan was to escalate the dose by 6 Gy total (2 Gy per fraction) in subsequent cohorts.

Stereotactic Body Radiation Therapy for Liver Metastases
Herfarth et al. [9] at Heidelberg University reported a phase I/II dose escalation study of single-fraction SBRT for hepatic metastases in which 37 patients participated. The median tumor volume was 10 cm^3 (range, 1–132 cm^3), and the dose was safely escalated from 14 to 26 Gy in 1 fraction. At the time of that report, the overall actuarial freedom from local failure at 18 months for the entire group was 67%; failures occurred predominantly in patients treated with lower doses. Wulf et al. [10] from the University of Würzburg reported a series that included 23 patients who received SBRT for liver metastases. The typical dose was 30 Gy in 3 fractions.

The actuarial rates of local control at 1 and 2 years were 76 and 61%, respectively. There was 1 case of grade 2 hepatitis at 6 weeks, which resolved after steroid treatment. No patient experienced grade 3 or higher toxicity of any kind.

Schefter et al. [11] from the University of Colorado and elsewhere conducted a phase I trial of liver SBRT, electing to use a 3-fraction regimen. Eligible patients had 1–3 discrete liver metastases, had had no prior radiotherapy to the liver, and had not had any chemotherapy for at least 2 weeks prior to SBRT. The aggregate tumor diameter (sum of all maximum individual tumor diameters) had to be less than 6 cm. The dose was escalated according to a standard 3 + 3 phase I study design. The first cohort received 36 Gy in 3 fractions (12 Gy/fraction), and for subsequent cohorts the total dose was increased by 6 Gy (2 Gy/fraction). Dose-limiting toxicity was defined as any grade 3 liver, gastric, small bowel, or spinal cord toxicity or any grade 4 toxicity from SBRT. It was preordained within the protocol that the maximum dose escalation would be to a total dose of 60 Gy in 3 fractions, even if the maximum tolerated dose had not yet been reached.

Dose was prescribed to a planning target volume (PTV) that included the gross tumor volume (GTV) plus at least a 5-mm radial and 10-mm superior-inferior margin. Respiratory control (abdominal compression or a breathing coordinator) was used. SBRT was administered with 6- to 15-MV beams through either dynamic conformal arcs or a combination of multiple noncoplanar static beams. The 3 fractions of SBRT could be given on consecutive or nonconsecutive days within a 2-week span. Prophylactic antiemetics were allowed at the discretion of the treating radiation oncologist.

A simplified form of the 'critical volume' model, initially proposed by Yaes and Kalend [12], was applied to construct the normal liver dose restriction in the University of Colorado trial. The essence of this model is that for a given irradiated organ, it is necessary to preserve a minimum 'critical volume' of cells with the capacity to regenerate so that organ function can be preserved. Based upon literature regarding surgical resection, it was estimated that if a 'critical volume' in the range of 500–600 cm^3 of normal liver were preserved, there should be adequate reserve to allow repopulation and maintenance of normal liver function.

It was also known from prior studies of whole-liver radiotherapy that a dose of 30 Gy in 20 fractions was expected to be well tolerated [13]. If an alpha/beta ratio of 3 is assumed, the biologically equivalent dose (BED) of this regimen may then be calculated as 45 Gy$_3$. Therefore, it was hypothesized that if an extraconservative 'critical volume' of at least 700 cm^3 of normal liver received a BED of less than 45 Gy$_3$, adequate reserve capacity should be preserved. Additional caution was applied in restricting the dose to the 700-cm^3 'critical volume' to a maximum of 15 Gy in 3 fractions, which yields a BED of 40 Gy$_3$. The use of dose-volume histogram (DVH) information to assess compliance with a critical volume-type restriction has not been commonly done in the past (an illustrative example is provided in fig. 1).

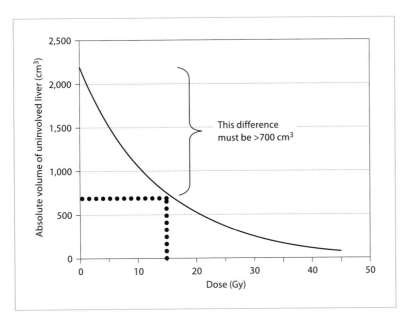

Fig. 1. Representative normal liver DVH, with indicated critical volume restriction whereby no more than 700 cm³ may receive more than 15 Gy. The horizontal and vertical dotted lines converge upon the point on the curve indicating the volume of normal liver that receives 15 Gy or more; thus, the difference between the total normal liver volume and the volume receiving 15 Gy or more, here indicated by a brace, must be more than 700 cm³.

Eighteen patients participated in the University of Colorado phase I liver SBRT study. A trend of asymptomatic elevation in serum liver enzymes was noted within the first few months after SBRT, but no patient experienced a dose-limiting toxicity. The dose was therefore safely escalated to 60 Gy in 3 fractions. Typically, well-defined regions of hypodensity in the normal liver tissue around the GTV were observed on CT scans obtained within the first few months after SBRT, similar to what has been reported after single-fraction SBRT [14]. The etiology of this phenomenon is not yet completely understood; a lymphocyte-mediated mechanism has been hypothesized [11]. Regardless of the mechanism, the important clinical relevance is that it is extremely difficult to evaluate tumor response within the first few months radiographically on account of this effect. Therefore, in clinical trials of liver SBRT in which tumor response is a primary endpoint, it is advisable to set the time point of radiographic response analysis at least 4–6 months after SBRT.

It should be appreciated that observations of the tolerance of normal liver to SBRT cannot be converted into assumptions regarding the tolerance of the gastrointestinal tract mucosa, generally assumed to be constructed in radiobiologically serial architecture, where the maximum point dose is the major

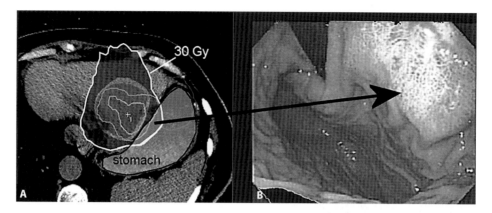

Fig. 2. A Cross section from the case study planning CT scan showing the 30 Gy isodose contour (thick white line) overlapping the stomach (labeled, outlined in black, and shaded in transparent gray). Other contours represent the GTV and PTV, and higher isodose contours are shaded regions inside the 30-Gy contour. **B** Image from an upper endoscopy approximately 8 weeks after liver SBRT. The arrowhead indicates an area of pale, denuded mucosa within the region that received more than 30 Gy.

limitation rather than the mean dose. It is likewise not known whether there is an equivalent application of critical volume-type dose constraints that would be appropriate, as seems to be the case for liver tissue. The following case study is illustrative.

Case Study 1
Stereotactic Body Radiation Therapy Tolerance Dose in the Gastrointestinal Mucosa
A 64-year-old female with metastatic colon cancer who had initially been treated with SBRT to lesions in the lung more than 2 years previously developed a new liver metastasis and was evaluated as a candidate for the phase I liver SBRT study. However, after a planning CT scan was obtained, it was evident that it would not be possible to treat her to the full prescription dose of the available cohort (54 Gy in 3 fractions) without exceeding the maximum point dose allowed by the protocol to gastrointestinal mucosa, i.e. 30 Gy in 3 fractions. Nevertheless, in an effort to give aggressive therapy to the patient who had had a generally favorable clinical course, the liver PTV was treated to a dose of 45 Gy in 3 fractions despite the inclusion of a section of the medial stomach within an isodose volume that received more than 30 Gy (fig. 2A).

The patient complained of dyspepsia within a month after treatment. Despite medical therapy with antacids, the discomfort persisted and worsened to pain requiring narcotic analgesics. Approximately 8 weeks after SBRT, an upper endoscopy revealed a region of pale mucosa that appeared to be poorly vascularized (fig. 2B). Proton pump inhibitor therapy was then added. Within 1 more month, repeat endoscopy revealed that the lesion had progressed to a shallow ulceration. Within another 2 months, the lesion gradually healed and symptoms abated with continued medical management.

It is possible that if an endoscopy had been performed earlier, initially the changes would have resembled a straightforward mucositis, with redness progressing to a pseudomembranous covering. However, the observed endoscopic changes were strongly suggestive of devas-

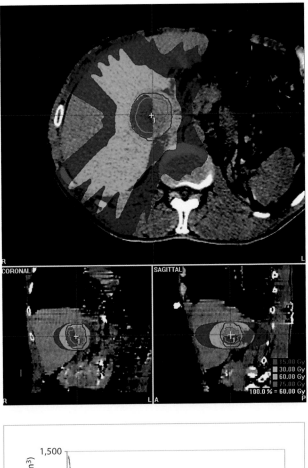

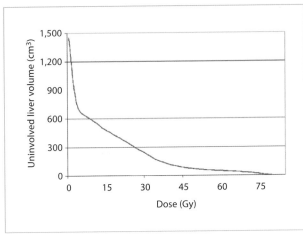

Fig. 3. Case study showing axial, coronal, and sagittal views of the isodose distribution super-imposed on CT images. Also, the DVH of uninvolved liver is shown.

cularization, potentially consistent with small vessel occlusion as a primary injurious event. The observations in this case underscore the need to proceed with particular caution when nearby gastrointestinal mucosa is positioned within a high-dose region. One possible solution would be a more fractionated course of therapy, perhaps administering similar doses in 6–8 or more fractions to a modestly lower dose.

Case Study 2

Patient. A 51-year-old man who 2 years ago underwent neoadjuvant chemoradiation and subsequent esophagectomy for a clinical T3N1M0 adenocarcinoma of the esophagus. He later developed liver metastases and achieved a good response from chemotherapy, but now he has clinical and radiographic evidence of a solitary 2.5-cm brain metastasis and a 3-cm liver metastasis.

Treatment. The patient elected stereotactic radiosurgery to the brain metastasis, deferral of any whole-brain radiotherapy, and enrollment on a phase II study of SBRT to the solitary liver metastasis. A dose of 60 Gy was given in 3 fractions using dynamic conformal arcs.

Result. From a pre-SBRT level of 450 ng/ml, the carcinoembryonic antigen decreased to 273 ng/ml 1 month following SBRT, indicating a favorable early response. No acute SBRT-related complications were observed. The patient will continue periodic surveillance (fig. 3).

Stereotactic Body Radiation Therapy for Renal Cell Cancer

SBRT has a potential role in the management of renal cell carcinoma (RCC), either as an alternative to surgery to the primary site or as cytoreductive therapy directed toward metastatic sites. First, considering the primary site itself, it has been demonstrated that nephrectomy has a proven role in extending overall survival, even in the setting of metastatic disease. The Southwestern Oncology Group and European Organization for the Research and Treatment of Cancer studies included a total of 331 patients with metastatic RCC who were randomized to either nephrectomy plus interferon-α_{2b} or interferon-α_{2b} alone [15]. The primary endpoint for each trial was overall survival. A combined analysis of these 2 trials revealed a 5.8-month increase in median survival from nephrectomy, representing a 31% decrease in the risk of death (p = 0.002). This effect was independent of patient performance status, the site of metastases, and the presence or absence of measurable disease. Given the proven clinical advantage of cytoreduction of the primary site, for patients medically unfit or otherwise unwilling to undergo nephrectomy, SBRT may serve as an appealing noninvasive alternative.

Regarding the use of SBRT to metastatic sites of RCC, the rationale is based in part upon the various reports documenting encouraging rates of long-term survivorship following surgical resection for selected patients with a limited burden of metastatic disease [16]. Until recently, the only systemic agent approved by the FDA for use in patients with metastatic RCC was interleukin-2, though no survival advantage has ever been demonstrated from the use of this agent or any

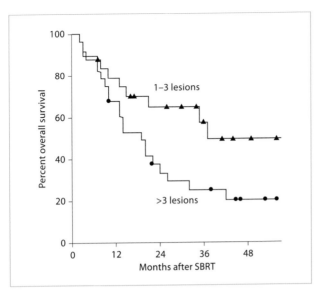

Fig. 4. Actuarial survival after SBRT for metastatic renal cell carcinoma, Karolinska Hospital experience. Patients with 1–3 lesions (n = 22) are compared with patients with >3 lesions (n = 28). Redrawn from Wersäll et al. [18].

other form of immunotherapy. In December, 2005, the FDA approved sorafenib (Nexavar®), a multikinase inhibitor, for use in patients with metastatic RCC on the basis of a randomized study that demonstrated an 83-day increase in median time to progression with the use of sorafenib. Only 2% of patients actually manifested a confirmed partial response to sorafenib, and a trend toward improved overall survival had not reached statistical significance at the specified time of analysis [17]. Thus, although the sorafenib results are a clear sign of progress, there remains room for improvement in outcome overall. Given that cytoreduction at the primary site confers a survival advantage, it is reasonable to postulate that effective cytoreduction in metastatic sites might likewise provide a survival advantage by delaying the time until a patient suffers from a lethal systemic burden of disease.

The largest published experience in the use of SBRT for RCC originated from the Radiumhemmet, at the Karolinska Hospital in Stockholm, Sweden. Wersäll et al. [18] reported the clinical outcomes for 58 patients with metastatic or inoperable primary RCC treated with SBRT between 1997 and 2003. The doses given to the PTV generally ranged from 30 to 45 Gy in 3–5 fractions, administered within 1 week. Among metastatic lesions treated with SBRT, there was a 30% rate of complete response and a 35% rate of partial response. Overall survival for patients with 1–3 metastatic lesions versus >3 metastatic lesions is shown in figure 4. The actuarial 4-year overall survival was approximately 50% for patients with fewer lesions, versus 20% for patients with a higher number of lesions.

The clinical outcomes of the 8 patients treated with SBRT to the primary site were likewise encouraging. Only 1 of the 8 developed an in-field recurrence after SBRT. Notably, the group of patients with metastatic disease included 5 patients with lesions treated in the remaining contralateral kidney after prior nephrectomy, and these patients tolerated SBRT well and experienced sustained disease control. The authors did, however, include a cautionary note of a single instance of grade 5 toxicity suffered by a patient treated for a metastasis to the pancreas. The patient died from gastric bleeding; no additional details of the treatment dosimetry were given.

Stereotactic Body Radiation Therapy for Retroperitoneal Tumors

Because of the proximity of intestinal tissue, with susceptibility to injury from SBRT as noted in the examples mentioned in previous sections, SBRT to retroperitoneal targets must be considered with special caution. Some locations, for example the adrenal gland and the lateral aspects of the spleen, are relatively well separated by at least a few centimeters from the nearest surface of the intestinal tract, and high-dose-per-fraction SBRT may be administered easily. In other situations, for example mesenteric nodes or tumors within the small or large intestines themselves, the unavoidable proximity of the intestinal tract renders it difficult to administer high doses in a hypofractionated course. Besides the obvious alternative of using conventionally fractionated radiotherapy when faced with such challenges, there are at least 2 other remedies that can be considered in selected cases.

The first, and more straightforward, is the surgical placement of a tissue expander or similar space-occupying material that displaces the bowel away from the tumor to be treated. A thickness of even just 1–2 cm or so can often provide a useful opportunity to construct a safe dose gradient between the edge of the tumor and closest critical structure. The second, and more case-specific, is the considered application of a highly heterogeneous dose distribution within the tumor, with planned hotspots in safer regions and lower doses along edges in closer proximity to sensitive normal tissues.

Although several reports have addressed key technical issues of patient setup reproducibility in the stereotactic treatment of retroperitoneal tumors, typically the clinical observations are restricted to individual anecdotes [19]. One exception is the experience reported by Wulf et al. [20] from Würzburg, in which 21 patients with inoperable abdominal and pelvic tumors were treated with an SBRT boost of 10–15 Gy in 2–3 fractions after a course of conventionally fractionated radiotherapy to a total dose of 45–50.4 Gy. Eleven of the 21 patients had a recurrent gynecologic tumor, and the authors note in their discussion that the selection of dose to be given was largely modeled on the well-documented safety profile of high-dose-rate brachytherapy in this setting, where it is known that small volumes of adjacent bowel and bladder can safely tolerate several single-fraction doses in the range of 5–7 after 45–50 Gy of conventionally fractionated radiotherapy. The patient population also included 4 others with pelvic recurrence of prostate or rectal cancer and 6 with either local recurrence of RCC, local recurrence of pancreas cancer, or paravertebral metastasis of soft tissue sarcoma.

Actuarial local control at 2 years was 70%, and treatment was generally well tolerated. There were 2 cases of intestinovaginal fistula observed as a late effect in patients treated for vaginal stump recurrence of cervix cancer and a paravaginal recurrence of endometrial cancer; however, the authors noted that in these 2 cases, the pretreatment imaging had revealed evidence of suspected tumor infiltration into the adjacent bowel. Furthermore, the tumors were large (50 and 144 cm^3, respectively), and it is likely that if the boost had been given via interstitial brachytherapy instead of SBRT, there would have also been a high chance of fistula given the likely preexisting compromise to the structural integrity of the bowel wall at baseline.

Conclusions

SBRT is currently under active study at numerous centers for clinical application in the management of patients with primary or metastatic tumors of the liver, primary or metastatic tumors of the kidney, and selected other retroperitoneal tumors. Its capacity to serve as a potent cytoreductive intervention offers potentially curative therapy for certain primary lesions and potentially valuable salvage therapy in other cases, where tumor shrinkage can lead to a favorable palliative effect and perhaps even prolonged survival by contributing to the prevention or delay of the time when a patient succumbs to an overwhelming systemic burden of disease.

References

1 Kelsey CR, Schefter T, Nash SR, Russ P, Baron AE, Zeng C, Gaspar LE: Retrospective clinicopathologic correlation of gross tumor size of hepatocellular carcinoma: implications for stereotactic body radiotherapy. Am J Clin Oncol 2005;28:576–580.

2 Dawson LA, Eccles C, Bissonnette JP, Brock KK: Accuracy of daily image guidance for hypofractionated liver radiotherapy with active breathing control. Int J Radiat Oncol Biol Phys 2005;62:1247–1252.

3 Fuss M, Salter BJ, Cavanaugh SX, Fuss C, Sadeghi A, Fuller CD, Ameduri A, Hevezi JM, Herman TS, Thomas CR Jr: Daily ultrasound-based image-guided targeting for radiotherapy of upper abdominal malignancies. Int J Radiat Oncol Biol Phys 2004;59:1245–1256.

4 Chiba T, Tokuuye K, Matsuzaki Y, Sugahara S, Chuganji Y, Kagei K, Shoda J, Hata M, Abei M, Igaki H, Tanaka N, Akine Y: Proton beam therapy for hepatocellular carcinoma: a retrospective review of 162 patients. Clin Cancer Res 2005;11:3799–3805.

5 Bush DA, Hillebrand DJ, Slater JM, Slater JD: High-dose proton beam radiotherapy of hepatocellular carcinoma: preliminary results of a phase II trial. Gastroenterology 2004;127(5 suppl 1):S189–S193.

6 Mornex F, Girard N, Merle P, Beziat C, Kubas A, Wautot V, Khodri M, Trepo C: Tolerance and efficacy of conformal radiotherapy for hepatocellular carcinoma in cirrhotic patients. Results of the French RTF1 phase II trial (in French). Cancer Radiother 2005;9:470–476.

7 Shim SJ, Seong J, Han KH, Chon CY, Suh CO, Lee JT: Local radiotherapy as a complement to incomplete transcatheter arterial chemoembolization in locally advanced hepatocellular carcinoma. Liver Int 2005;25:1189–1196.

8 Blomgren H, Lax I, Naslund I, Svanstrom R: Stereotactic high dose fraction radiation therapy of extracranial tumors using an accelerator: clinical experience of the first thirty-one patients. Acta Oncol 1995;34:861–870.

9 Herfarth KK, Debus J, Lohr F, Bahner ML, Rhein B, Fritz P, Hoss A, Schlegel W, Wannenmacher MF: Stereotactic single-dose radiation therapy of liver tumors: results of a phase I/II trial. J Clin Oncol 2001;19:164–170.

10 Wulf J, Hadinger U, Oppitz U, Thiele W, Ness-Dourdoumas R, Flentje M: Stereotactic radiotherapy of targets in lung and liver. Strahlenther Onkol 2001;177:645–655

11 Schefter TE, Kavanagh BD, Timmerman RD, Cardenes HR, Baron A, Gaspar LE: A phase I trial of stereotactic body radiation therapy (SBRT) for liver metastases. Int J Radiat Oncol Biol Phys 2005;62:1371–1378.

12 Yaes RJ, Kalend A: Local stem cell depletion model for radiation myelitis. Int J Radiat Oncol Biol Phys 1988;14:1247–1259.

13 Russell AH, Clyde C, Wasserman TH, Turner SS, Rotman M: Accelerated hyperfractionated hepatic irradiation in the management of patients with liver metastases: results of the RTOG dose escalating protocol. Int J Radiat Oncol Biol Phys 1993;27:117–123.

14 Herfarth KK, Hof H, Bahner ML, Lohr F, Hoss A, van Kaick G, Wannenmacher M, Debus J: Assessment of focal liver reaction by multiphasic CT after stereotactic single-dose radiotherapy of liver tumors. Int J Radiat Oncol Biol Phys 2003;57:444–451.

15 Flanigan RC, Mickisch G, Sylvester R, Tangen C, Van Poppel H, Crawford ED: Cytoreductive nephrectomy in patients with metastatic renal cancer: a combined analysis. J Urol 2004;171:1071–1076.

16 Wersäll PJ, Kavanagh BD: Stereotactic body radiation therapy for renal cell carcinoma; in Kavanagh BD, Timmerman RD (eds): Stereotactic Body Radiation Therapy. New York, Lippincott Williams & Wilkins, 2005.

17 Sorafenib (Nexavar®) product prescribing information; available at www.nexavar.com.

18 Wersäll PJ, Blomgren H, Lax I, Kalkner KM, Linder C, Lundell G, Nilsson B, Nilsson S, Naslund I, Pisa P, Svedman C: Extracranial stereotactic radiotherapy for primary and metastatic renal cell carcinoma. Radiother Oncol 2005;77:88–95.

19 Buatti JM, Meeks SL, Howes TL: Stereotactic body radiation therapy for retroperitoneal and pelvic tumors; in Kavanagh BD, Timmerman RD (eds): Stereotactic Body Radiation Therapy. New York, Lippincott Williams & Wilkins, 2005.

20 Wulf J, Hadinger U, Oppitz U, Thiele W, Flentje M: Stereotactic boost irradiation for targets in the abdomen and pelvis. Radiother Oncol 2004;70:31–36.

Dr. Brian D. Kavanagh
Department of Radiation Oncology
University of Colorado Comprehensive
Cancer Center
Anschutz Cancer Pavilion, 1665 N. Ursula St.
Suite 1032, PO Box 6510, Mail Stop F706
Aurora, CO 80045 (USA)
Tel. +1 720 848 0156, Fax +1 720 848 0222
E-Mail Brian.Kavanagh@uchsc.edu

Author Index

Subject Index